c/o Dr. N. Gledhill
Room 356 Norman Bethune College
4700 Keele Street
Toronto, Ontario M3J 1P3
Phone and Fax No.: (416) 736-5794

Occupation Specific Fitness, Vision & Hearing Assessment For Firefighter Applicants

Most municipalities require applicants for firefighting positions to provide, at some point in the application process, a recently dated certificate which indicates that they are capable of meeting the physical demands encountered in firefighting. Prospective firefighter applicants can book appointments with York University - Fitness to undergo the Occupation Specific Fitness, Vision and Hearing Assessment at their own expense, and successful candidates receive the required certificate which provides an evaluation of the participant's performance in each of the areas assessed. A physical examination by a medical doctor and an electrocardiogram are generally not conducted on these occasions. However, vision and hearing assessments are administered. The certificates are signed and sealed with a corporate impression and provided to the participants for submitting to fire departments. Below is an overview of the test components, booking information, the associated fees and instructions.

Screening of Selected Health/Medical Items	Aerobic Fitness Test	Job Simulation Performance Tests
Visual Acuity (minimum 20/30 in each eye uncorrected) Depth Perception (Stereopsis Test) Colour Vision (City University Test or Farnsworth D-15 Test) Normal Unaided Hearing (Audiometer) Normal Resting Lung Function	Aerobic fitness (treadmill test with direct expired air analysis)	Acrophobia (ladder climb- pass/fail) Claustrophobia (search confined area - pass/fail) Ladder lift (56 lb - pass/fail) Rope pull (50 lb - timed) Hose carry/stair climb (85 lb - timed) Simulated hose advance (150 lb - timed) Victim drag (200 lb - timed)

FOR THE DATE OF THE NEXT TESTING SESSION PHONE (416)-736-5794 MONDAY TO FRIDAY DURING REGULAR OFFICE HOURS: 8:30 am - 4:30 pm

Cost And Booking Information: The all-inclusive fee for testing is $160.00. Phone to find out upcoming test dates, then make a reservation by mailing a *non-refundable* **$60.00 CERTIFIED cheque or money order (payable to "York University - Fitness")** to the above address. Be sure to include your complete mailing address AND TELEPHONE NUMBER along with the test date. Upon receipt of your deposit, you will be contacted by telephone to confirm your test reservation. Since there are limited spaces available per testing day, it is advisable to reserve your testing appointment as soon as possible. The remaining $100.00 of the testing fee is to be paid by **CERTIFIED cheque or money order (payable to "York University - Fitness"), or cash** on the day of the testing. Additional certified copies of your results can be ordered for $2.50 each on the day of your testing. "PAR-Q", and "Consent For Exercise Testing" documents will be completed on the day of testing.

Instructions: The testing will take approximately four and a half hours. Changing and showering facilities are available. Please bring a towel, exercise clothing and running shoes (an extra top is a good idea). It is also recommended that you bring a fluid bottle (not sports drinks, which are frequently regurgitated) and a snack. It is advisable to eat a light meal up to two hours prior to the testing, but do not smoke or drink caffeine-containing beverages on the day of the test. In addition, you should not exercise heavily or consume alcohol for **24** hours prior to the testing.

The location of the testing facility on the university campus and the location of York University in Metropolitan Toronto are indicated on the attached maps. Enter the university via North West Gate off Steeles Avenue. You can park in lot 5A along the East side of North West Gate for a parking fee of approximately $7.00. The testing takes place in Room 120 Norman Bethune College.

PHOTO IDENTIFICATION WILL BE REQUIRED ON THE DAY OF THE TESTING

Revised January 2001 - Implementation Spring 2001

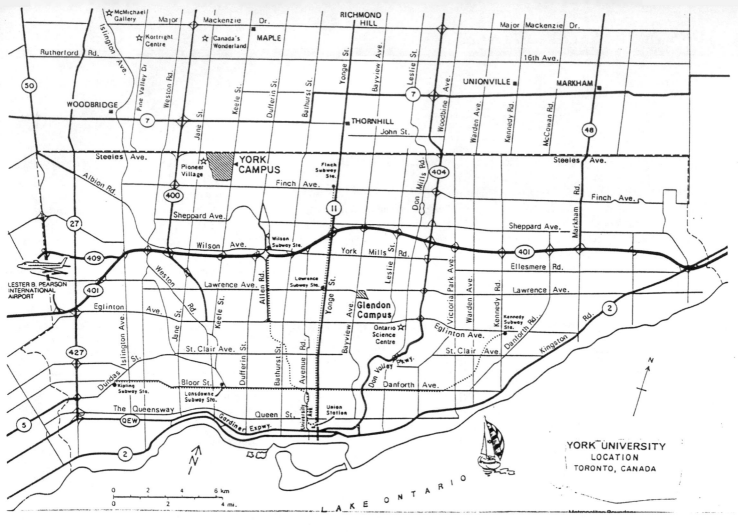

York University Location
Toronto, Canada

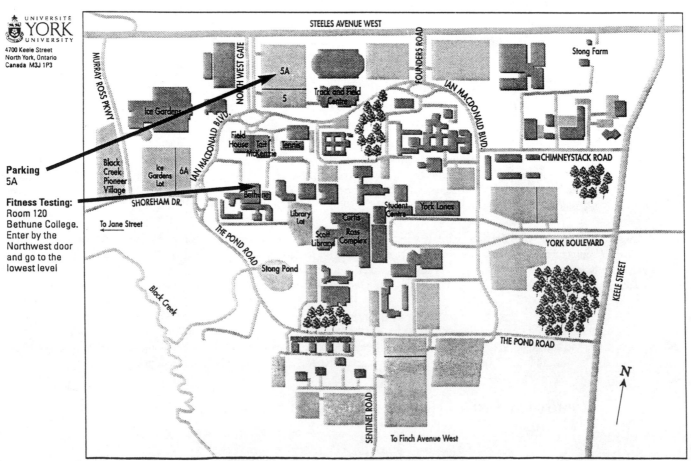

UNIVERSITÉ
YORK
UNIVERSITY

4700 Keele Street
North York, Ontario
Canada M3J 1P3

Parking
5A

Fitness Testing:
Room 120
Bethune College.
Enter by the
Northwest door
and go to the
lowest level

Vehicle Rescue and Extrication

Ronald E. Moore
RESQUE-1, Inc.
Montour Falls, New York

with **548** *illustrations*

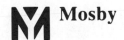 **Mosby**

A *Harcourt Health Sciences Company*
St. Louis Philadelphia London Sydney Toronto

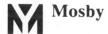 **Mosby**

A *Harcourt Health Sciences Company*

Editor Dave Culverwell
Assistant Editor Claire Merrick
Project Manager Carol Sullivan Wiseman
Production Editor Linda McKinley
Design Candace Conner

The author is not affiliated with any rescue tool manufacturer or sales organization. To the best of his ability, the author has been fair to all parties that manufacture or sell rescue tools and equipment.

Mosby, Inc.
11830 Westline Industrial Drive, St. Louis, Missouri 63146

Library of Congress Cataloging-in-Publication Data
Moore, Ronald E.
     Vehicle rescue and extrication/Ronald E. Moore.
          p.   cm.
     Includes index.
     ISBN 0-8016-3351-6
     1. Traffic accidents.   2. Crash injuries.   3. Rescue work.
  4. Transport of sick and wounded.   I. Title.
     [DNLM: 1. Accident Prevention.   2. Accidents, Traffic.
  3. Equipment Safety.   4. Wounds and Injuries — prevention & control.
  WA 275 M823v]
  RC88.9.T7M66 1991
  617.1'028 — dc20
  DNLM/DLC
                                                            89-12502

EG/VH/VH 9 8

Dedication

I want this text to serve as a tribute to Jim Yvorra, a very special friend of mine, who is alive today only in my memories. Jim served as Assistant Chief of the Berwyn Heights Fire Department, Prince Georges County, Maryland, until January 29, 1988. On that day, Jim was struck and killed by a passing automobile as he was surveying the scene of an accident. Jim was one of 139 firefighters to die in 1988.

I had met Jim years before in Pennsylvania when we were members of the South Williamsport Fire Department, First Ward Fire Company. He impressed me with his love and devotion to the fire service, his progressive thinking, and his never-ending dedication and professionalism. Although considered an expert in his field, Jim was such a down-to-earth guy that he never saw himself as an expert and never placed himself above those he worked with or trained in classes or seminars.

I worked with Jim as a book reviewer when he was an editor for the Robert J. Brady Company, Bowie, Maryland. He was always willing to listen to my suggestions, readily accepted new ideas, and placed a great deal of confidence in my review work. When it was my turn to be the author, I turned to Jim for guidance. He became an invaluable source of infor-

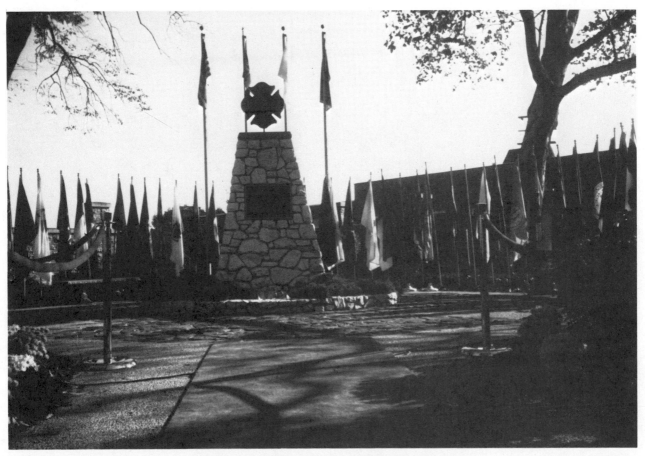

The Fallen Firefighter's Monument, Emmitsburg, Md.

mation and was a great personal strength to me as he coached, guided, and directed me through the complex and somewhat confusing world of technical publishing. His keen insight into the publishing industry and his vision of what my book should be were important to me when I was first exploring the possibility of writing a vehicle rescue book. Jim constantly inspired me as those first thoughts and ideas became words and sentences, and those first feeble sentences grew into pages and then chapters. I was not sure what I was getting myself into, but he knew what I could do and most important, believed that I could do it. When I faltered, Jim's encouraging words always seemed to come at the right time to inspire me and get me back on track.

Word reached me of Jim's tragic and senseless death as I was passing the halfway point in writing the book. At first I felt abandoned and alone without him being just a phone call away. My silent partner in this seemingly massive undertaking had now left me without even saying goodbye. I nearly abandoned the entire project. As time passed and the pain of his loss subsided, my mind cleared and I began to realize that Jim Yvorra is still with all of us in the emergency services field. His spirit lives on, guiding those of us who, like him, strive to serve others in their time of need.

I do not want my efforts here to be a memorial to Jim — he would not have wanted it that way. Rather this text should serve as a tribute to Jim and all others who have given the supreme sacrifice. The Berwyn Heights (Maryland) Fire Department and the entire emergency service community of this country have lost one of the great ones. His short life proved to me that each of us, alone and working together, can make a difference in this world.

I miss you, Jim. We all do!

Ronald E. Moore

Preface

This text is intended to serve as a source of information; it is not an authority. You should choose the meaningful portions and use this information to better yourself and your organization. Information that is not directly relevant to a specific individual or organization should still be considered. Have the courage to accept and try a new concept. Modify these suggestions to change or improve your existing procedures. Remain open-minded to new ideas, tools, and techniques. If you like a suggestion or concept in the text, understand the reasons you like it and its advantages and disadvantages. If you disagree with an idea, have definitive reasons why you feel as you do.

The contents have been specifically designed to address the important aspects of vehicle rescue and patient extrication. The information is of interest to all emergency service personnel, regardless of their agency affiliation. The common theme remains emergency service personnel safety above all else.

In the first chapter the reality of the challenges of modern-day vehicle rescue is presented. Features of vehicles posing a threat to personnel safety are explained. Chapter 2 details the Vehicle Rescue Life Cycle, the most comprehensive and systematic approach for fulfilling all responsibilities at an accident scene. Chapter 3 addresses personnel safety at motor vehicle accident incidents, and Chapter 4 focuses on the safety concepts that supervisory personnel must consider. Incident scene management, command and control, and size up are included to assist command personnel in creating a safer and more efficient rescue environment. Chapter 5 discusses the special needs of motor vehicle accident trauma patients. This chapter explains concepts such as mechanism of injury, trauma patient size up, and other EMS concerns related specifically to vehicle rescue. Chapter 6 classifies vehicle rescue tools into basic groupings according to their function and details the operating characteristics of each family. Tool and component identification, safety considerations, and preventive maintenance information are also discussed. Chapter 7 organizes vehicle rescue evolutions into categories such as stabilization, access, interior patient disentan-glement, and hazard control measures. The many options that are available for accomplishing a safe and efficient vehicle rescue are also presented.

My reward in completing this 4-year project will be up to you. I want to see this text stimulate an exchange of new thoughts and ideas. Your success in the field will not be easy unless you study many sources of information on vehicle rescue, become proficient with available vehicle rescue and emergency medical equipment, and practice the medical and rescue evolutions until they become second nature. At the emergency scene, make your strategic and tactical decisions based on everything you have ever learned through your training and your experience. Do not rely on this one source of information.

This text is not a free-standing program and is not meant to set a standard of operations. This work is a sharing of ideas and experiences. It is up to you to judge the merits of these ideas and this information. It is your responsibility to stay up to date with accepted vehicle rescue and medical procedures and to follow your organization's operating procedures and guidelines. To truly save lives, you must apply the presented information to your best advantage.

"People trapped" to me means that I and the rescue crew with whom I work and train are once again being challenged in a physical and emotional test in which the final outcome will be measured in life-and-death terms. It means that all my countless hours of studying and researching and the repetitive training sessions at the station come together to give me the courage and the ability to act and act correctly. I want to do the best I can as safely and efficiently as I can and set an example of professionalism in both my attitude and my actions. I want to survive this call to duty and return home safely to my wife and children.

In writing this text, I hope that I have done something to make those who work in the field or are just getting involved in it better able to serve. I thank everyone I have had the opportunity to meet in my career in the fire service, and I look forward to working with those of you I have yet to meet. Thank you for using this text.

About the Author

Ronald E. Moore currently serves as a Fire Protection Specialist I with the New York State Office of Fire Prevention and Control and is assigned duties at the New York State Academy of Fire Science, Montour Falls, New York.

He is the president and founder of RESQUE-1, Inc., a firm that provides training and consultant services to fire, rescue, and emergency medical agencies worldwide. His firm specializes in automobile and bus vehicle rescue training programs.

He has degrees with honors in the field of graphic arts and photography and in fire protection technology. He is New York State certified as a Level 2 Fire Officer, Level 2 Fire Instructor, Hazmat Responder (Operations Level), and a Code Enforcement official. In 1984, he received the coveted George D. Post Instructor of the Year award from the International Society of Fire Service Instructors. Mr. Moore is also an active fire officer with the Montour Falls (New York) Fire Department and a member of their rescue squad.

Contents

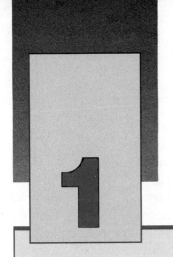

New Technology

Safety is more than just a word; it is the difference between life and death. For persons injured in an automobile accident, survival often depends on the type and quality of care they receive in the first 60 minutes following the accident. If fire, rescue, and emergency medical personnel rendering emergency care are injured themselves while operating at the scene, the rescue's success, as well as the very survival of victims and emergency service providers, can be jeopardized.

Common accident scene hazards include leaking gasoline and other fuels, unstable vehicles, sharp metal, broken glass, and hazards involving the vehicle's battery or electrical system. Many other dangerous conditions and situations are potentially as deadly to emergency service personnel, who must be completely familiar with all of today's vehicle rescue hazards and trained to quickly identify each one present at an accident. Certain emergency service personnel must also be proficient in mitigating the threats posed by these hazards.

Responding emergency personnel are trained to recognize totalled vehicles and dismantle a vehicle with trapped occupants (Fig. 1-1, A). Changing technology creates new indicators for determining a totalled vehicle (Fig. 1-1, B). Rescue personnel must be as aggressive when performing extrication of the trapped occupants in Fig. 1-1, C, as they would with the vehicle in Fig. 1-1, A.

The phrase *new technology* describes both the safety hazards that vehicles present and the steadily growing list of important features found in, on, and around today's vehicles. Each of the new technology items in this chapter affects the safety and survival of emergency service personnel during vehicle rescue activities at an accident scene.

ENERGY-ABSORBING BUMPER SYSTEMS

In 1973, a U.S. government requirement for a more crashworthy automobile in low-speed collisions brought the development of an early prototype energy-absorbing bumper system. Although in the first production year (1973 models) energy-absorbing bumper systems were installed only on front bumpers, since 1974 they have been installed on both the front and rear of passenger automobiles. Energy-absorbing bumper systems are not yet found on trucks, vans, or commercial-plate vehicles, but this is likely to change because the government is now considering including these vehicles under current automobile safety equipment standards.

The first energy-absorbing bumper systems for automobiles were designed to withstand a 5 mph frontal or rear-end collision with little or no damage to the vehicle itself. Variations of the unit created by various auto manufacturers used either a leaf spring

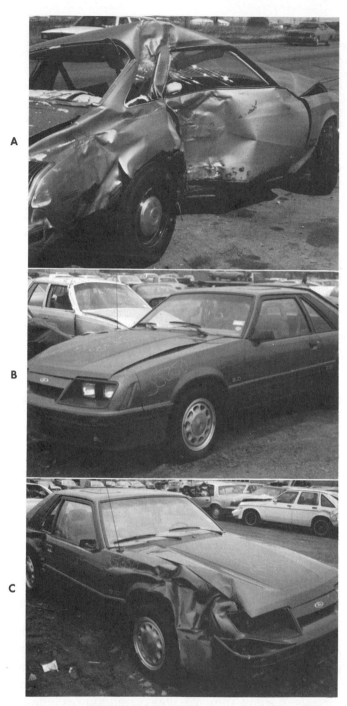

FIG. 1-1 A, This vintage 1970s automobile was totalled in a side collision into a tree. **B and C,** Appearance is no longer a reliable indicator of a totalled vehicle. This Mustang GT was also involved in a passenger-side collision and was "written off" by the insurance company because the undercarriage structure sustained irreparable damage.

type of assembly (Fig. 1-2, *A*) placed horizontally behind the front bumper, a two-piece sliding metal assembly with a rubber cushion acting to absorb impact energy (Fig. 1-2, *B*), or the basic design that would eventually become most prevalent, the fluid-filled, pressurized piston unit.

Each energy-absorbing piston unit (there are now four units per vehicle) consists of a metal tube secured to the bumper that telescopes inside a larger tube mounted into or along the side of the vehicle frame (Fig. 1-3). A floating disk inside the tubes separates the front and rear sections of the piston assembly. The smaller front tube is typically filled with an inert pressurized gas such as compressed nitrogen; the larger tube contains a small quantity of lightweight hydraulic fluid. As the bumper of the vehicle is impacted in a low-speed collision, the small tube moves inside the larger tube causing the fluid and the compressed gas to work together to absorb impact energy (Fig. 1- 4). The piston tubes are intended to return to their original positions after a low-speed impact.

Bumper System Hazards

When a vehicle with an energy-absorbing bumper system is involved in a collision or fire, emergency service personnel arriving on the scene must anticipate the possible presence of some special safety problems (Fig. 1-5). If an intact piston unit is exposed to heat, under the right conditions it may violently explode, propelling loose parts off the vehicle. The entire bumper may even detach itself and move a considerable distance away from the vehicle. Emergency service personnel must thus be constantly on the alert for the sudden "launching" of any portion of an energy-absorbing bumper system as they arrive at an emergency scene and find a vehicle on fire (Fig. 1-6). A burning vehicle should be approached from a vantage point other than the front or rear of the vehicle. This area, called the *bumper strike zone,* presents the greatest risk if a bumper system component should rupture and launch off the vehicle.

Launching of bumper components because of heat exposure is further complicated when the automobile is an older model. As the vehicle ages, rust and corrosion can develop at the mounting brackets connecting the piston tube to the bumper of the auto. In an accident situation, the mechanical impact of a collision may be strong enough to fracture this mounting bracket assembly, mechanically disconnecting the bumper from the piston tube. If the vehicle were to be

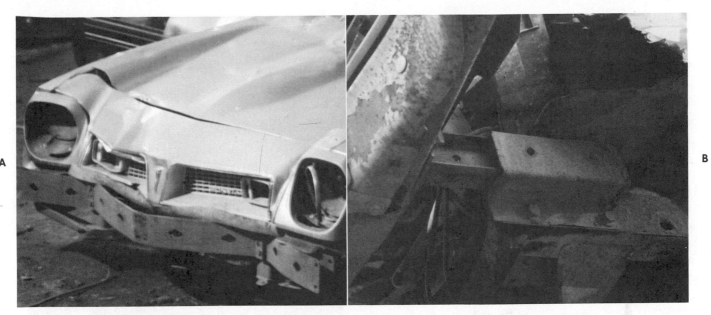

FIG. 1-2 Original energy-absorbing bumper systems include both **A,** the leaf-spring assembly and **B,** the rubber cushion assembly.

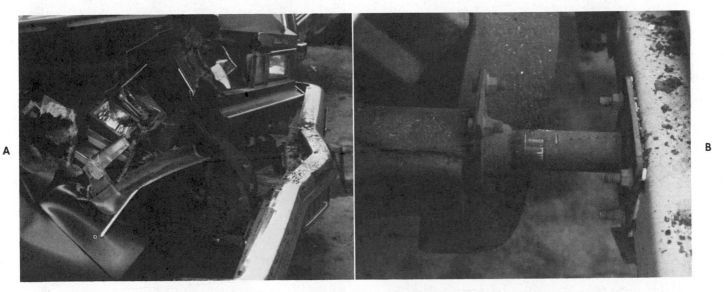

FIG. 1-3 A, Hydraulic piston unit. **B,** Small piston is secured to the front or rear bumper mounting plate. Larger portion of the unit attaches inside or along the vehicle's frame structure.

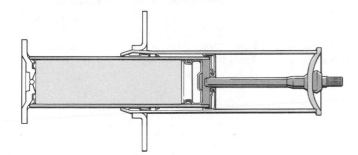

FIG. 1-4 The small tube moves inside the larger tube causing the fluid and compressed gas to work together to absorb impact energy.

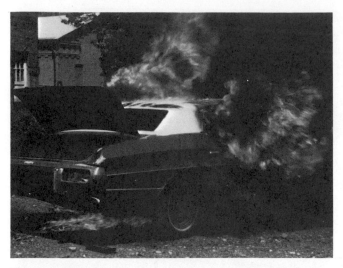

FIG. 1-5 Emergency service personnel arriving on the scene of a vehicle fire must anticipate the possible presence of some special safety problems.

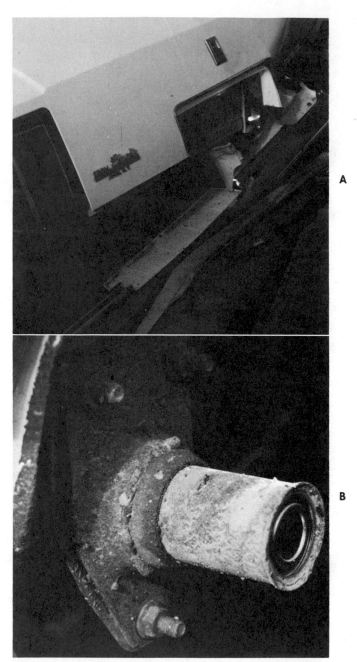

FIG. 1-7 A, This seemingly minor fender-bender accident has sheared off the piston at the bumper mounting plate. **B,** If exposed to heat from a fire, this unrestrained piston tube will readily launch off the vehicle.

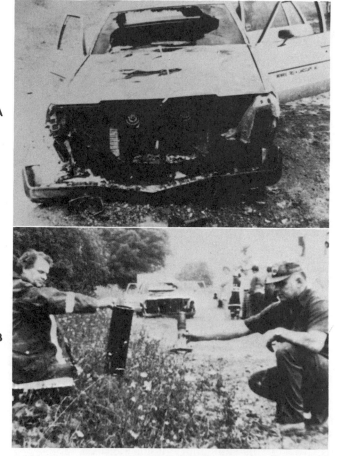

FIG. 1-6 A, An intact energy-absorbing bumper system has the potential of instantaneously launching off the vehicle if exposed to heat from an impinging fire. Note the completely detached bumper and the piston unit in front of this fire-damaged vehicle. **B,** This 2½-lb piston launched itself 187 feet from the vehicle.

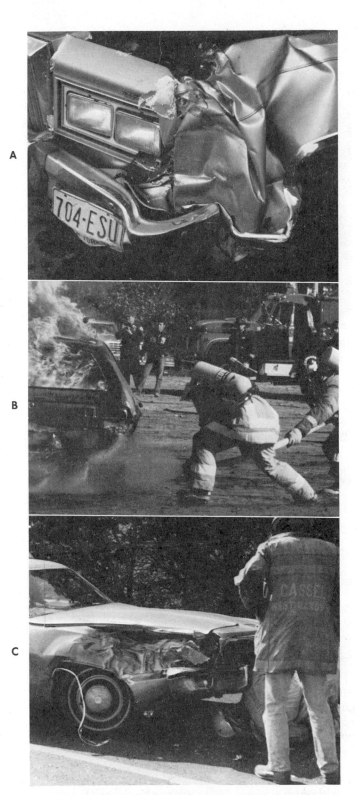

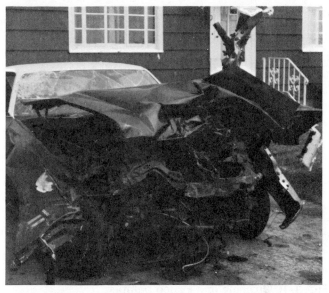

FIG. 1-9 During a head-on collision, this mechanically loaded bumper released and impacted the driver's side of the car. The bumper pivoted vertically along the front fender.

FIG. 1-8 A, A bumper found in this condition is an example of a loaded bumper. **B,** Firefighters should approach a burning vehicle from outside the strike zone and spray the bumpers to cool them down. **C,** The strike zone should be kept clear of all personnel until the status of both bumpers can be determined. The firefighter kneeling in front of this damaged vehicle is in an extremely unsafe location.

involved in fire, the heat could launch the unrestrained piston tube assembly, with a potential travel distance of over 300 feet.

Bumper system safety concerns are not limited to vehicle fire situations. Personnel must always consider bumper systems as a potential threat. In collisions at less than 5 mph impact speed, the pistons are designed to return to their original positions. If the collision forces against the bumper are greater than 5 mph, the piston may compress initially and fail to return to its original position because of vehicle body or frame damage (Fig. 1-7). The collision may mechanically hold the bumper piston in its compressed or *loaded* position. The piston and bumper can suddenly pop out to the original preaccident position.

There have been cases where loaded bumpers did not release until after medical and rescue activities were underway. When the bumper releases, anyone near it may be in jeopardy (Fig. 1-8). The size of the strike zone area directly in front of the bumper varies from several inches to more than 10 feet. This strike zone extends to the sides of a vehicle in an arc at the front or rear of the vehicle equal to the length of the bumper. A released bumper may travel into this side strike zone if one piston unit on a bumper completely releases and the other remains intact. The stationary piston acts as a pivot point as the released piston scribes the arc of danger (Fig. 1-9).

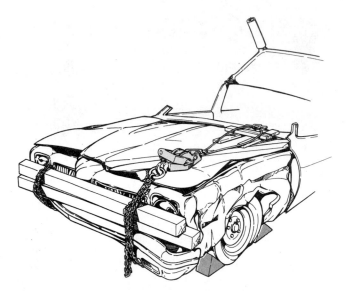

FIG. 1-10 Chaining of a loaded bumper.

FOR SAFETY, CHAIN IT OR VENT IT

Two actions may be taken to reduce the threat of injury from a loaded bumper, both of which assume that all personnel will avoid the strike zones while they are being rendered safe. The most successful method is to use 12- to 15-foot lengths of rescue chain to restrain the bumper to a solid portion of the vehicle's undercarriage (Fig. 1-10). Lengths of 9/32-inch or ⅜-inch diameter alloy quality chain are appropriate. This procedure restrains the bumper in its compressed position and limits any travel if the piston unit should release.

An alternate safety method suggested by some automobile manufacturers is to use a hand-held drill, preset with a ¼-inch drill bit, to bore a hole through the small piston tube of the compressed energy-absorbing unit. As this venting takes place, the tube hisses and hydraulic oil squirts out from the hole being drilled in the tube, which relieves the piston of its dangerous compression forces (Fig. 1-11).

Since the 1983 automobile production year, manufacturers have been permitted to reduce the impact-absorbing capability of their bumper systems from 5 mph to 2.5 mph. The smaller units resemble the originals in design and function and present the same hazards to emergency service personnel. Some vehicle manufacturers, however, have instead opted for a crushable plastic or styrofoam "egg crate" bumper and vehicle frame design (Fig. 1-12). Others, such as the Ford Motor Company, have continued to produce cars with the full 5 mph bumper systems at both the front and rear of their vehicles.

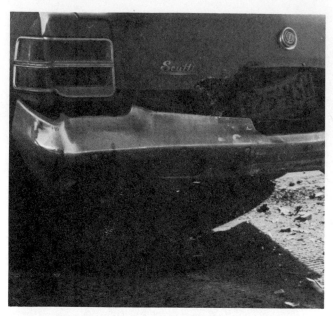

FIG. 1-11 The end result of venting the piston of dangerous compression forces. Note the small quantity of hydraulic fluid that escaped from the piston as it was drilled by rescue personnel.

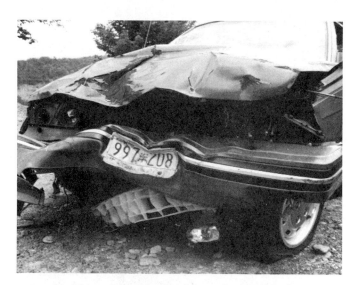

FIG. 1-12 Alternate methods of complying with the current 2.5 mph bumper standard exist. This Renault's egg crate, energy-absorbing bumper design is in compliance with the standard and eliminates the hydraulic piston units entirely.

Although these systems vary, the 2.5 mph system can be just as dangerous as the full-size system and requires the same degree of awareness and respect at an accident scene. All bumpers should be considered potentially lethal until identified as safe or until being rendered safe by the direct actions of emergency service personnel.

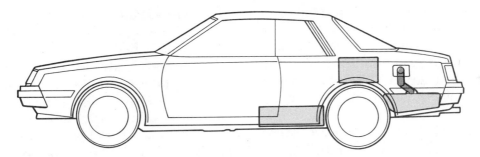

FIG. 1-13 Examples of potential fuel tank locations. The fuel tank of an automobile may be positioned under the floor of the trunk, within the trunk, at the back of the rear seat, within a rear wheelwell, or under the vehicle between the axles.

FUEL SYSTEMS

As vehicle technology advances, the problems and hazards that confront emergency service personnel continue to multiply. The fuel system has always been a focal point of vehicle hazard discussions. Rescue personnel must understand the function of the various components of the fuel system and the effect of each on safety at the scene of a vehicle fire or rescue incident.

A typical automobile fuel system consists of the fuel tank, the fuel filler neck and cap, fuel lines, vapor lines, various filters, and the fuel pump. The development of higher emission control standards for vehicles produced since the 1975 model year and the introduction of unleaded fuel have added vapor recovery devices and a modified filler neck opening to the basic system.

Fuel Tanks

Emergency service personnel were made keenly aware of the possibility of fuel tank rupture, explosion, and fire with the Ford Pinto and Mercury Bobcat problems in the 1970s. A 1978 recall of 1.5 million 1971 to 1976 Pinto and 1975 to 1976 Bobcat sedans was due to the high incidence of vehicle fires resulting from rear-end accident damage and fuel tank rupture.

With the fuel tank located behind the rear axle, two problems developed during these rear-end collisions. The fuel tank itself would move forward, disconnecting the fuel filler neck from the opening at the fuel tank. As the fuel tank continued to be pushed forward by the collision, the tank then hit underbody components like the rear shock absorber units or the rear axle. Recalled vehicles were provided with a plastic deflector shield in front of the vehicle tank to minimize rupture possibility and with a replacement fuel tank filler tube with a longer neck.

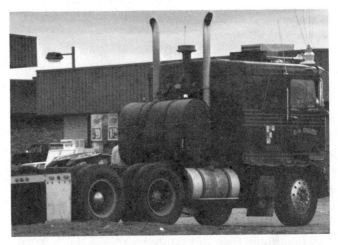

FIG. 1-14 Auxiliary fuel tanks may potentially be found on any type of vehicle. It is important for rescuers to note the material the tank is made of, the location of the tank, and the quantity of fuel. This unapproved auxiliary fuel tank installation consists of a 275-gallon capacity home fuel oil tank secured to the truck with bungie straps and blocks of wood.

The fuel tank of a passenger automobile is commonly constructed of lightweight metal. Fuel tank capacities on small-size automobiles range from 10 gallons to upward of 25 gallons of fuel. The tanks are generally located toward the rear of the car behind the rear axle (Fig. 1-13). Beginning with 1987 models, there has been a definite trend by automobile manufacturers to locate fuel tanks between the front and rear axles, which puts them in a less vulnerable position in the event of a rear-end collision.

Many newer fuel tanks are constructed of blow-molded, high-density polyethylene plastic. Vehicles likely to have these plastic fuel tanks include pickup trucks, some full-size automobiles, and recreational vehicles; most owner-installed auxiliary fuel tanks are also plastic (Fig. 1-14). The National Highway Transportation Safety Administration notes that although plastic fuel tanks perform as well or better than metal tanks in resisting punctures in crash situations, they react differently when exposed to fire or high heat conditions. The plastic material is likely to soften or melt completely through, spilling the liquid fuel it contains.

The fire service recorded its first known vehicle fire involving a plastic fuel tank in November 1976. In that incident, a 1974 crew-cab style pickup truck was operating with a hole in its exhaust pipe. Hot exhaust gases escaping from the pipe melted a hole in the nearby plastic fuel tank. The leaking fuel ignited, causing a fuel tank failure that destroyed the vehicle.

In a fire test conducted by the Federal Highway Administration, U.S. Department of Transportation, a plastic fuel tank exposed to a ground fire condition began to noticeably sag within 2 minutes of the ignition of the exposure fire, at which point drops of molten plastic were noted. The fuel tank failed, completely dumping its contents, 2 minutes and 30 seconds after initial fire exposure. In another test conducted by the Fire Department in Scranton, Pennsylvania, an automobile with a plastic fuel tank was burned. At 30 minutes into the test, the plastic fuel tank itself began to burn. After another 4 minutes and 30 seconds, the fuel tank failed as the contents of the tank were dumped to the ground. Flames instantly shot 20 to 25 feet into the air. By contrast, substantial quantities of gasoline are often recovered from metal fuel tanks of vehicles that have been totally consumed by fire. Fire-suppression personnel must consider the potential for the melting of the plastic fuel tanks and must quickly control the vehicle fire to reduce the risk of fuel tank failure.

Fuel Pumps

Important changes have also been made in the vehicle fuel pump, which moves the liquid fuel from the tank where it is stored to the carburetor of the engine where it is burned. In most automobiles, the fuel pump unit is located along the vehicle undercarriage area near the engine, with fuel lines running from the tank to the pump and from the pump to the engine.

Powered electrically whenever the car's ignition system is in the "on" position, the pump draws fuel from the tank and pushes it to the engine for burning. A recent trend, however, has been to locate the fuel pump completely inside the fuel tank itself, where it

forces the fuel through the fuel lines to the engine at up to 90 psi pressure. Since it is located inside the tank itself, the fuel pump can remain undamaged, although the vehicle may have sustained severe front or side damage. If the electrical system of the vehicle is still energized after a collision and the ignition system is in the "on" position, it is possible for the electric fuel pump to continue to operate. Manufacturers have installed inertia switches to cut the power to the fuel pump as a safety feature. If the fuel line is broken, it can result in a very pronounced fuel leak at the accident scene. Emergency service personnel who gain initial access to the driver's front-seat area should do what is necessary to get the ignition to the "off" position.

Fuel Emission Control Systems

Anyone who has ever removed the fuel filler cap of a late-model automobile on a hot summer day knows that it hisses as the cap is loosened. This sound is caused by pressure created by the vehicle's fuel evaporation control system and the new sealed fuel systems. Along with the introduction of some emission control equipment, significant changes occurred with automobile and light-duty truck fuel systems in the mid-1970s. The new system is comprised of a sealed fuel tank, a vapor-holding canister, and vapor recover lines. In this evaporative emission control system, the escape of gasoline hydrocarbon vapors or fumes to the outside atmosphere is virtually eliminated.

Unfortunately, for emergency service personnel responding to automobile emergencies — particularly fires — this new fuel system has had a dramatic effect on safety. The holding canister, which is usually located near the engine block, has been added to the sealed fuel system to act as a vapor reservoir. When the automobile is not being used, vapors that would normally have escaped to the outside are collected by the charcoal element within this canister, resulting in a concentration of fuel vapors in a sealed container. During the operation of the engine, air is used to empty the canister, forcing the vapors into the intake manifold so that the engine may burn the vapors.

Other vapor lines include inverted horseshoe-shaped vapor lines also located within the trunk area just behind the back of the back seat. These lines serve as liquid/vapor separators and contain fuel vapors at all times. When these lines are damaged or rescue operations must take place near this area, caution must be exercised. Unintentional damage to these lines may release hazardous vapors.

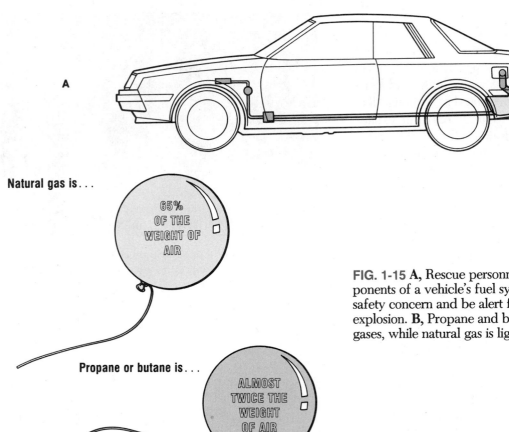

A

B

Natural gas is . . .

65%
OF THE
WEIGHT OF
AIR

Propane or butane is . . .

ALMOST
TWICE THE
WEIGHT
OF AIR

FIG. 1-15 A, Rescue personnel must consider all components of a vehicle's fuel system as a potential area of safety concern and be alert for possible leak, fire, or explosion. **B,** Propane and butane are heavier-than-air gases, while natural gas is lighter than air.

Alterations in the fuel filler tube include the unleaded fuel neck reducer flange and a hinge valve within the filler neck. This clapper device is designed to minimize spilling of fuel in a rollover collision. The newer fuel filler caps have a vacuum relief built into them, set to operate at ⅜ psi pressure. An additional pressure relief device operates at 1 psi.

When exposed to enough heat from a vehicle fire, this new sealed fuel system can increase gasoline vapor pressures to above-normal levels, triggering the explosion of any component of the fuel system. Emergency service personnel must consider the entire fuel system as a potential hazard and be fully aware of the potential for vapor leak, spill, fire, or explosion at an accident scene. These hazards must be identified and quickly controlled.

Fuels
FUEL TANK QUANTITIES

Fuel safety concerns rise in proportion to the quantity of fuel that is present. Recent consumer demand for extended travel distance between fill-ups has increased the number of vehicles with additional "auxiliary" fuel tanks, which may be factory-installed or installed after the vehicle's original purchase.

Auxiliary fuel tanks are usually plastic and range from 20- to 100-gallon capacity or more. Locations of these additional tanks are not standardized. In passenger automobiles, they are commonly installed in the trunk. Pickup truck fuel tanks may be a pair of saddle tanks, one metallic and the other plastic, or one large additional tank installed in the bed of the truck near the back of the passenger compartment. Although commercially available auxiliary fuel tanks may be purchased through auto parts catalogs for vehicles as old as 1965 models, those that fit in the trunk can be added to the fuel system of any vehicle. An owner with a disregard for safety can install any size, shape, or type of container in any location that it fits. This means that rescue personnel must search for auxiliary fuel tanks on each and every vehicle involved in an accident and anticipate the additional hazards presented by additional quantities of fuel (Fig. 1-15).

FUEL TYPES

Types of vehicle fuels have also changed in recent years. Unleaded gasoline was introduced in the mid-1970s in compliance with more stringent emission control regulations. Gasoline with alcohol added is known as gasohol. Although limited in its availability, gasohol's use is intended to limit harmful exhaust emissions and reduce the drain on the world's petroleum reserves. Personnel involved in suppression of fires involving these unleaded gasoline and alcohol fuel mixtures have discovered that, under the right conditions, some foam-extinguishing agents lose their ability to combat the fire. Currently available foam concentrates approved for use on hydrocarbons at a 3% proportioning rate can also perform satisfactorily at a slightly higher rate of 6% with spill fires involving gasohol or alcohol fuels.

ALTERNATE FUELS

The technology of vehicle fuels has always been an active research field, especially as alternate vehicle fuels gained attention during the oil embargo of the 1970s. Commercially available systems using natural gas, propane, or butane in compressed gas form are available for a wide variety of vehicles such as passenger cars, school bus and city transit bus vehicles, and trucks. Natural gas fuel industry experts estimate that there are 500,000 natural gas-fueled vehicles on U.S. highways. The National LP-Gas Association claims that there are over 1.5 million vehicles presently operating in the United States on liquified petroleum gas as a motor fuel. These alternate fuels have been present in vehicles since propane as a motor fuel was first used back in 1938.

A vehicle accident can expose these fuel systems to severe physical damage or high heat conditions. Emergency service personnel must be able to detect the presence of an alternate-fuel system and understand the processes necessary to reduce hazards posed by the system.

Emergency service personnel are often perplexed about the technology surrounding these special fuel systems. How does their presence affect medical and rescue activities at an auto accident or vehicle fire? Do they compromise the rescuer's safety? Answers vary. The fuel industry has developed these systems with the utmost regard for safety. Relief valves are present to minimize, but not totally eliminate, the possibility of container failure. The containers themselves are closely scrutinized during their manufacture. The installers of the alternate-fuel systems are safety-

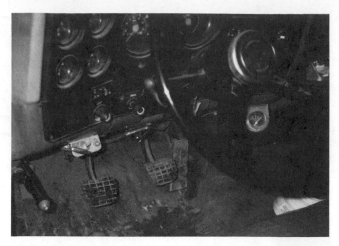

FIG. 1-16 Change-over control mechanism on dual-fueled truck allows the engine of the vehicle to run on propane or gasoline.

conscious professionals who comply with applicable standards for system installation. Still, problems can arise.

It is important for emergency service personnel to have a basic understanding of alternate-fuel systems, of which the two most common are *compressed natural gas* and *propane or butane*. Personnel should note that an alternate fuel vehicle may operate on two distinctly different types of fuels. These vehicles are equipped with two completely separate fuel systems, one for natural gas or propane and the second system for gasoline, for example. The fuel being used by the engine is determined by operating a manual fuel selector switch in the driver's compartment (Fig. 1-16).

Liquified petroleum gas (LP-Gas), known as propane, and its close relative, butane, are fossil fuels. They are stored and transported as a liquid under moderate pressure that, upon release from the container, becomes a dry gas, expanding 270 times its liquid volume. Propane has a flammable range of 2.4% to 9.5% air-to-fuel mixture, has an ignition temperature of 871° F, and is 1.5 times heavier than an equivalent volume of air. Compressed natural gas, also a fossil fuel, has a combustion range of 4% to 14% air-to-fuel ratio, and requires a 1300° F heat source for ignition compared with approximately 800° F for gasoline vapors. Natural gas weighs only 65% of an equivalent volume of air, is non-toxic, and important for emergency personnel, is odorized with the familiar scent of domestic natural gas.

FIG. 1-17 A, Locations of alternate fuel system cylinders vary from one vehicle to another. This compressed natural gas cylinder has its shutoff valve located under the plastic shroud material. **B,** The propane/butane fuel system cylinder is secured into the bed of this pickup truck. Note the cylinder's fill, shutoff, and relief valve components.

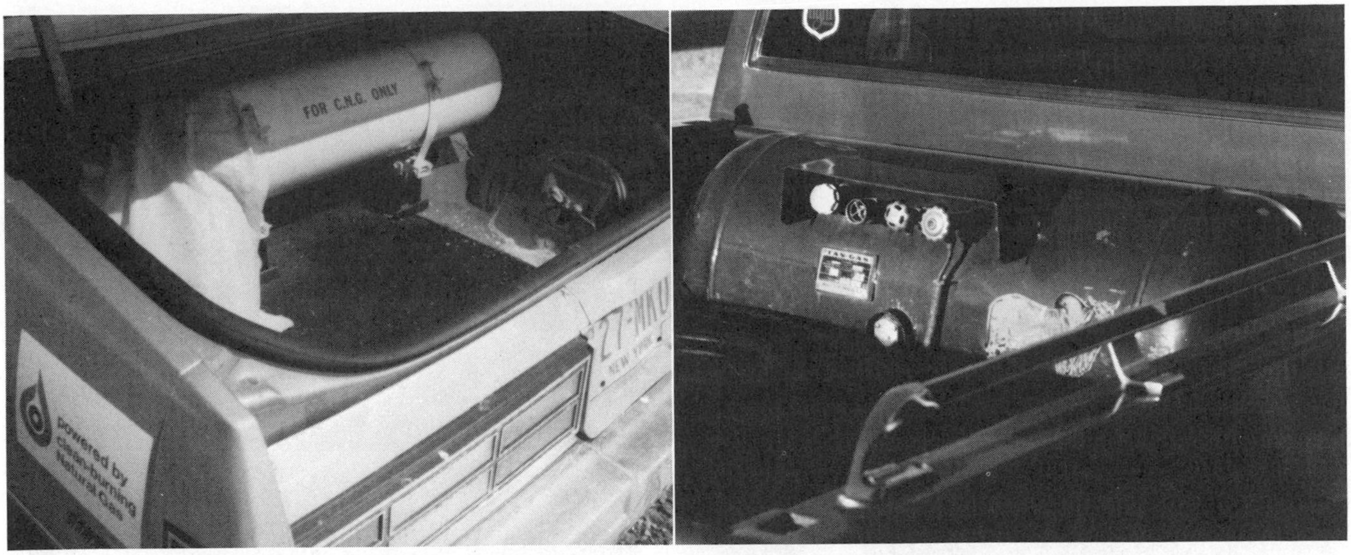

All alternate-fueled systems have one or more storage containers (Fig. 1-17). These containers may be located in the trunk, in the bed of a pickup truck, or under the floor of the vehicle. Fuel storage tanks installed on vans are generally mounted inside, behind the driver, or in the rear cargo area. A typical storage cylinder can be up to 13 inches in diameter with a length of up to 10 feet.

Compressed natural gas is stored in approved cylinders at a pressure up to 2400 psi at 70° F ambient temperature. Liquified propane or butane is stored at a normal working pressure of 175 psi. Storage cylinders for propane or butane systems are constructed of heavy gauge steel in accordance with federal, state, and local codes. Industry sources state that in the event of a collision, propane tanks have over 20 times the resistance of a gasoline or diesel fuel tank. Natural gas fuel-storage cylinders may be constructed of steel or a composite reinforced aluminum. The latter are fabricated from extruded aluminum alloy tubes; their sidewalls are reinforced by a high-strength fiberglass wrap.

A pressure relief valve located at the storage cylinder protects the alternate fuel system against container explosion, yet it is possible for a failure to occur. The valve may not function as designed or may be inadequate to relieve excessive pressure buildup in the gas system. In all installations a manual screw valve or ¼-turn Hoke shutoff valve is provided in the high-pressure system as a means of shutting off the fuel supply from the storage cylinder feeding the rest of the alternate fuel system. Valve locations may be on or in close proximity to the storage cylinder or under the hood near the engine. When natural gas cylinders are mounted in the passenger compartment, the cylinder valve ends are enclosed within a flexible vinyl bag. The shutoff valve is located within this bag. The piping or tubing used for distributing fuel to the vehicle's engine is either high-pressure steel tubing or braided flexible rubber hose, depending on the fuel used. Additional pressure reducers or regulators may be located in the engine compartment to allow for normal burning of the alternate fuel by the engine.

A Warning for Responders

Some cities and states now require visible identification on the outside of alternate-fueled vehicles. New York State, for example, passed legislation in January 1984 that requires placing a reflective two- by four-inch decal on the driver's side of the rear bumper of every alternate-fueled vehicle, regardless of owner, operator, or the vehicle's size or shape. The intention is to provide a visible early warning to first-arriving response personnel at an emergency incident involving that vehicle (Fig. 1-18). Although the decal is a step in the right direction, experience has shown its effectiveness to be somewhat unreliable. In an accident the collision can destroy or obstruct the bumper decal and

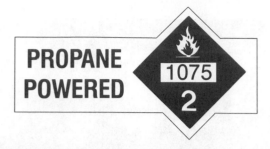

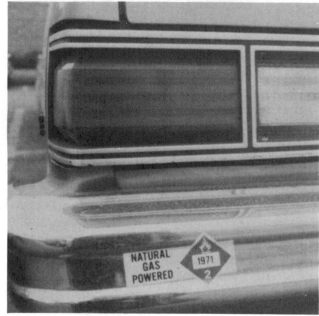

FIG. 1-18 **A,** Example of mandatory decal used to identify alternately fueled vehicle in New York State. **B,** Decal in place on automobile.

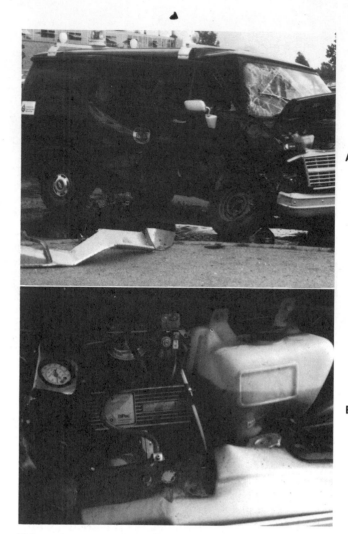

FIG. 1-19 **A,** T-bone collision involving natural gas-powered van owned by a local utility company that caused entire contents of the van's four storage cylinders of natural gas to leak out at the accident scene. **B,** Collision damage to natural gas components inside engine compartment is evident.

under adverse weather conditions, dirt, mud, and snow can completely obscure it. In an alternate-fueled vehicle fire emergency, flames can quickly scorch and blister the tape decal. The best indications of the presence of alternate-fueled vehicles may thus be the sights, sounds, and smells noted by the observant emergency responder when initially surveying the accident scene.

Emergency Procedures
Leaks

Collision damage may cause leaks in natural gas, propane, or butane systems that allow fuel to filter into the vehicle or escape into the atmosphere, where the vapors can become a serious ignition and explosion hazard (Fig. 1-19).

If the positive shutoff valve is on or near the cylinder and the cylinder is in the trunk, the leaking fuel system cannot be shut down without opening the trunk. Only

manual operation of this valve by emergency response personnel can stop the flow of vapor from a leaking system.

The odor of propane, butane, or natural gas in or near a vehicle involved in a fire or collision emergency denotes the possible presence of a dual-fueled or alternate-fueled vehicle. Action must be taken to shut off the fuel leak at the supply source, eliminate possible sources of ignition, and quickly ventilate the confined spaces of the vehicle to a vapor concentration below the flammable limits of the leaking fuel. If the fuel line from the storage cylinders to the engine develops a leak and personnel are unable to reach or operate the shutoff valve, water spray can be used to disperse the gas vapors.

Fires

Fire situations present additional safety hazards. An engine compartment fire involving only leaking natural gas or propane can be controlled by shutting off the engine and shutting off the fuel supply valve, bearing in mind that although the valve has been closed manually, it may take some time for the residual fuel in the lines to be consumed, depending on the size of the supply line and the size of the leak. For more involved engine compartment fires, fire suppression would be by conventional means. When fuel storage cylinders are exposed to heat from a fire, water should be applied at the point of contact to cool the cylinder, concentrating on the cylinder's upper vapor area.

It is important to determine the condition of the relief valves at the supply cylinders or near the engine compartment. Until the situation is stabilized, non-essential personnel should be kept clear of these areas. If the relief is not adequate for the situation, a boiling liquid expanding vapor explosion (BLEVE) becomes a very real possibility. All precautions inherent with compressed cylinders under potential BLEVE conditions should be undertaken.

Final Word

The likelihood of a dual-fueled or alternate-fueled vehicle being involved in an accident or fire incident becomes more common every day. The presence of sealed and pressurized containers within vehicles is also becoming a frequent occurrence. Additionally, nitrous oxide boosters, campers with propane cylinders for cooking or heating, even acetylene or oxygen cylinders for cutting torches or welding outfits can be found at an accident scene. Safety for responding emergency service personnel depends on quick detection of such items and decisive action to render them safe. Alternate-fueled systems for vehicles should be thoroughly studied and necessary actions preplanned to ensure safe and efficient operations at the emergency scene.

Catalytic Converters

In 1970, Congress passed the Clean Air Act, which calls for major reductions in U.S. air pollution. Beginning with the 1975 automobile production year, manufacturers complied with regulations by introducing the catalytic converter, a pollution control device for automobile exhaust emissions (Fig. 1-20). Emergency service personnel must understand the operating characteristics of different catalytic converters, be able to quickly identify them on vehicles, be aware of the fire and safety hazards, and be able to render them safe for operating personnel working nearby.

Catalytic converters are metal vessels of various shapes and sizes located in vehicle exhaust systems, anywhere from the rear tailpipe to a location under the hood. Although most automobiles have only one converter, some have more. The 1990 Chevrolet Corvette, for example, is equipped with three units, one on each side of the engine block, and a third integrated into the exhaust pipe system.

Inside the shell of the converter lies a ceramic glass substrate coated with platinum. This glass element may be in small pellet form (General Motors vehicles) or in a honeycomb structure with up to 600 cells per square inch density (Chrysler and Ford vehicles). Hot exhaust emission gases from the engine pass through the platinum-coated ceramic glass as they exit from the rear tail pipe. The platinum changes (catalyzes) the exhaust pollutants into carbon dioxide and water vapor. Hydrogen sulfide and sulfur dioxide gas vapors are also present in the exhaust emission.

For the converter to work properly, the glass catalytic element must reach a relatively high and sometimes dangerous operating temperature; its normal operating temperature may approach 1300° F. The exterior of the metal catalytic converter shell typically reaches a temperature of 1000° F. Shields and insulation are installed on the vehicle to keep converter heat out of the passenger compartment and away from other vehicle components. The catalytic converter's greatest heat management problem occurs when a rich fuel and air mixture is inducted into the catalyst, with little or no cooling air flowing around the outside of the converter shell. A misfiring engine or a stationary vehicle with its engine running may cause the converter's surface temperature to reach or exceed 2000° F.

One obvious hazard associated with the catalytic converter and its high heat yield is the possibility that it will ignite leaking vehicle fuel vapors. If the vapors contact the converter in the correct fuel-to-air mixture, with the shell temperature above the ignition temperature of the fuel, instantaneous ignition of the vapor results in fire and explosion. Emergency vehicles that are catalytic converter-equipped must exercise caution when arriving on an accident scene. The catalytic converter on an emergency vehicle, whether police car, ambulance, or private automobile, may ignite leaking fuel vapors from accident-involved vehicles.

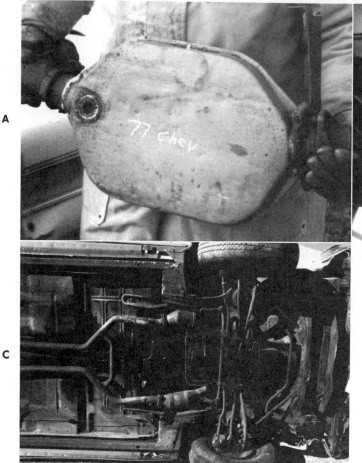

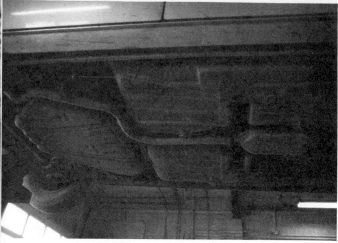

FIG. 1-20 A, A typical catalytic converter from a General Motors vehicle. **B,** Catalytic converters are always located somewhere in the exhaust system. They may be at the exhaust manifold, in the engine compartment, or anywhere along the exhaust piping. **C,** Vehicle may be equipped with up to three catalytic converters. View of the undercarriage reveals dual converters positioned on each side of the transmission.

Direct contact with the converter produces grotesque, even fatal burn injuries, to which anyone trapped under the vehicle is susceptible. Emergency service personnel working at an accident scene, particularly one in which a vehicle has rolled onto its top or side, must thus avoid exposure to the hot converter shell because even state-of-the-art protective garments will deteriorate at 2000° F surface temperatures.

Another catalytic converter hazard is best summed up by the statement: "Catalytic converters eat air bags!" These powerful and effective rescue tools, which are gaining increasing popularity among rescue teams around the world, are generally constructed of abrasion-resistant neoprene rubber, which will permanently scorch at 220° F and destructively melt at 330° F. Rescue personnel working close to the catalytic converter must exercise extreme caution when placing an air bag or air cushion rescue tool. Even momentary contact with the converter shell can damage or destroy the integrity of the air bag unit. Contact with a fully inflated bag or cushion can yield an explosive failure of the rescue tool. Repositioning air bags away from the heat source, shielding them from the converter, or applying water to cool the converter shell may be necessary before the rescue can proceed.

VEHICLE DRIVE SHAFTS

The oldest new technology item, the vehicle drive shaft, is becoming less common as the number of front-wheel drive automobiles increases. Trucks and buses will continue to use drive shafts as part of their power train, as will cars built with rear-wheel drive.

The basic change in drive shaft design took place many years ago. Drive shafts on early-model American cars were constructed of solid metal. They are now hollow but of heavier gauge than the metal that makes up the body panel areas. Circular metal end plates are welded at each end of the shaft making a closed-tube design.

If the drive shaft of a vehicle needs to be removed during a vehicle rescue incident, personnel can readily disassemble it by sawing or chiseling or by cutting it with power rescue system cutter units. The hollow design is actually a benefit to rescue personnel operating at an accident because it aids drive shaft removal.

The safety concern with drive shafts is limited to fire exposure, either along the entire length of the drive shaft or at any particular point. Although the shaft is hollow, it is not empty. Moisture may be present due to simple condensation or pinhole openings that may have developed at the weld, allowing moisture inside. When the shaft is heated, the internal pressure can build to dangerous levels and cause sudden explosive failure of the casing of the shaft, tearing open along its length. Although this results in a loud, muffled sound, the drive shaft rarely produces loose flying pieces of metal. Instead, it flattens out, remaining attached to the automobile. The portions that tear open may poke up through the vehicle floor pan, exposing sharp metal and endangering anyone near the floor area above the drive shaft. Loose items around the shaft may be scattered during the explosion.

This possible rupturing of the drive shaft is an additional reason for quickly spraying cooling water low along the undercarriage during automobile firefighting operations. Take away the heat and you take away the explosion possibility.

VEHICLE SUSPENSION SYSTEMS

Automobile suspension systems are currently undergoing significant change. Standard systems of the last 50 years are being replaced by systems that use no coil or leaf springs and have no standard hydraulic shock absorbers. These new *active suspension* systems are important to understand because of the possible fire explosion hazards and safety concerns they present.

Vehicle suspension systems are typically made of metal leaf springs on the rear axle and coil springs and hydraulic shock absorbing units on the front. With the popularity of front-wheel drive automobiles, the MacPherson type of strut suspension system has become almost an industry standard for front suspension systems (Fig. 1-21). The strut, sometimes referred to as an Iso-Strut, is located in each front fender well. The piston-like shock-absorbing unit contains hydraulic fluid and compressed gas and is surrounded by a coil spring held under a compressive load. The

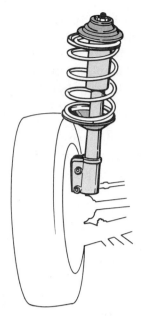

FIG. 1-21 The MacPherson strut suspension system has become an industry standard.

strut and spring unit is generally 14 to 18 inches in overall height.

The sealed and pressurized units, poised at the front wheels only inches from the actual engine block, can overheat to the point of explosive failure during a vehicle fire. The strut piston can rupture with enough force to blow the wheel and tire off the car, right over the lug nuts. The hood may fly up, and the fender and body trim near the strut may fly off the vehicle's front and sides.

When the older style of standard shock absorber unit failed because of heat exposure, there was a loud bang. Today, with the pressurized strut units "poised on the launch pad," whoever is close to the vehicle may not survive to hear the bang.

With the exception of the suspension systems of tractor-trailer trucks and some city and commercial bus vehicles that have used compressed air in rubber bellows units since the early 1960s, automobile suspension systems remained relatively unchanged until General Motors produced a "load leveling" suspension system in the late 1970s for their Cadillacs. Beginning in 1984, selected luxury models from the Ford Motor Company and its Lincoln Mercury Division were available with computer-controlled air suspension systems. The new units, which are similar in function to those found on trucks and buses, use air bellows units, an onboard air compressor unit, and a computer to monitor vehicle handling functions

(Fig. 1-22). When the active suspension sensor units detect road bumps — even vehicle lean or sway during curves in the road — the computer acts to inflate or deflate the appropriate air bellows. This seemingly instantaneous action gives the occupants of a luxury car the smooth ride they have come to expect.

This new technology air suspension system presents problems to emergency service personnel responding to motor vehicle fires or accidents. It is impossible to memorize the suspension systems of each and every make of vehicle. Personnel must understand the hazards that each system can present and be able to quickly control potential problems through prompt, safe, and effective vehicle stabilization efforts.

Active suspension systems (such as the air suspension equipment for automobiles) literally hold the body of the vehicle off the chassis or frame with a cushion of air. Any action that disrupts the integrity of the air bellows units, such as heat from a vehicle fire or a puncture of the bellows due to a collision, removes this layer of air. If the air goes out, the car goes down, sometimes instantly.

Fire suppression crews should not subject themselves to the possibility of becoming pinned or trapped under any portion of the vehicle should the bellows suspension unit fail. The firefighter with the nozzle must not reach under fender wells or the bottom of the vehicle at any time to sweep fire from that area. The suspension system collapse potential makes this an unsafe act. Rescue, fire, and medical personnel must not place their hands, arms, feet, or head under a vehicle at an incident until it has been declared properly and fully stabilized.

During rescue incidents, when the metal of a vehicle is being pushed and pried around by rescue personnel, an air bellows suspension unit may inadvertently be punctured. When this happens, the air releases and the body of the vehicle drops between 3½ and 5 inches. This crushing action can be instantaneous. Like a guillotine of medieval times, the falling vehicle could sever an arm or leg caught beneath it.

To prevent injury, personnel must keep the vehicle from moving at all. The stabilization routine practiced by many rescue personnel is to simply *chock the wheels*. This blocking action at the front and rear tires is intended to prevent the tire, and thus the vehicle, from moving. However, additional stabilization work is required to eliminate the potential for the vehicle to move up and down. Complete stabilization procedures, explained fully in Chapter 7, involve placing blocking or similar stabilization equipment under the rocker panel or frame area on each side of the vehicle. This added support minimizes side-to-side sway in the vehicle and decreases the likelihood of collapse because of failure of the suspension system.

Since the 1950s, a gas-over-hydraulic suspension system used by several vehicle manufacturers, including the original developer Citroen, has seen limited production. This system, which is receiving renewed attention from Lotus Cars Ltd. of Great Britain, Volvo, General Motors, and other manufacturers, is expected to be available in expensive production automobiles by 1991. This complex active suspension system does not use standard hydraulic shocks, springs, torsion bars, or compressed air. Instead, a system of sensors and hydraulic actuators linked to a computer built into the automobile moves each of the four wheels up or down in response to road surface and vehicle dynamics.

The hydraulics of the system react within $3/1000$ second and can cycle 1500 times a minute. To accomplish this, the computer changes the actual hydraulic pressure in each advanced design individual shock absorber-type unit. This new computer-controlled, high-speed hydraulic suspension is yet another reason for not trusting an automobile's suspension system but instead developing a standard stabilization procedure to properly block and support the undercarriage as well as chock the wheels.

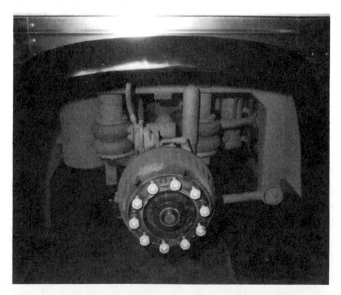

FIG. 1-22 Air suspension units may now be found on automobiles, trucks, buses, and even some motorcycles. The donut style of bellows unit on this commercial coach is pressurized to 120 psi air pressure. (Passenger front wheel and tire have been removed for clarity.)

Whenever the body of a car moves, whether it is back and forth or up and down, emergency personnel and their patients can be injured. By eliminating unwanted or unexpected vehicle movement, we decrease injury potential and increase safety for vehicle occupants. Emergency service personnel must develop renewed respect for both today's suspension systems and those of tomorrow. Every vehicle *must* be stabilized every time.

SPLIT RIMS

What has enough explosive force to lift a 2000 lb object 8 feet into the air or hurl a cannonball 2000 feet? The answer is not a new military weapon but a split rim — a method of connecting the halves of a metal wheel of a vehicle to hold a tire under pressure. All emergency service personnel must be familiar with the features of this wheel and mounting system, be able to recognize and identify its presence, and be fully aware of the hazards it presents.

In contrast to the familiar single-piece automobile wheel, the split rim has two separate wheel halves joined together to form a complete wheel assembly. The rubber tire is then mounted around the split wheel and inflated. Split rims can generally be identified by looking at the edge of the metal wheel where it meets the rubber tire. A solid wheel has a continuous round edge, but a split rim has a slit or separation between the halves of the rim that may be visible along its junction with the tire.

The split-rim design was first used on heavy vehicles such as tractor trailers, buses, and construction equipment that used pneumatic (pressurized air) tires. As wheel design technology progressed, these systems became available for smaller, lighter-duty vehicles. Today, split rims can be found on a variety of recreational vehicles, vans, and pickup trucks with oversized tires or heavy load-rating capacities, as well as on "big rig" trucks and construction equipment.

Although no emergency service personnel are known to have been injured or killed by split-rim wheel designs, there have been accidental deaths among mechanics in tire service centers and repair garages. During tire dismounting or repair, a worker would usually stand on or next to the tire and wheel. While a mechanic attempted to disassemble or "break down" the tire from the large split-rim wheel, the tire assembly would explode without warning, launching the heavy metal rim halves and maiming or killing the worker instantly.

Split rims can also fail when exposed to heat, either from a vehicle fire or from overheated brakes. There may be no visible flame or smoke to warn of impending wheel failure. The importance of recognizing this hazard and taking the precautions to avoid necessary injury or death cannot be overstated. Any vehicle on the road today, with the exception of the passenger automobile, should be suspected of having split-rim wheels until proven otherwise.

When the rim fails, the greatest danger area is straight out from the face of the wheel, in line with the axle. The tire or halves of the split rim can travel a great distance with great force in this direction, endangering any person in their path. Manufacturers of heavy construction equipment place this prime strike zone as far as 1500 feet from the wheel itself. Another shorter strike zone lies directly ahead of or behind the wheel in the direction the tire would travel if it were to roll forward or backward.

Firefighting forces making a fire suppression attack on a vehicle that might be equipped with split-rim wheels must consider the travel distance of the flying wheel halves and tires if the wheel explodes and approach the vehicle at an off-angle to the strike zones. Until wheel, tire, and all nearby components can be safely cooled well below any possible failure point, these strike zones must be respected. The explosion is so sudden, so violent, and so powerful that anyone struck by the failed split rim would probably never know what happened. Be aware; you may not get a second chance.

BATTERIES

Of all the safety hazards that may be present at an accident scene, the battery and fuel tank are the most familiar to rescuers. However, there are many misconceptions about batteries. Because many traditional methods of dealing with the battery and vehicle electrical system are no longer safe or effective in today's rescue environment, clearly it is time for emergency service personnel to catch up with today's battery technology.

Emergency service personnel must be fully aware of the operating characteristics of a typical vehicle electrical system, be able to anticipate the hazards it can present, and be able to render the battery and electrical system of a given vehicle safe for operating personnel and accident victims.

A typical vehicle has a generator that creates electrical power, large amounts of electrical wiring to carry

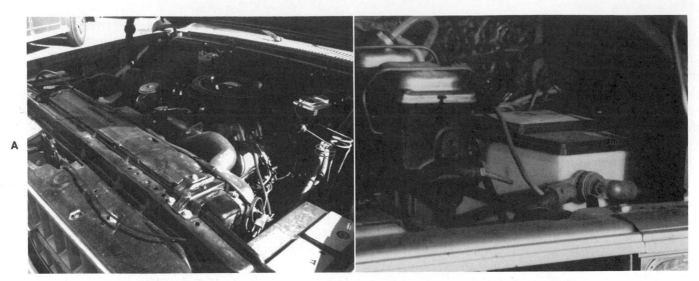

FIG. 1-23 A, Any vehicle encountered at an emergency incident can have the potential for multiple batteries. The diesel-powered pickup truck has a battery at each front corner of the engine compartment. **B,** The presence of dual batteries may be realized because they will be connected together by dual hot cables.

electrical impulses throughout the vehicle, and an enormous number of electrical switches and connectors to complete the electrical circuits. A battery stores energy for starting of vehicles and powers certain electrical equipment when the engine is not in operation.

All automobiles used to have one battery. This one battery had two posts: one typically a positive or hot terminal and the other a negative or ground terminal. Each battery post also had only one cable attached to it with a clamp type of device.

Many automobiles now have dual batteries. Excluding trucks and buses, there are still millions of vehicles that need dual batteries for daily operation, usually because they are diesel fueled. When diesel engines were used exclusively in trucks and buses, emergency personnel expected to find several batteries (usually in a tray or compartment somewhere) only on the big rigs. However, an increasing number of small vehicles are now diesel-powered, increasing battery hazards accordingly.

Multiple Batteries

Any vehicle in an emergency incident may have multiple batteries but finding them can be difficult because they may not be located next to each other. One battery is commonly located in the standard battery mounting bracket and tray on one side of the engine. A companion battery may be located on the opposite side of the engine, connected only to the first battery by a second power or hot cable (Fig. 1-23). If a design problem prevents placing the second battery under the hood or near the engine, the manufacturer may decide to place it in a remote location. For example, a new GMC van ordered with a factory-installed diesel engine has one of its two batteries located in the standard position, under the short hood on the driver's side of the engine. The second battery, too large to fit anywhere under the hood, is located outside the van in a small metal compartment under its floor pan. The battery box is on the driver's side of the van behind the driver's area.

The only clues to the existence of the other battery are markings identifying the vehicle as diesel-powered and a second power cable connected to the positive terminal of the front battery. Failure to locate and control this second battery may lead to serious problems.

A battery that has three battery terminals is available. One of the terminals is the negative or ground, and the remaining two are hot power terminals. The battery is actually two batteries in one, separated internally so that one circuit is connected to the starter and the other is used for all other electrical requirements.

A battery can have two terminals but have three or more cables connected to it. This is common on

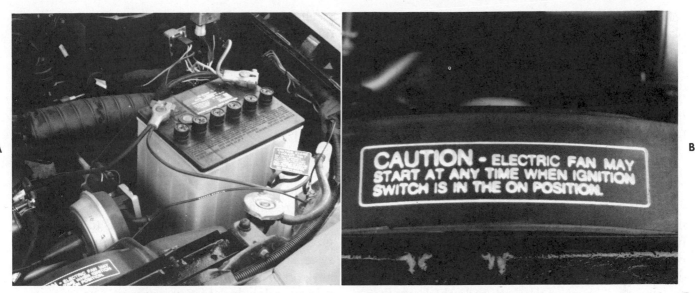

FIG. 1-24 A, Rescuers should ensure that the electrical systems are completely disconnected. Note the dual ground cables present on this battery. **B,** Electric-powered fans may or may not display warnings to rescuers. They may operate independently of the vehicle's engine, running until rescue personnel disable the electrical system.

newer automobiles. Two ground cables are provided to ground the vehicle; both are attached to the same negative terminal. One ground cable is attached to the engine block or frame, while the second is connected to a different grounding location, usually the body or chassis. Emergency personnel must be alert to the possibility of multiple cables because cutting or disconnecting just one cable may not completely interrupt the electrical circuit, thereby leaving an unsuspecting crew member with an electrical system that may still be energized (Fig. 1-24).

Battery Explosion

At a vehicle emergency, it is possible for the battery to explode. This can happen if there is a massive short circuit of the system, if a surge of electrical current hits the battery, or if it is exposed to heat. The liquid sulfuric acid inside the battery is a dangerous corrosive material that can injure an unprotected person. Sealed "maintenance-free" batteries that never need water have no means for excess pressure to vent to the outside, which makes them a sulfuric acid "bomb" waiting to go off in your face. Under fire conditions, if the battery does not actually explode, it is common for its outer casing to melt away. As the top of the battery disintegrates, the liquid battery acid and lead cells are exposed.

Personal protection at the emergency scene must include full body protection from head to toe, especially for personnel working near or with any battery; they must wear safety eyeglasses and full face shields. The smaller Bourke flip-down eye shields provide inadequate eye and face protection. When an accidental spill or explosion occurs, there is no time to put on gloves or don safety glasses. By the time you know what hit you, it may be too late.

Electric Cooling Fans

Caution must also be exercised when working around the radiator and engine areas. Because the engine is turned sideways in front-wheel drive vehicles, they are equipped with electric cooling fans. The fans are powered entirely by electricity, with on and off cycles controlled by heat-sensitive thermostats.

Chrysler Plymouth's mini vans, for example, can have two electric cooling fans located within inches of each other; one cools the small engine, and the second cools the air conditioning condenser unit.

When the front engine area of a vehicle with electric cooling fans is not seriously damaged in an accident, the electric cooling fan or fans can still be found operating at full speed as the hood is opened. The engine may be stalled out or even shut off at the ignition switch. As emergency personnel work under the hood, they can be hit by the spinning fan's rotating blades, get their clothing tangled, or be splattered by leaking gasoline, hot antifreeze, or motor oil.

As soon as the hood is raised, whether the electric fan is operating or not, the power supply to the small electric fan motor must be disabled by quickly cutting, pulling, or disconnecting it. Don't trust your luck to an electric fan!

Disabling the Battery

Today's automobile is becoming a sophisticated machine with electricity playing a large part in its function. Work with the battery should be accomplished only after a complete vehicle survey is conducted. After personnel survey the overall situation, the electrical system of the damaged vehicle can then be disabled. There are two methods for accomplishing this and both involve working with the ground cable. Because some vehicles have negative electrical ground systems and others have positive systems, personnel must first identify the type of system by reading battery markings or physically locating the ground wires attached to the frame, engine, or body of the vehicle. The "ground" cable is worked with rather than the "hot" lead because it is less likely to develop a spark or arc.

The battery cable that serves as the ground can be cut or disconnected with bolt or wire cutters, which may produce a spark when the wires actually separate. Cutting also leaves the tip of the cable with bare wires exposed. If these wires accidentally contact bare metal, they may reestablish the electrical ground to the system, energizing the entire electrical system once again. If the decision is made to cut the ground cable, the free ends should be folded back onto themselves, wrapped with tape to insulate the wires, and secured in the folded position. Another option when cutting the negative ground cable wire is to make a second cut on the same cable, completely remove a section to minimize the possibility of bare wire contacting metal, and tape the cut ends.

The electrical system can also be disabled by disconnecting or "pulling" the ground cable off its battery terminal post with pliers, wrenches, or a battery cable puller tool. Again, the disconnected cable end should be folded back onto itself and securely taped to insulate it from any bare metal contact.

If vehicle rescue or fire suppression personnel have the necessary pulling or disconnecting tools readily available, disconnecting can be done as quickly and as safely as cutting. There generally is adequate time to disconnect the cable at most incidents. A spark may be produced, however, when the cable or clamp piece separates from the battery terminal and if the electrical system is under a load condition. Personnel should not work with batteries until the work area has been ventilated by opening the hood. The ignition should also be shut off, as should any electrical accessory devices such as headlights or turn signal flashers.

The advantages of disconnecting the ground cable are that it does very little permanent damage and allows reconnection of the cable during the rescue process if the electrical system needs to be re-energized. Connecting the battery back into the electrical system could be an advantage for example, whenever all doors of a vehicle must be unlocked and an electrical power door lock feature is present. The contents of the trunk can also quickly be checked by operating a remote electrical trunk-release mechanism.

In cold-weather rescue incidents, rescuers can turn the ignition switch of the damaged vehicle to the "on" position and operate the heater unit blower fan. The warm air from the residual heat in the radiator coolant may continue to warm the interior of the automobile for 5 to 10 minutes.

Because most accident situations involving people trapped in the wreckage require complex rescue and extrication efforts by personnel, it is advisable to disable vehicle electrical systems at an early stage of operations at the scene to reduce the risk of electrical short circuits, sparks, or fire ignition. Most air cushion passenger restraint systems (discussed in detail later in this chapter) function on electrical impulses. Accidentally activating these systems during the rescue process can have very serious consequences. If in doubt, disable the electrical system by cutting or disconnecting.

The many circumstances that enter into the battery decision-making process make it vital for emergency service personnel to have all the facts and be properly prepared before taking action. The method of choice is your decision, based on the circumstances of the specific incident.

WINDOW DEFROSTERS

Rear window defroster units have become commonplace. Their presence is readily identified by the heater wires bonded in the rear window glass and connecting busbars at each side of the window edge. Rear window tempered safety glass, even with these

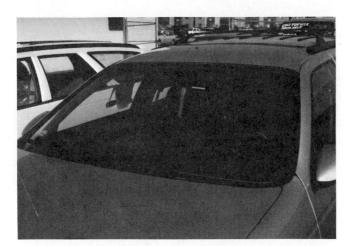

FIG. 1-25 Seventy volts of DC current are used to defrost windshield glass. The presence of these systems may be evident if rescuers observe a bronze-colored or peach-colored tint to the windshield or spot electrical busbars running along the bottom and top edges of the glass.

thin wires bonded to the glass, can still be removed with relative ease at fire or rescue incidents.

Front windshields with defroster heater elements integrated into the layers of the glass were first introduced by Ford with the 1986 Ford Taurus and Mercury Sable automobiles. Using the standard glass-plastic-glass lamination technique, Ford has bonded an ultra-thin conductive layer of zinc and silver oxide to one of the inner surfaces of glass. A thicker band of silver is painted around the perimeter of the windshield to serve as an electrical conductor. Two wires connected to the conductive silver band at the base of the "electric windshield" are supplied with electric current from the automobile's alternator. Seventy or more volts of DC current heat the conductive layer and defrost the windshield glass (Fig. 1-25).

Emergency medical and rescue personnel have been concerned about recognizing this defroster system and dealing with its operating characteristics. What happens to the victim of a head-on automobile collision thrust into the windshield during the collision? What hazards await rescuers if they contact the damaged windshield or forcibly remove it during rescue activities?

We need not worry, according to officials at the Ford Motor Company. Excellent safety features have been engineered into the system to protect both automobile occupants and rescue personnel. As an initial safety measure, the windshield is only charged with electricity when the automobile's engine is running. The engine must be running to provide alter-

nator output. Stop the motor, and the current stops and the electrocution hazard disappears. Second, if a crack develops anywhere in the windshield itself, as would occur during a collision, a small sensing resistor, mounted with a power relay switch, instantly cuts off the current used to power the windshield heater element.

Although broken glass is still a safety concern, it is refreshing for emergency service personnel to meet a new technology that poses no undue health or safety hazard to rescuers or automobile occupants.

DOOR COLLISION BEAMS

In 1986 the U.S. Commerce, Science, and Transportation Committee reported that more than 9000 Americans die each year in side-impact collisions, and another 20,000 are seriously injured. In response to the need for a more crashworthy passenger compartment for occupants of vehicles involved in these side collisions, the innovative door collision beam was developed.

Collision beams have been a component of U.S. passenger car doors since 1973. These beams vary in shape and size depending on the vehicle in which they are mounted. The most prevalent type is a steel beam, 7 inches high and approximately 2 inches thick overall. The multilayered metal beam, which resembles a guide rail along a roadway, is designed to increase the structural strength of the doors. Three layers of steel, folded and shaped in a corrugated fashion, give the beam rigidity.

The finished beam is located horizontally inside the door, attached at the hinge side and at the latch side. Regardless of the beam's size, shape, or thickness, the metal attaching it to the ends of the door is only one layer thick (Fig. 1-26). This one layer of steel at each end of the beam is attached to the door with spot welds.

The beam is designed primarily to prevent side-impact collision injuries by resisting or limiting penetration of the striking vehicle into the passenger compartment of the vehicle being struck, as in an intersection "T-bone" collision. Although the system is effective, it introduces several new safety concerns that must be dealt with by emergency services personnel. In a severe collision, particularly a side collision, the collision beam can bend or yield to the impact, actually piercing the interior door panel and injuring or even impaling the occupant seated near the door (Fig. 1-27). Medical personnel may find door

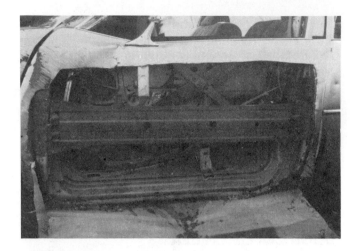

FIG. 1-26 Although three layers thick at its center, the side-door collision beam is only one layer thick at the point where it is spot welded to the door.

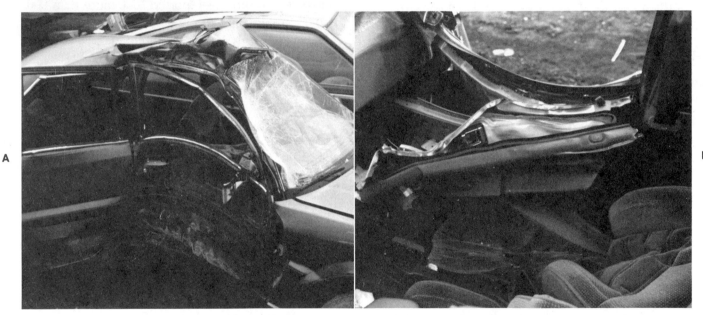

A   B

FIG. 1-27 A, The door collision beam may be forced through the interior panel of the vehicle's door, possibly injuring the occupant seated near the door. **B,** As the impact pushes the collision beam in toward the occupant, the inner door panel, arm rest, and window crank can contact the person seated closest to the door.

knobs, window cranks, handles, or the beam itself in contact with the victim and must therefore be alert to this potential injury problem.

It is also possible for injured and trapped occupants not initially injured or impaled by the door collision beam to be harmed by the actions of rescue personnel during the disentanglement process. Because for every action there is an equal and opposite reaction, a door that has already been pushed or bowed in by the impact may actually move further into the passenger compartment as it is being forced open with rescue

equipment. In this situation, rescue personnel, by failing to think out their actions in advance, can make things worse rather than better.

Two steps are recommended to minimize this danger during jammed door evolutions. First, remove all tempered glass from the door and its immediate vicinity. Second, place an immobilization type of wooden shortboard device vertically between the inside of every damaged and jammed door and the trapped occupant. The ¾-inch-thick shortboard, maintained in this position during the entire door-opening

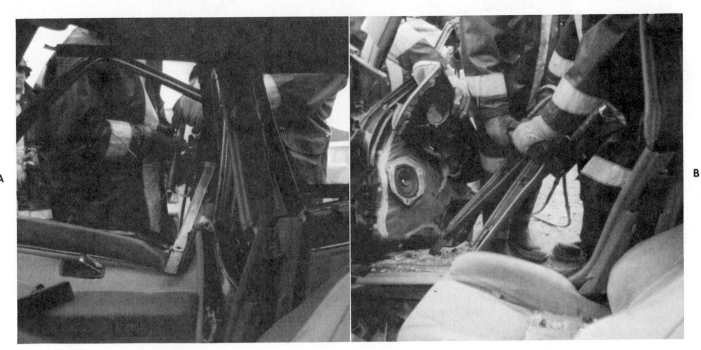

FIG. 1-28 A, The vertical crush door-opening evolution allows the impacted door to move down and out initially, away from the patient area inside. **B,** After the door is opened, it may be removed to increase access to the patient.

process, acts as a protective layer for all persons inside, including medical personnel.

Another approach, discussed in detail in Chapter 7, is use of the vertical crush door-opening technique, in which a spreading rescue tool is placed vertically in the window opening of the jammed and impacted door. As the rescue tool opens, the door is crushed down and out, away from the interior of the auto (Fig. 1-28).

STEERING COLUMNS

Another new technology challenges fire, rescue, and emergency medical personnel at the scene of a motor vehicle accident when steering wheel and column evolutions must be accomplished. New front-wheel drive vehicles have rack-and-pinion steering systems that use a slightly different arrangement for steering control than the systems used by those with rear-wheel drive.

Because of the front-wheel drive vehicle's transverse engine, the steering column is necessarily shorter and designed differently (Fig. 1-29). The *split steering column,* rack-and-pinion design is not, however,

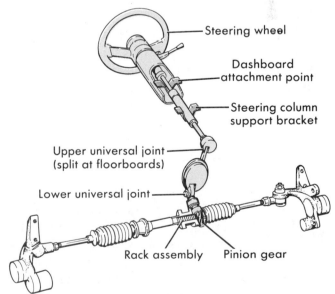

FIG. 1-29 The split steering column rack-and-pinion steering system consists of a multipiece steering column ending with a spiral pinion gear. Steering is accomplished as the pinion moves the notched rack of the front steering assembly.

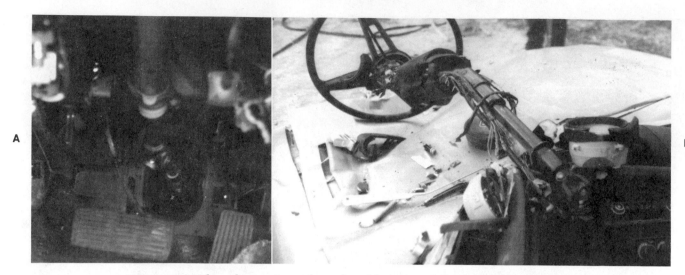

FIG. 1-30 A, The split-steering-column knuckle joint or joints located inside the passenger compartment near the floorboards may pose special problems when column movement is necessary. **B,** The rack-and-pinion column has been removed to allow for viewing of components of the split column.

limited to front-wheel drive vehicles. The rack-and-pinion steering column shaft is two to four separate and distinct sections coupled together by universal joints. The steering column of the rear-wheel drive Volkswagen Van, for example, consists of four separate pieces or sections of steering-column shafts.

It is important to note that at least one of the universal joints, typically a flexible knuckle joint that joins the multisection steering column shafts together, is actually located *inside* the passenger compartment area, just under the dashboard or instrument panel area in close proximity to the floorboards (Fig. 1-30). Where this assembly may wind up after a collision is impossible to predict, although its location can have an important influence on entrapment problems and rescue methods used to free the occupants.

During a vehicle rescue operation, it may be necessary to move the steering column away from any trapped front seat occupants. If done incorrectly, it is possible to make conditions worse for both trapped occupants and rescue personnel. To date, the most commonly used and widely known technique for moving a steering column involves a pulling action with air bags, come-alongs, or power spreader units placed across the hood of the vehicle. With a firm anchor at the front of the damaged vehicle and a chain or strap safely secured to the steering column near the dashboard, rescue personnel have until recently been relatively successful in moving the column.

Rescue personnel are becoming increasingly aware, however, that forces generated by rescue equipment operated in this horizontal pulling mode can cause problems with front-wheel drive vehicles involved in collisions. As the top steering wheel end of the column moves up and toward the front of the auto, the lower end of the split column near the floorboards can move down into or onto the driver's leg area. The effect is that of a child's seesaw, with the "action end" of the column moving up and away from the driver as the "reaction end," the portion of the split column nearest the floorboards, lowers itself (Fig. 1-31), further endangering patients near the column.

Stories are circulating among vehicle rescue instructors about the performance of split columns at accident scenes. The common belief is that the column can be pulled so far that the interior universal joints will fail and the column will snap in two. The free end, it is reported, will then launch itself into or onto a trapped occupant or the rescue personnel inside the auto. It is true that the column can be pulled hard enough and far enough for it to fracture. At that point the column can release, moving suddenly into the passenger compartment of the vehicle; in reality, the trapped occupant would be freed long before a split steering column would actually fracture at the universal joint.

Experienced rescue personnel know that the tilt-column feature found on more cars on the road today has a similar fracturing potential. As the rescue officer in the Film Communicators' 1974 rescue training movie *Collision Rescue* put it when responding to a question from a less-experienced firefighter, "Get on

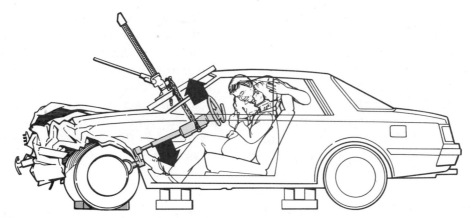

FIG. 1-31 Rescue personnel must monitor both the action and reaction movement of the rack-and-pinion split-steering column.

the high side of the knuckle joint and the wheel can actually pop up and take some of the driver's teeth with it!" If we've known about this problem for so long, why is there so much recent fuss about the columns on front-wheel drive cars?

Rescue personnel who run into trouble while applying the original method of using equipment across the hood for column movement may be victims of tunnel vision. When emergency service personnel at a rescue scene become swept up by the "emotion of the motion," problems develop. It is important to remember that rescue operations should only accomplish what is necessary to successfully complete the task. When the desired movement is achieved, the task is complete. There are no extra-credit points given for "hot-dogging" it. In vehicle rescue, an inch can be as good as a mile.

A major error that can result in split-steering column failure is wrapping the rescue chain or strap too high on the column. This causes stress near the top of the column and results in the unwanted "seesaw" action. It is best to place column strapping or chain as low as possible on the column, regardless of the rescue tool or technique used to free the trapped occupant.

Remember, it is the responsibility of all personnel directly involved with moving the column, including the rescue sector commander supervising this evolution, to detect any unwanted action of the column; the unwanted seesaw effect can be detected long before the column is stressed to its fracture point. The clues are there in time for alert rescue personnel to intervene. If the lower portion of the column does in fact move in and onto the trapped driver/occupant, column movement should be stopped and a different disentanglement procedure initiated. Important in-

gredients for success are the willingness to adapt and the ability to try new procedures. Rescue personnel must strive to keep ahead of the challenges presented by these special steering columns.

AIR BAGS

On rural Highway 175 near Milwaukee, Wisconsin, State Trooper John Leitner was on routine patrol operating his police vehicle's radar equipment when suddenly he clocked an approaching motorcyclist speeding past him at 99 mph. Officer Leitner began a pursuit that continued through two counties, at times reaching speeds of 115 mph. The chase ended abruptly for Officer Leitner when he lost control of his Chrysler-Plymouth vehicle on a turn, skidded, and crashed head-on into an earthen enbankment alongside the road. Under ordinary circumstances, the destructive impact collision would have seriously or even fatally injured the driver. This officer's injuries, however, amounted to only a few minor cuts and bruises. His life was saved because his police vehicle had been specially retrofitted with an air bag supplemental restraint system (SRS).

SRS-equipped vehicles are accumulating an impressive record of death and injury reduction as SRS automobile occupants continue to walk away from head-on collisions under what would once have been unsurvivable circumstances. SRS, when used with the lap and shoulder harness seatbelt designed into the vehicle, minimizes the injuries and deaths to vehicle occupants that emergency response personnel would otherwise encounter.

After years of being virtually unavailable, SRS equipment is increasingly being provided on automobiles sold in North America. The first SRS units, also known as air bags or passive restraints, were developed by engineers at Eaton Corporation, an automotive supply company in Cleveland, Ohio. The air bag concept was outlined as early as 1941, and the first patents issued in the 1950s. SRS units were first offered for sale by an American automobile manufacturer on selected General Motors Corporation automobiles during model years 1974 through 1976. Over 10,000 customers ordered the optional air bags then available on certain model Cadillacs, Buicks, and Oldsmobiles. Volvo and Ford Motor Company also participated during these early years. Today, SRS equipment is available from almost all major automobile manufacturers, both foreign and domestic.

For example, Mercedes Benz, a pioneering firm in automobile safety, has offered their driver-side SRS on selected models sold in the United States since the 1984 production year. All Mercedes Benz automobiles since 1987 come equipped with factory-installed, driver-side-only SRS equipment. Ford has provided 1 million air bag systems per year on 11 of their models, beginning with the 1989 model year.

In addition, the U.S. Supreme Court, finding SRS to be an "effective and cost-beneficial lifesaving technology," has instructed the U.S. Department of Transportation to require "automatic restraint" equipment in all new automobiles, with either automatic seat belts or SRS qualifying as automatic restraints. Federal Motor Vehicle Safety Standard 208 was promulgated by the department. The phase-in period mandated that automakers equip at least 40% of their 1989 cars with some type of automatic restraint equipment. Ford and Chrysler expect by the 1993 model year to also install driver-side SRS equipment on both their passenger automobiles and on their popular mini vans. Approximately 10 million automobiles are purchased each year in the United States; experts estimate that there are more than 3.3 million air bag systems on 1990 model vehicles.

SRS technology is here to stay as part of an evolutionary trend to more crashworthy and safer vehicles. The presence of SRS equipment in a vehicle involved in fire or damaged in an accident indeed affects the safety of all responding emergency service personnel. Present-day emergency scene operating procedures for medical, fire, rescue, and police agencies, as well as our vehicle fire and extrication training programs, must be changed and updated immediately to effectively answer the challenge of this "new kid on the block," the supplemental restraint system.

Emergency service personnel can meet the safety challenge of SRS vehicles in two ways. First, all personnel must be made aware of the design and operation of SRS equipment and be trained properly so that they can quickly *detect the presence* of such systems. Second, if an accident or fire involves an SRS vehicle, emergency personnel must be able to safely and efficiently *render the system safe* to minimize any safety hazards present that are attributable to the SRS equipment.

Air Bag Systems

The two basic types of air bag SRS designs now available differ primarily in their method of air bag activation. Both systems consist of impact sensors, an air bag module or modules, necessary wiring, instrumentation, and diagnostic devices. Of the two basic designs, the more prevalent system activates itself by electrical impulses, while the second type uses a purely mechanical device for activation. The electronic activation SRS produced by several system manufacturers typically requires that three electronic sensor devices be installed on the vehicle. These sensors are present inside boxes smaller than a pack of cigarettes and are positioned on the automobile in locations such as the sides of the engine compartment, the firewall, transmission tunnel area, or inside the passenger compartment. The sensors contain movable metal contact points and are wired together in series. For an SRS air bag inside the vehicle to deploy, the sensors must receive the energy of an impact equivalent to a 12 mph or greater collision into a solid wall (Fig. 1-32). *It is crucial that emergency service personnel realize that this impact energy is designed to come only from a head-on or a near head-on crash, not a side, rear-end, or rollover collision.*

Once triggered, the small sensors use electricity to send an impulse to the SRS module located inside the passenger compartment. This results in the burning of the air bag chemical sodium azide, producing almost pure nitrogen gas, which deploys and fully inflates the air bag.

The Breed Corporation, a firm in Lincoln Park, New Jersey, is researching, field testing, and tooling up for volume production of a mechanical activation SRS unit. The potentially low-cost Breed system is designed with a sensor located in the steering wheel assembly that contains a steel ball held in a cylinder by a spring-loaded lever. Deceleration of more than four Gs (four times the force of gravity acting on the ball) is required to overcome the lever's spring. (Even under emergency braking, most vehicles cannot approach one G of deceleration.) When a crash generating sufficient G forces acts on the ball in the steering wheel sensor, a mechanical firing pin is released. The pin ignites the chemical tablets, which generate the needed nitrogen gas for air bag inflation.

The actual air bag used in both systems is typically about two cubic feet in volume at maximum inflation and is constructed of neoprene-coated nylon or vinyl. The bag, with several large vent holes or flaps located at its base, is folded and packed securely inside its container in the steering wheel hub for a driver-side-only system and under the dashboard area for a full, front-seat occupant protection system.

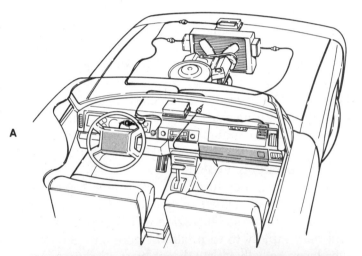

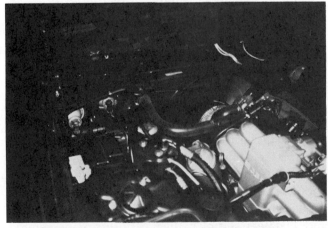

FIG. 1-32 A, Electronic or mechanical impact sensors detect forces of 12 mph or more. The air bags are contained within the steering column assembly and in the glove compartment area if a full front occupant air bag system is provided. **B,** Typical locations for the SRS impact sensors are shown along the top fender and wheelwell area of this BMW automobile.

Along with the air bag module is the gas generator module containing a mixture of salts, inorganic pigments, sulfur compounds, and additives in a sealed metal container. Approximately 90 grams of sodium azide in pellet or powder form serve as the main gas generator ingredient; the azide pellets resemble white aspirin tablets. Sodium azide, a hazardous material, is classified as a flammable solid. Once charged with an electrical impulse, the lightweight fabric, pillow-like air bag(s) is instantaneously filled with the gas generated from the reaction of the sodium azide composition with an oxidizer as the propellant. The entire event — from initial impact to full deployment — takes approximately 55 milliseconds. In comparison, it takes 100 milliseconds to blink an eye. Vehicle occupants protected by the SRS are cushioned from impact with interior components of their automobile during the first critical second of their collision. Within 1 second of the primary collision, the side vent openings on the now fully inflated air bag have unfolded, and the air bag begins to deflate, venting the slightly warm nitrogen gas into the interior of the vehicle. The deflation of the bag occurs in less than 1 second; the entire inflate/deflate cycle occurs in less time than the duration of a sneeze.

SRS DEPLOYED

One safety concern for emergency personnel that arises when a system has activated is direct skin contact with the deflated air bag itself. A chalky white powder will be found on the bag, possibly the front chest and face area of the vehicle occupant it cushioned during the crash, and the area around the individual's feet. This powder is slightly alkaline and may cause minor irritation to an individual's skin, nose, and eyes, although it is considered nontoxic. Whenever a deployed air bag is handled, adequate hand and body protection should be provided along with approved safety glasses or safety goggles. If the chalky residue does come in contact with skin, the contaminated area should be flushed with cool water. Rescue personnel may consider removing the bag to minimize exposure of operating personnel or patients to this residue. If the deployed air bag is removed, it should be placed in a plastic bag, sealed, and disposed of properly.

SRS NOT DEPLOYED

An additional safety hazard that SRS vehicles may present to emergency service personnel arises when an SRS vehicle is involved in a fire, accident, or rescue situation and the air bag does not deploy. Emergency service personnel must be trained and ready to identify this condition and to initiate appropriate safety measures at the emergency scene.

System designs share certain safety concerns that personnel must recognize. Ford Tempo or Lincoln-Mercury Topaz SRS vehicles, for example, carry several important labels that can begin to provide answers to the health and safety questions posed by emergency personnel. They are intended for use by service and maintenance technicians when working on the vehicle in repair facilities under controlled circumstances.

One service label, mounted on the hub of the steering wheel, states the following:

WARNING: This restraint module cannot be repaired. Use Ford-published diagnostic instructions to determine if the unit is defective. If it is defective, replace and dispose of the entire unit as directed in instructions. Under no circumstances should diagnosis be performed using electrically powered test equipment or probing devices. Tampering or mishandling can result in personal injury. For special handling instructions, refer to the Ford Air Bag Shop Manual.

A second label, located in the engine compartment, states the following:

WARNING: This vehicle is equipped with a supplemental driver-side air bag system. Tampering with or disconnecting the air bag system wiring could deploy the bag or render the system inoperative, which may result in human injury.

The most critical information on the Ford system is contained in a third service information label located on the rear of the air bag module itself. The information on this label is vitally important for emergency service personnel. The label states the following:

Contains sodium azide and potassium nitrate. Contents are poisonous and extremely flammable. Contact with acid, water, or heavy metals may produce harmful and irritating gases or explosive compounds. Do not dismantle, incinerate, bring into contact with electricity, or store at temperatures exceeding 200° F.

FIRST AID

"If contents are swallowed, induce vomiting. For eye contact, flush eyes with water for 15 minutes. If gases from acid or water contact are inhaled, seek fresh air. In every case, get prompt medical attention."

Another bulletin, this one from Chrysler Corpora-

tion, is intended to serve as a hazard information sheet to Chrysler personnel who work with large quantities of air bag units in one place. The Manufacturing Technical Instruction bulletin on the subject, *Safety, Packaging, Storage, and Security of Driver Airbags,* (10/1/87, Series SMI, Number 100), advises company employees that a potential health hazard exists if sodium azide dust or gas is inhaled. Symptoms of irritated mucous membranes, lowered blood pressure, headaches, and dizziness can result from low-level exposure. Higher concentrations can yield more serious results. Skin contact or eye contact with the dust or vapor can also produce health problems for the exposed individual. (It should be noted that once the sealed metal sodium azide inflator unit is installed in a vehicle, the chemical is isolated and the quantity small enough to pose only a minimal threat of exposure to operating personnel.)

The unreacted sodium azide chemical can react with acid to yield hydrozoic acid gas, which reacts with metals and may explode. The pellets or powder, if dislodged from their sealed container, should be kept away from bromine, selected metals, sulfuric acid, water, strong acids or alkali, fluorine, and chlorine. The actual sodium azide chemical should be kept away from sparks, open flame, electrical arcs, and temperatures exceeding 300° F. The inflator chemical, if exposed to such temperatures, can auto-ignite. If still contained within the inflator system when ignited, the sodium azide will not explode but will burn rapidly to form almost pure nitrogen gas, which can actually inflate the air bag.

DETECTING SRS EQUIPMENT

The first step in ensuring safety for operating personnel at incidents where an SRS vehicle is involved is *rapid detection* of the presence of the SRS. Indications of an SRS vehicle are easiest when the air bag has activated before the arrival of emergency service personnel. Rescuers arriving at a vehicle collision scene might observe the deflated synthetic bag hanging from the horn button or dashboard area. In a vehicle fire situation, however, detection is slightly more difficult because the bag may already have inflated, deflated, and then been shrunk by heat exposure or incinerated by flame contact or obscured by smoke from the fire.

If the SRS unit has not activated before the arrival of emergency crews, it is described as a "loaded" system and, like a loaded handgun, should be considered armed and dangerous. To detect a loaded SRS is much more difficult than one that has been activated. It is important to remember that the system is not designed to function in side, rear-end, or rollover collisions and that in a fire or rescue emergency with occupants trapped, accidental deployment will be sudden and unpredictable and may yield tragic results.

There is no readily recognizable feature or visible identification system to inform emergency service personnel that they are operating on an SRS vehicle. Safety concerns for emergency responders appear not to have been considered in designing any of the SRS units. The most reliable visual clues when checking for the presence of an SRS unit on a vehicle are a large steering wheel hub and an extra-thick padded lower dashboard area called a knee bolster. The large hub unit is necessary to accommodate the air bag and the inflator module contained within it, and the lower dashboard knee-level padding improves occupant survival in a crash. The problem is that the large hub, which may be readily identifiable in American-made automobiles, is common among the stylish interior designs of European automobiles. Regardless of make or model, personnel must be trained so that when they observe a large steering wheel hub (about the size of a child's lunch box) inside the steering wheel ring, they assume that the automobile is SRS equipped unless proven otherwise.

Mercedes Benz SRS vehicles offer another clue to the presence of air bag equipment with special embossed "SRS" lettering approximately ½-inch high on the front cover of the steering wheel hub. Although small, this lettering, similar to that used by several other auto manufacturers, may help to detect the presence of air bag equipment.

All electrically activated systems have a small instrumentation light located somewhere within the instrument cluster or on the dashboard itself that monitors the readiness of the SRS components. It is doubtful, however, that emergency service personnel would be able to locate this indicator light under real-world conditions. Beginning with the 1990 model year, Ford Motor Company has added a dashboard air bag label along the left edge of the dashboard to identify an SRS vehicle. Arriving in 1985, Mercedes Benz's 1986 and later models have an additional label attached to their VIN plate. In some crashes or vehicle fires, it is hard enough to find the dashboard itself, let alone a series of small numbers on a metal plate. To date, there is no universally recognized reliable method by which emergency services personnel can readily determine whether a vehicle is or is not SRS equipped. This is an important area of concern that needs to be fully addressed by fire, medical, and rescue services.

SRS ACCIDENTAL ACTIVATION

There is cause for concern by emergency service personnel about the possibility of accidental activation of a loaded SRS in a vehicle. An intact and active system is sensitive enough to electric impulses to be accidentally activated at the emergency scene by actions of the emergency personnel. The electrical impulse can come from stray electrical surges that might occur during fire suppression or vehicle rescue operations. An active SRS vehicle (one with an intact and uninflated air bag unit aboard) must be considered a hazard to operating personnel and vehicle occupants until rendered safe.

The output of the gas generator, measured in BTUs, reportedly equals the explosive energy of ½ cup of gasoline. Not only could accidental inflation prove harmful to medical or rescue personnel working inside the vehicle, a sudden jolt from the inflated air bag striking the trapped or injured patient could have similar results. The legal ramifications of determining the cause of the accidental activation of an SRS unit after the initial accident are likely to be very complex. This issue has yet to be addressed in a court of law.

All SRS units that operate on electrical impulse have a time-delay electrical storage capacitor integrated into their circuitry. Should the initial vehicle collision destroy the vehicle's battery or electrical system, internally stored energy in the capacitor would immediately be available to activate the sodium azide and inflate the air bag.

With the electrically activated SRS design, the only method available for emergency service personnel to deactivate the entire air bag system safely is to disconnect the vehicle's battery early into the incident and allow the time necessary for the stored energy to discharge. The "drain" time on most SRS vehicles would be a brief 8 seconds after the negative or ground cable has been disconnected. It should be noted that service technicians working on General Motors 1990 model year SRS vehicles are advised by GM to allow 10 minutes of drain time before proceeding with any work on the vehicle. According to the GM information, it is not safe for their technicians to work on the vehicle until all of this electrical energy has discharged.

Emergency service personnel who undertake safety measures on SRS vehicles must therefore access the interior of the vehicle to quickly turn the ignition switch to the "off" position and immediately (or simultaneously) disconnect the negative or ground cables of the electrical system. The sooner the better because as the storage capacitors within the system discharge, the system disarms itself. Until the necessary time has elapsed and the stored energy has drained, the potential for accidental SRS deployment is very real indeed.

ACTIVE SRS VEHICLE ON FIRE

Experts acknowledge that sodium azide, the chemical that generates the nitrogen gas, is a substance that requires special but simple attention. Direct contact with the chemical should be avoided as should any ingestion into the body. Sodium azide is a Class C explosive propellant with an auto ignition temperature of 600°F. This means that the chemical, when heated sufficiently, can ignite by itself. Bonfire testing done to study the gas generator reaction to heat produced a "loud report" when this spontaneous ignition occurred. Standard fire suppression activities that include 100 gallon-per-minute or more fireflow in handlines, safe approach positioning, full protective clothing, and mandatory breathing apparatus for operating suppression personnel will decrease hazards to personnel attacking SRS vehicle fires.

SRS TRAINING: THE TIME IS NOW

The report of a vehicle fire or auto accident with people trapped has been considered a "bread and butter" call for fire, rescue, and medical personnel. Technology is calling us now, and it is challenging emergency service personnel with more than we expected. The time to find out about SRS and their impact on our safety at the scene of the emergency is now. Automobile dealers who offer SRS in their new vehicles are generally cooperative in explaining the particular features of their systems and may well allow detailed inspection of actual vehicles in their showrooms. If access can be gained to the dealerships' service departments, service technicians who have been specially trained for SRS work can provide valuable insight into the inner workings of their particular system design. Ask about permission to view manufacturers' technical service bulletins and whether they have video tapes produced specifically for training repair technicians that might be available for viewing. All emergency service personnel have to do is care enough to ask, and the time to ask is now!

All emergency service personnel must be fully trained to detect the presence of supplemental restraint systems and be proficient in choosing the correct procedures to follow in an SRS vehicle emergency. For vehicle occupants, supplemental restraint system technology may well be one of the biggest advances in auto crash survival to date. Air bags work, and lives will be saved because of their presence. As emergency service personnel, we must learn to work with this life-saving equipment and understand what we can and cannot do at an SRS incident. There is an air bag out there waiting for you; your turn is coming. Prepare now so that your safety and the safety of others can be ensured.

ANTILACERATIVE WINDSHIELDS

Efforts to improve the type of antilacerative windshield glass accepted for installation in vehicles in the United States have finally succeeded. A new second layer of clear plastic polyurethane film is now available to be bonded to the inside surface of the basic high-penetration resistant, laminated safety glass currently in use for motor vehicle windshields.

Pioneered by the French firm Saint-Gobain Vitrage, the trade name product Securiflex Inner Guard windshield is expected to drastically reduce the painful and disfiguring facial lacerations that commonly result from frontal motor vehicle collisions. Automobile accident victims who hit the inside of the improved windshield will come in contact with an extra layer of plastic rather than the raw edges of broken glass, the "nest of razor blades" commonly found with the standard laminated windshield.

Although the improved windshield has only been in limited U.S. vehicle production since the 1987 model production year, increased production and installation are expected to turn the tide in the battle against severe facial lacerations and disfigurement of front seat occupants.

Emergency service personnel responding to motor vehicle accidents involving vehicles equipped with the new antilacerative windshield will still find the windshield glass fractured in the familiar "spider web" pattern. They may note, however, that the vehicle safety inspection sticker is located on a side window instead of on the windshield. (The additional plastic layering on the windshield precludes scraping off expired stickers.) But the real surprise will come when medical personnel survey the patient who has contacted the windshield and fractured the glass and discover that they have been spared the severe lacerations of what once was an extremely nasty, injury-producing accident. The viable condition of the accident victim will be living proof of the differences in windshield construction designs.

Rescue personnel who have to remove these improved antilacerative windshields during motor vehicle accident entrapment situations may note a slightly thicker windshield. In cold weather the new windshield may be somewhat stiff and more resistant to forcible removal. The windshield removal techniques detailed in Chapter 7 should be used for standard or antilacerative windshields.

SEAT BELTS

The slogan "Let's Get it Together... Buckle Up" is now becoming commonplace in our thinking about auto safety. Seat belts may be more appropriately called "life belts." Lap and shoulder belt systems do save lives and reduce injuries, as reported time and time again in government and private industry studies and in real-world crash experiences (Fig. 1-33). The Insurance Institute for Highway Safety reports that seat belt legislation in the province of Ontario, Canada, reduced highway fatalities by 11%. The motor vehicle departments of many states report

similiar reductions in fatalities in the months following enactment of mandatory seat belt legislation.

A recent seat belt-use program sponsored by the General Motors Corporation confirms the validity of seat belt-use documentation. The program began on April 16, 1984, when it was announced that after that date, each new GM car and light truck sold in the United States and Canada would have in its glove box a $10,000 Safety Belt User Insurance Certificate. This certificate provided that for one year from the date of purchase of the automobile, $10,000 would be paid to the estate of any occupant of that vehicle who suffered fatal injuries while properly wearing a GM seat belt. The GM program, administered through their affiliate Motors Insurance Corporation, concluded at the end of production of their 1986 model vehicles. During the brief time the special GM insurance policy was in effect, it was provided to 17 million vehicles. From April 1984 through November 1986, the covered vehicles traveled an estimated 198 billion miles and a total of 540 death benefit claims were paid, 465 in the United States, and 75 in Canada. General Motors estimates that belt usage in the covered GM vehicles saved some 360 lives and prevented thousands of serious injuries.

Because of the publicity surrounding the GM pilot project, buyers of new automobiles equipped with

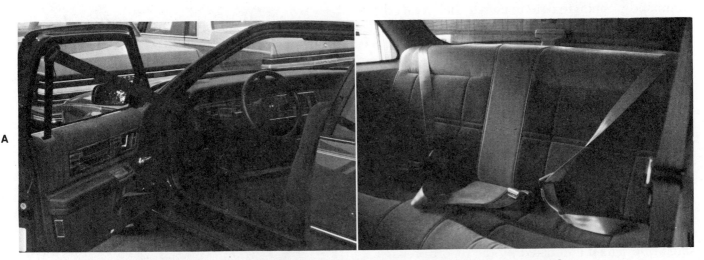

FIG. 1-33 A, One lap/shoulder restraint system locates the belt anchor point and recoiler spool inside the structure of the door. If the door opens during the collision, occupants may be ejected from the vehicle. Rescue crews must be alert to disconnect or cut the seat belt before opening doors in entrapment situations. **B,** Car manufacturers are installing lap/shoulder harness restraint systems in the outboard rear seats to increase occupant protection. Some manufacturers provide a three-point system for even the middle rear-seat position.

automatic restraints can obtain insurance discounts on their medical insurance premiums and on the personal injury protection offered by many leading insurance companies. Some insurance companies have developed seat belt death benefit policies that can be purchased along with a conventional auto insurance policy. Many of these private policies state that the belted occupant does not have to be found "dead on arrival" to qualify for the death benefit payment. In some cases the family of an injured person who later dies can still qualify for up to 3 years from the date of injury. This stipulation underscores the need for emergency services personnel to document whether or not each patient had a seat belt on at the time of the collision.

For the estate of a deceased accident victim to collect the safety belt user insurance money, it must provide the insurance carrier with two important documents. The first is proof of death. The second, which is just as important to the claim, is a police agency report or *other reasonable proof* stating that at the time of the accident the deceased was wearing a seat belt. This aspect of the insurance claim may require emergency service providers, particularly rescue or medical personnel, to appear in court to confirm or deny the wearing of seat belts by accident victims.

All agencies responding to motor vehicle accidents should immediately implement a written documentation system for seat belt use. The effort must be made by each and every emergency service person in a command position to determine whether in fact the injured occupants of a vehicle are or were wearing their seat belt equipment. This information should be corroborated by another witness, an EMS partner, for example, or a law enforcement official. A statement confirming whether or not seat belts were worn at the time of the accident should appear on the patient's treatment record sheet and on the official report of the response to the incident by each agency involved. Some state medical incident reports now have space provided specifically for such seat belt-use documentation. The vehicle make, model, and year and the location of the injured occupants in the auto at the time of the collision can also be recorded. The report should be signed and dated by the report preparer with all necessary information included.

The most important reason to document a patient's seat belt use and log this information on the patient treatment report is that the information will be of value to the staff at the medical facility as they understand and treat the accident victim's injuries.

Seat belt-use documentation is becoming increasingly important in the total of services provided by the emergency community to an individual involved in an accident. Medical and rescue personnel must now take the time and make the effort to observe and record the use or nonuse of seat belts at all vehicle accident incidents.

CHILD SAFETY SEATS

Although infant and child safety seats cannot be called a new automotive technology, their use in vehicles is increasing. All 50 states now have laws requiring the use of safety seats for select age groups of children while in passenger automobiles. Of the more than 45,000 persons killed each year in the United States in motor vehicle accidents, nearly 1000 are children under the age of 4. In fact, the leading cause of death for children under 4 in the United States is fatal injuries sustained as passengers in automobiles. For each preventable death, the U.S. Department of Health, Education, and Welfare reports that thousands more are injured, many suffering serious, permanent injuries. Motor vehicle accidents are also the number one crippler of children in the United States.

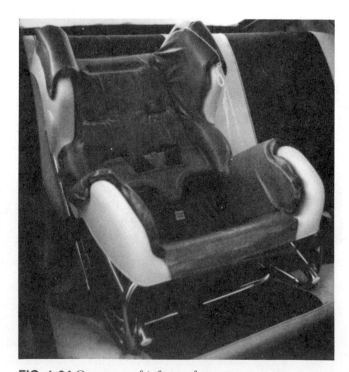

FIG. 1-34 One type of infant safety seat.

The U.S. National Transportation Safety Board reports that almost two thirds of these disabling child injuries could have been prevented by proper use of child safety seats (Fig. 1-34). According to the Gerber Products Company, safely constructed, properly anchored restraints can reduce the probability of fatal injury for children involved in accidents by more than 95%.

In response to the need to decrease child fatalities and injuries caused by vehicle accidents, state governments passed laws mandating the use of car safety seats. Typical state legislation requires the use of a car safety seat for all front- or rear-seat child passengers under the age of 4. The state of New York, which was the first state to enact mandatory seat belt legislation, additionally requires the use of a seat belt or shoulder belt harness equipment for children in the front or rear seat up to the age of 10. Safety seat legislation and, more important, compliance with such legislation can greatly reduce the daily toll of childhood deaths and injuries that result from automobile accidents.

EMS Concerns

Child safety seat legislation is having an important and noticeable impact on the patient handling standard operating procedures employed by emergency medical personnel. When adults are victims of automobile collisions, they are immobilized by medical personnel using portable shortboard equipment. This equipment —the boards, immobilization devices, straps, and collars — is carried by the medical or rescue team. Consideration must now be given to the growing likelihood that medical personnel arriving at a motor vehicle accident scene will find a child or infant secured within a car safety seat and possibly injured.

Experience has shown that child car seat occupants are likely to survive an automobile accident. Restrained infants and children can still be injured, however, most often when struck by flying glass or other objects inside the vehicle. Improper use or incorrect installation of the car safety seat itself also contributes to child injuries in vehicle accidents.

These special patients present special challenges to medical and rescue personnel. Most EMS organizations do not carry equipment for spinal immobilization of young collision victims. Specially designed child immobilization and treatment equipment is just now becoming available for this application. By using tools similar to those used to immobilize adults, medical personnel may also be able to effectively and efficiently immobilize children by using the existing structure of the car safety seat as a patient spinal immobilization device. If the seat has been grossly deformed or broken (as with an all-plastic infant seat), its use for immobilization is diminished and not recommended. Once immobilized, the infant can usually be brought out of the accident vehicle in the seat by rescuers cutting or unbuckling the straps or belts.

If this car seat immobilization technique is accepted by the local authority having jurisdiction, practiced during training sessions, and presented during medical training programs, this relatively new concept will quickly become an accepted routine and will save the lives of infants and children.

CAR DOORS AND LOCKING MECHANISMS

"Station 11...a rescue call...child locked in an automobile...engine running. Vehicle located in the driveway of 15 West Mountain Avenue. Time out 07:45."

Calls requesting a fire department, rescue squad, or medical crew to respond to a vehicle lockout such as this used to be rare. Car doors in the 1960s and 1970s were easy to unlock with a few simple tools and a little patience. Recent changes in the automobile industry's thinking regarding vehicle security now make the locked vehicle nearly impossible for the average person to open.

Antitheft Design

In recent years, both foreign and domestic auto manufacturers have increased the theft-resistance of their automobiles. Early changes included redesigning the standard "mushroom" door lock buttons and replacing them with slim, tapered "antitheft" knobs. This design essentially relegated the "coat hanger around the knob" routine to history. Then the manufacturers designed the flush-mounted door lock button, which, when locked, stays even with the top surface of the door panel.

Still later design changes moved the entire locking button device to the side door panel, making locked door entry techniques even more difficult for rescuers. Emergency service personnel are now confronted by levers or knobs that must pivot to lock or unlock the door.

A flat piece of flexible metal with notches cut in the bottom end, commonly referred to by the trade name Slim-Jim or Lok-Jok, has been used by personnel to move internal door lock or latch linkages. In recent years, however, a metal plate or shield device has been installed just above the door lock and latch to prevent access to these linkages. When an unlocking bar is unable to contact any of the necessary linkages, which is usually the case, the tool becomes useless for unlocking the doors of newer vehicles.

Another theft-deterrent system has been pioneered by General Motors. Best described as the *break-away* system, its main purpose is to make doors even harder to unlock. Thin plastic linkages included as part of the door lock-and-latch linkage system are designed to break when contacted by the force of a door-unlocking tool, which makes them useless on those vehicles as well. To make matters worse, the door needs the broken parts replaced.

The continuing introduction of theft-deterrent equipment on automobiles has produced the keyless electronic door-locking system. The conventional key has been replaced by buttons that must be pushed in a prescribed sequence to unlock the door. Chevrolet has developed and put into selected automobiles a door lock system that also requires the door to recognize a small coded magnet pellet within the key before it will unlock.

The new technology of flush-mounted door lock buttons, theft-deterrent plastic door linkage mechanisms, and keyless locks calls for thorough reevaluation of the procedures used by emergency service personnel responding to a vehicle lockout. These lock-and-latch assemblies are doing nothing to make our job easier. Recommended practices and procedures for emergency service personnel to use at vehicle lockout situations encourage action to be taken only in life or death circumstances and specify that forcible-entry work be accomplished by breaking tempered safety glass.

CHANGES IN VEHICLE SIZE, DESIGN, AND CONSTRUCTION

Since 1973, some very important changes have been made by automobile manufacturers in the size, weight, body-construction materials, and assembly techniques of vehicles being produced. Each of these developments has a tremendous impact on the activities of emergency service personnel operating at a vehicle emergency.

The first *down-sized* automobiles appeared from the foreign import market, many of them in response to the oil crisis of the early 1970s. As these first compacts hit the streets, personnel in the rescue field found existing tools and rescue techniques becoming less and less effective when used on these smaller, lighter vehicles. The little cars crumbled more than other models. When rescue equipment was used to pry against the vehicle, its structure would rip or tear away. When personnel attempted to pull, the small vehicle would simply fold. Certain rescue tools and techniques could no longer be relied on to solve all problems encountered.

The latest cause for concern among emergency response teams is represented by the Yugo, a mini subcompact vehicle from Yugoslavia. This vehicle, more than any other new generation mini subcompact, personifies the extreme challenges that we are only today beginning to recognize. The Yugo's metal frame and outer body skin are as thin as can be used (Fig. 1-35). The total vehicle wheelbase is just 85 inches; the vehicle weighs a mere 1832 pounds. Anything that is not necessary is not there. If the part can be plastic, it is. Industry sources claim that within 2 years, some 15 manufacturers will be offering mini subcompact automobiles for sale in North America.

The National Highway Traffic Safety Administration (NHTSA) in an extensive study of selected crashes that occurred between 1980 and 1983 found that in crashes between a subcompact and a full-size

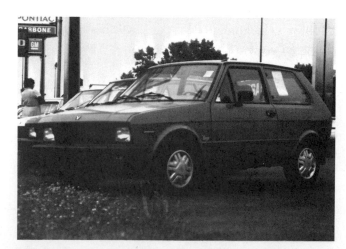

FIG. 1-35 New automobile technology is producing even lighter weight vehicles than this mini subcompact two-door Yugo.

vehicle, the driver of the small car was 14 times as likely to be killed as the driver of the bigger car. The NHTSA predicts a rise in the proportion of fatal accidents involving subcompact cars from 41.2% in 1981 to 47.5% by 1990. This means that every other accident incident that rescue, fire, and emergency medical personnel respond to will involve a small, lightweight vehicle.

Vehicle Construction: Materials

Emergency service workers responding to vehicle accident and fire situations are painfully aware that the "iron" of automobiles has gone the way of the rumble seat. Many automobile construction materials are now plastic and aluminum. What was once a frame with heavy channels bolted together with great precision is now a frameless, lightweight shell constructed by robots that arc, spark, or glue with computerized precision (Fig. 1-36).

In 1953 the Chevrolet Division of General Motors Corporation introduced the first Chevrolet Corvette, a car with a fiberglass body construction that has spawned today's lightweight plastic and fiberglass automobile body components. Plastic injection molding processes developed now allow mass production

of totally plastic body components to meet mass assembly demands. General Motors' all-purpose van (APV) was introduced in the 1990 model line as the Chevrolet Lumina APV, Pontiac Trans Sport, and Oldsmobile Silhouette. These APVs represent the first mass-produced, plastic-body van. They consist of composite, plastic body panels glued to a steel cage framework (which resembles a squirrel cage), and the steel and plastic work in harmony to hold the entire vehicle together. Industry analysts report that a similar manufacturing process will also be used on GM's Saturn line, ensuring the future for high-volume, mass-produced, plastic-bodied vehicle technology.

It is chilling to think about the outcomes when a plastic vehicle collides with a tractor-trailer truck or hits a bridge abutment in a frontal collision. The plastic vehicle can be expected to literally explode on impact. What will rescue personnel find left at the scene to push, pry, or pull (Fig. 1-37)? Many familiar rescue techniques must be changed to be of value in the new world of plastic automobiles, and new techniques must be developed to meet this need. In certain situations, powerful, brute force rescue tools will be less valuable than smaller tools that permit a degree of finesse in their use.

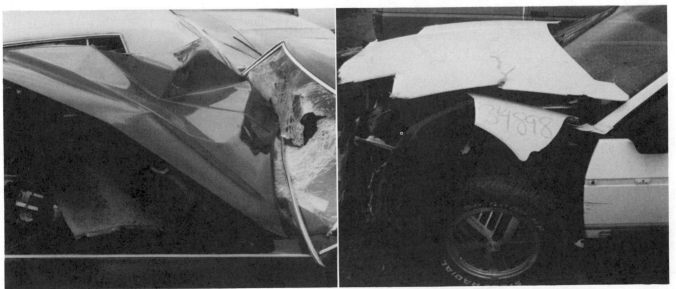

FIG. 1-36 A, What was once a heavy metal frame and body structure that would bend and fold on impact is often a frameless, lightweight body shell today. **B,** Rescue crews have less substantial structural strong points to use during rescue evolutions with plastic-bodied vehicles.

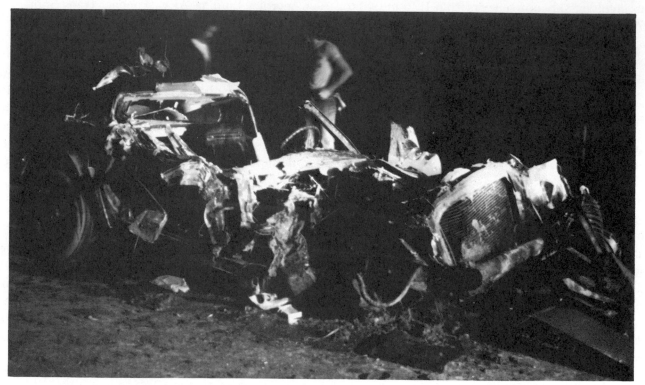

FIG. 1-37 This Chevrolet Corvette struck a utility pole at high speed. The impact energy completely disintegrated the body of the vehicle. The driver was critically injured but survived. (All damage was due to the collision and necessary extrication work — there was no fire.)

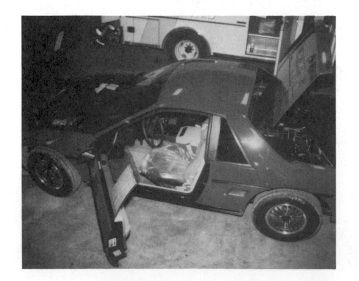

FIG. 1-38 The midengine design of Fiero remains popular, although production was halted after the 1988 model year.

Vehicle Body Construction: Midengine

When GMs Pontiac Motor Division introduced the first Pontiac Fiero 2M4 automobile in the fall of 1983, it received considerable consumer attention. As the most popular American-made automobile of both 1984 and 1985, the Fiero was a first in American auto manufacturing as the first American-built two-seater (2), mid-engine mount (M), 4-cylinder engine (4) automobile ever mass produced. Fiero production halted at the end of the 1988 model year, although the two-seater, mid-engine design remains popular. The critical factor for emergency response personnel is to know exactly how this automobile is designed (Fig. 1-38).

The engine is not in the front; a trunk is under the hood. The engine is not in the rear; there is a small trunk there also. The engine is literally in the back seat. In a midengine vehicle, the engine is located just behind the driver and passenger, near the middle of the car. Behind the front-seat passenger is the battery. Between the driver and passenger, on edge, is the 14-gallon fuel tank. Just below the driver's seat area, under the car, is the catalytic converter. All this is contained in about a 24-inch radius.

The new APV and the Fiero employ a new frame technology known as space frames. This cagelike steel structure differs from the two most common vehicle frame designs (full frame and unit-body/uni-body) in that it employs steel frame members to form a load-bearing cage frame to carry vehicle stresses and loads. The Fiero space frame carries all the load of the vehicle (the car can be driven without the skin), but the APV space frame shares some load-carrying capabilities with the glued-on plastic body panels.

The rescue and extrication concern lies with the lightweight space frame structure, which collapses on impact, and the fiberglass/plastic body panels. Experience with the Fiero vehicle in real-world incidents has shown that the plastic panels are also prone to failing on impact and offer none of the strength necessary for vehicle rescue tools (Fig. 1-39).

Of even greater concern is how these breakable plastic body panels react during a car fire incident. Firefighter Roger Garner of the Mason (Michigan) fire department described an incident that his department responded to in the March 1986 issue of *Fire Command* magazine, a publication of the National Fire Protection Association. Firefighter Garner reported on a vehicle fire involving a 1984 model Pontiac Fiero, and follow-up questions were posed by his fire

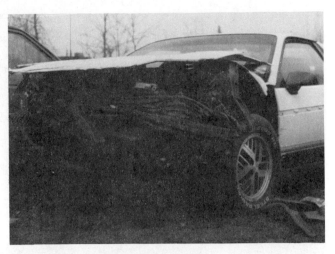

FIG. 1-39 Plastic body panels, lightweight space frame structure, and midengine design of the Fiero produced the lowest crash test dummy impact forces recorded during the 1984 government-sponsored new car assessment.

department to sources within the automobile industry in the Detroit area regarding the unusual destruction of the vehicle during the fire. All emergency responders need to know what the Mason Fire Department discovered.

The Fiero's body is comprised of a plastic derivative known by the trade name Enduraflex. This body panel plastic contains the compound isocyanate. When a Fiero burns, the isocyanate decomposes and releases highly toxic hydrogen cyanide gas. Although Firefighter Garner reports that the amount of gas given off during the fire is estimated to be relatively small, even a small amount of the deadly poison gas can be fatal if inhaled or absorbed through the skin (Fig. 1-40). Enduraflex has since been incorporated into the design of several conventional automobiles.

A vehicle fire is no longer just a simple fire. It is a potential killer in many ways. Awareness of fire hazards like those posed by Enduraflex is a first step in improving our safety and survival at the emergency scene. Recommended operating procedures for handling vehicle fire incidents are presented in Chapter 2.

Vehicle body sizes, weights, construction materials, and processes have changed significantly in recent years. Emergency service personnel must be constantly on the alert for the potential safety hazards associated with each of the new technology vehicle body changes.

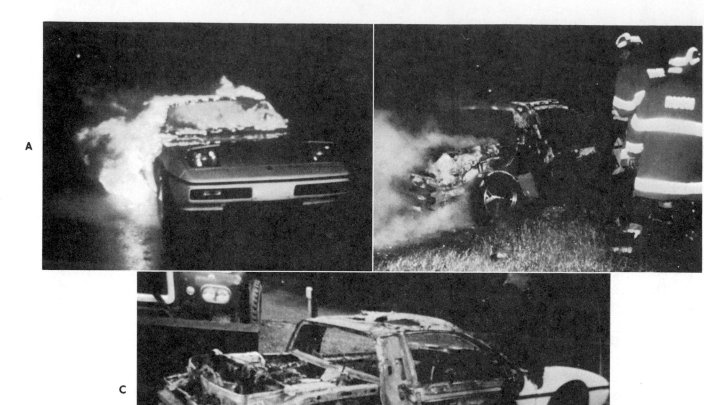

FIG. 1-40 A, A burning Fiero, which has the newer plastic body, gives off toxic gases as fire "meltdown" occurs. Enduraflex, a plastic derivative, produces extremely poisonous hydrogen cyanide gas that can be fatal if inhaled or absorbed through the skin of unprotected firefighters. **B,** As fire knockdown is accomplished, the smoldering vehicle continues to release large volumes of gases and fumes. Firefighters must use self-contained breathing apparatus until toxic gases completely dissipate. **C,** The aftermath of the fire reveals vehicle's mid-engine design, space frame structure, and complete incineration of portions of the plastic body.

America's New Station Wagon

The popular image of the family station wagon is changing. We no longer think of a station wagon as simply an automobile with no separate luggage compartment, a rear tailgate, and one or more seats that fold flat to accommodate large objects.

In late 1983 a new vehicle style was born: Chrysler Corporation unveiled their new mini van, a cross between a truck, a station wagon, and a car. Chrysler's original models, the Plymouth Voyager and Dodge Caravan, were quickly imitated by foreign and domestic competitors (Fig. 1-41).

Several significant features of mini vans warrant the attention of emergency service personnel. The occupant load of the mini van, depending upon the make, model, and seating package provided, can be as high as seven to nine seated individuals. The concept of the first due medical team providing total care for one or two patients per vehicle, as with a typical automobile

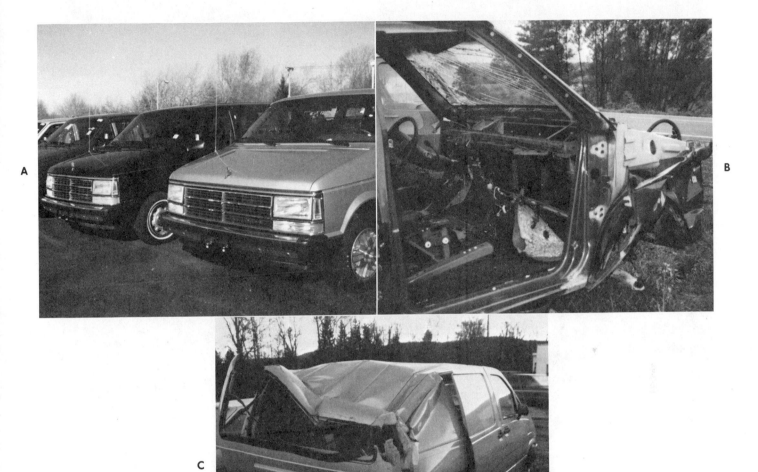

FIG. 1-41 A, In 1984 the Plymouth Voyager and Dodge Caravan introduced the North American fire and rescue service to the "station wagon of the future," the mini van. **B,** Typical mini van is constructed of metal structure and covered with sheet metal panels. **C,** In a collision the sheet metal body panels fold and crumble on impact. Note fiberglass rear hatch on Ford Aerostar mini van.   *Continued.*

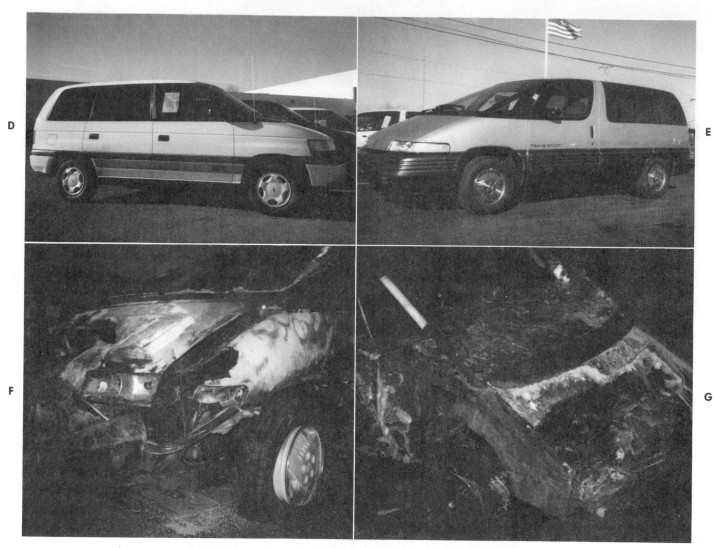

FIG. 1-41, cont'd D, Competition in mini van market has produced many diverse manufacturers of the popular van. Vehicle shown is Mazda's MPV. **E,** General Motor's second generation mini van, the Trans Sport, Lumina, or Silhouette, first introduced during the 1990 model year, features composite fiberglass and plastic body panels glued to spot-welded steel space frame structure. **F,** Pontiac Trans Sport mini van involved in fire shows extensive damage to both the interior and exterior. **G,** Plastic instead of steel eliminates many structural strong points routinely used as push, pull, or pry points during the most common vehicle rescue tasks.

accident, is no longer valid in the context of this multiple casualty potential. When patient needs exceed the resources and capabilities of initial response personnel, emergency service personnel, particularly those with medical responsibilities, must immediately reclassify the incident as a multiple casualty incident and proceed accordingly.

When a medic cannot care for a victim on an immediate, almost individual basis, as is clearly impossible when there are seven or more patients and only two or three medical personnel, injuries must be sorted out and initial care prioritized. This basic triage operation will be needed far more frequently as vehicle carrying-capacities increase.

HIGHER HIC?

The head injury criteria (HIC) is a key component of the system by which the U.S. government numerically rates the forces that impact the head of a crash test mannequin in new car assessment programs each year. Recent test results are alerting emergency service personnel to high HIC ratings on certain mini van

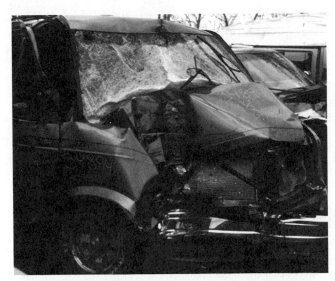

FIG. 1-42 Flat-nosed mini van after a head-on collision. Front seat occupants can be trapped by pedals, floorboard, dash, steering wheel and column, and windhsield.

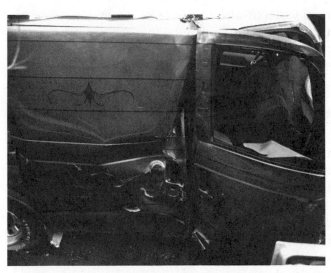

FIG. 1-43 Forcible entry may be a problem if door structure, hinges, or slide tracks are damaged.

makes and models. In these tests a low number means a low level of potential head injury; 1000 is the highest acceptable rating above which the would-be occupant would suffer fatal injuries in a real-world collision. In 1985 the GM Astro/Safari mini van, as an example, rated an HIC of 2202 and had the worst driver chest deceleration score of any of the vans tested; the Volkswagen Van Wagon mini van HIC score was 1905. Chrysler's 1984 Voyager/Caravan had an HIC rating of 973.

FLAT-NOSED MINI VANS

Rescue personnel must also anticipate the special rescue evolutions needed to free front-seat occupants trapped in a mini van. In a serious front collision when the driver is trapped, the steering wheel and column may have to be moved or removed. Efforts to complete the task by placing tools across the hood are frustrated by the sloping front of the vehicle, which is generally so blunted that what was once horizontal has become nearly vertical (Fig. 1-42). Moving columns by placing equipment across the windshield or working from inside the vehicle are effective solutions to difficult disentanglement problems (see Chapter 7).

SLIDING DOORS

Mini van occupants enter and exit the vehicle through two standard front doors and a third sliding door. Rescue personnel who must force entry into the interior of a mini van must understand the operating characteristics of this new generation side-sliding door. The door has at least one rated safety lock-and-latch unit and may have additional safety lock-and-latch devices at both the front and back edges. In forcible entry evolutions involving a jammed sliding side door, both the front and rear safety lock-and-latch mechanisms must be free at the same time for the door to open, but it may not open even then. Because the door must slide along the body of the van, two swivel arms of heavy cast white metal construction slide along the body of the van on guides or tracks (Fig. 1-43). Forcible-entry problems may be encountered if the sliding tracks or swivel pivot arms are damaged in the collision.

It is worth noting that the latest models of the Nissan Motors Company Sentra station wagon have two conventional front-hinged doors and two sliding doors, one on each side for rear-seat occupants. The latch-and-lock mechanisms on the sliding door are located along the top and bottom edges of the door instead of along the sides as with a conventional sliding door. Rescue personnel must learn the specific techniques that open these sliding doors when they are jammed. Several tool options and rescue techniques should be practiced in anticipation of the various scenarios that may be encountered. In rescue situations, initial access may be as simple as glass removal. An alternate opening into the interior of the mini van may also be made by totally removing the roof or by cutting open the thin sheet metal sidewall on the driver's side of the van, exactly opposite the sliding side door, to provide quick and effective access for rescue work and patient extrication.

SPECIAL CONSIDERATIONS

Mini van vehicle collisions call for accurate assessment of patients with special attention to possible head injuries, prior knowledge of the vehicle's special features, and an available arsenal of primary and alternative disentanglement techniques to achieve the safest and most efficient possible rescues. Rescue personnel need to familiarize themselves with APV vehicles such as the Pontiac Trans Sport, more conventional mini vans such as Chrysler's Caravan and Voyager models, General Motors' Astros and Safaris, Ford's mini vans, and the mini vans manufactured by such familiar names as Toyota, Mitsubishi, and Nissan. Emergency service personnel should make the effort now to inspect the major brands of mini vans so that they understand their design and operation before they face the new technology challenge of a mini van rescue situation.

Light Trucks and Vans

According to a study by the U.S. General Accounting Office (GAO), one of every four light-duty vehicles built in the United States is a light van or truck. The study refers specifically to vehicles having gross weights below 10,000 pounds. This includes jeep vehicles, light trucks, and vans.

Among the many government rules and regulations that apply to motor vehicles are the Federal Motor Vehicle Safety Standards. These standards cover such items as vehicle braking distance, side door strength, roof crush resistance, impact-absorbing steering columns, interior padding, passenger head restraint devices, and automatic frontal crash protection. These features, which are required on automobiles, are taken for granted by most automobile owners. Unfortunately, this safety equipment either is not required on light-duty vehicles or is regulated by a less stringent requirement (Fig. 1-44). However, consideration is now being given to extending Federal Safety Standard coverage to include both multipurpose and light-duty vehicles.

In accident data collected by the GAO from 10 states over a period of 2 years, the percentage of fatal accidents to total accidents was "consistently higher" for the light trucks, vans, and jeep vehicles. The government report concluded that the "vehicle's occupants face a greater risk of severe injury in collisions than passenger car occupants." Medical personnel may therefore expect to find occupants of vans, jeeps, or light trucks more seriously injured than their counterparts in passenger automobiles.

In motor vehicle accident size-up activities, rescue personnel may also find that occupants of these vehicles face greater entrapment problems. In head-on collisions, the nonenergy-absorbing steering column may trap the driver, and doors that do not have the side collision beams required in passenger automobiles will be more susceptible to crushing and jamming from collision forces.

Pickup trucks used as work vehicles by road highway crews, construction companies, or farmers, for example, may have auxiliary fuel tanks mounted in the bed area. These diesel or gasoline tanks can rupture during a collision or be completely dislodged from the vehicle. Heavy cargo objects in the bed of a pickup truck can slam into the passenger cab area, crushing the cab and trapping the occupants. Long slender cargo may even impale occupants. Vans outfitted as recreational or customized vehicles often contain small refrigerators, wet bars, or even tables and chairs.

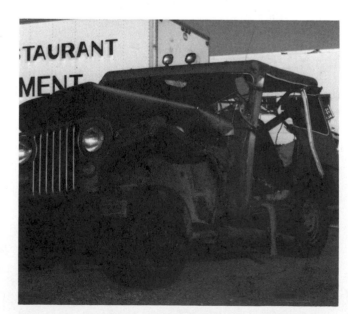

FIG. 1-44 Many safety features required on automobiles by government regulation are not currently required on vehicles such as jeeps, vans, mini vans, or pickup trucks.

Unfortunately, many passengers in the rear customized area of the van, seated in soft swivel bucket seats, fail to wear seat belts. During the dynamics of a collision, these unrestrained people and their loose personal objects become flying objects both inside and outside the vehicle.

Utility Vehicles

Vehicles such as the famous Jeep from American Motors are classified as utility vehicles. Not only do these vehicles lack many of the safety features found on passenger automobiles, they may even be missing some standard features. A utility vehicle designed with a convertible option could have a soft vinyl or plastic top, plastic walls and doors, and no side or rear window glass. The safety roll cage or roll bar system added by the manufacturer is a metal tube assembly designed to limit the crushing of the front seat passenger area in a rollover accident. The roll cage, however, can only withstand impact forces up to a point; depending on the severity of the collision and the direction in which the force hits the roll cage, the tubing can be bent off to the side, crushed downward, or even broken at a welded connection.

Emergency response personnel should study the designs and construction of roll cage assemblies used on pickup trucks and jeep vehicles in terms of the potential need to move or remove portions of the tubing by cutting, prying, or disassembling. Appropriate techniques should be practiced to allow for these types of evolutions if necessary at an accident scene.

These trucks, vans, and utility vehicles are very popular. Because we are increasingly likely to encounter them at accident scenes, we must understand how different they are — in both design and construction — and be prepared for the special problems they present in vehicle accidents.

SUMMARY

The first and most important incident priority at any emergency is life safety. The predominant life safety concern is ensuring the safety of the responding emergency services personnel. The first step in effectively dealing with any safety hazard encountered at a motor vehicle accident or fire incident is recognition and awareness of its potential. When every member of the emergency service teams has a clear picture of the specific challenges and how to meet them, safe and effective operations can be ensured.

Rescue personnel sometimes rationalize that they can react in time to avoid a problem — that they will "get out of the way" if anything goes wrong. But vehicle design and construction are changing at too rapid a pace for this attitude to make sense. These rescuers may not even know what new technology hazard hit them since many of these innovations give their victims no time to react.

The challenge of new technology in automobile extrication and fire suppression is growing. Our skills in anticipating problems and dealing with them have become crucial to our survival. Ultimately, mastery of this technological challenge will affect everything we do at automobile incidents. Our ability to act and our skills in carrying out the correct actions lie in the balance.

The real bottom line is that our patients receive the best possible care in the most efficient possible manner. Everyone involved in the rescue and extrication process works in a safer environment when they truly understand the hazard potentials. In this field, what you do not know can *really* hurt you.

The difference between training and no training can be the difference between life and death.

2 Life Cycle

All of the activities and events that take place at a typical vehicle rescue incident can be categorized into basic stages or steps. Once they have been identified, these steps can be arranged into an organized sequence. Our term for the suggested sequence of events necessary for safe and successful vehicle rescue operations is the *vehicle rescue life cycle*, which updates and expands the study of earlier rescue systems. This new life cycle is an in-depth organization of the rescue-related activities that evolve before, during, and after an accident (Fig. 2-1).

Each responding agency has its own vital role to fulfill if the life cycle is to be complete. The efficiency of the overall rescue operation depends to a large extent upon how well the responding agencies work together as they complete various elements. The life cycle is intentionally depicted as a flow chart to emphasize that the final stage, termination, flows or cycles directly into the first stage, readiness.

The vehicle rescue life cycle is a logical explanation of our overall rescue and extrication activities. Although each accident presents its own individual situations, the actual sequence of the life cycle rarely changes, and no steps are ever omitted. In the case of a simple rescue where, for example, access to the patient is gained by opening an undamaged door, it may seem that a certain step in the cycle was not accomplished or even considered. In essence, opening the door accomplishes the patient access stage. Although one step or stage may be more critical or take more time than another, *all steps are considered at all times for all incidents.* No portion of the sequence should ever be omitted.

This guide, which is designed as an advisory, is based on the experiences of many years of vehicle accident rescue experience by many different organizations in North America. If there is a discrepancy between what is suggested here and what one is instructed to do at an actual accident scene, the orders of the command officer at the scene must be followed. The real-world circumstances we work under will differ, but we all need to accomplish the same result: delivery of a viable patient to a medical facility within a given period of time. We want to save lives. The vehicle rescue life cycle is a comprehensive technical analysis of the steps needed to accomplish this goal.

READINESS STAGE

The first step in the procedural guide for proper vehicle rescue is the readiness stage. This important step has several elements, each of which has its own individual components. The readiness stage begins when the emergency service organizations within a community accept the challenge to provide a quality vehicle rescue service to their citizens. The individual steps of this stage include readiness of personnel, equipment, and apparatus. Each component depends on the others because it takes all three to achieve full rescue readiness (Fig. 2-2).

Personnel readiness means the availability of adequate numbers of trained working crew members and command personnel for supervision and safety. To meet the rigors of today's vehicle rescue operations, these individuals should be physically and mentally fit for their tasks. Physical fitness training on

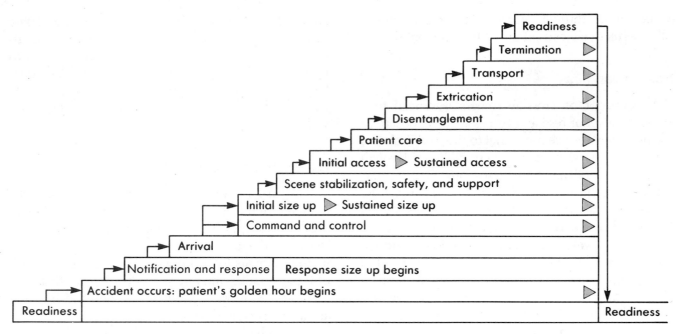

FIG. 2-1 The vehicle rescue life cycle flow chart is a comprehensive and systematic visual representation of activities that take place before, during, and after a rescue incident.

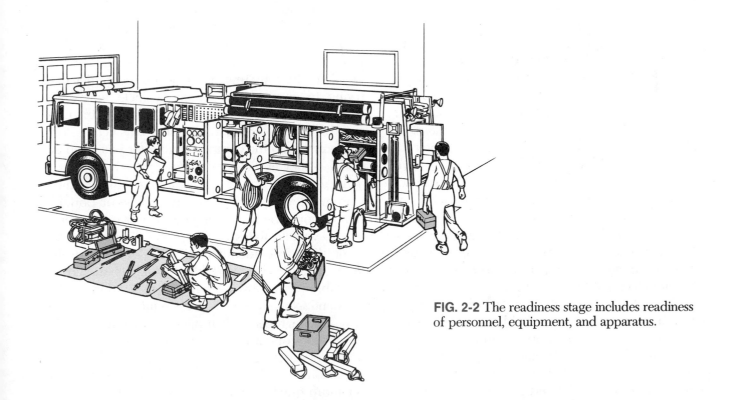

FIG. 2-2 The readiness stage includes readiness of personnel, equipment, and apparatus.

a departmental basis or as a personal endeavor is highly recommended because it increases the individual's chances of performing without being injured.

Mastering the actual rescue techniques to be used is another component of the readiness stage. The proper practices and procedures must be learned through training and rehearsed until they become second nature. In times of stress, the actions that have become second nature through effective training programs will be effectively carried out at the accident scene.

Cross-Awareness

The concept of cross-awareness is crucial to a successful level of rescue readiness. The exposure of all emergency service personnel to fire, medical, and rescue specialty areas can be accomplished through multi-agency drills and training sessions. These important training endeavors will serve to maximize the efficiency of any rescue operation. Personnel trained in the field of emergency medical service must, for example, be aware of and cross trained in the principles and practices of fire and rescue personnel, just as the operators of vehicle rescue equipment must be trained in the principles and practices of medical care providers. Cross-trained crews, knowledgeable in fire safety, vehicle rescue, and emergency medical services, must be present at each accident scene.

Equipment

The second component of readiness is tool and equipment readiness. Equipment should be equal to the tasks at hand, well maintained, and preconnected where feasible so that each responding organization can safely, effectively, and efficiently meet its responsibilities at an incident scene. It should be available in several basic categories and in sufficient quantities. (A recommended tool inventory appears in Chapter 6.) The goal of any equipment inventory is to have enough equipment available so that trained personnel can accomplish their rescue tasks without tools becoming a limiting factor.

Quantities should be sufficient to handle a two-vehicle accident where persons are trapped in each vehicle. Working two similar rescue tasks on two different vehicles at the same time is a very realistic possibility. Duplicate equipment also anticipates the tool failure problems that inevitably occur at an incident. Enough medical equipment and personnel to handle multiple patients, enough fire personnel and resources for dealing with multiple hazards, and enough rescue equipment and personnel to work on multiple vehicles simultaneously should be the rule in rescue equipment planning.

Each organization's equipment inventory should have one primary tool and a backup tool for each potential rescue task. For lifting a portion of an object

like a car, for example, the primary tool (the tool they plan to use) could be a low-pressure, air-cushion lifting system. The backup tool, possibly a standard hydraulic jack, is what they know is available in their tool inventory that will also accomplish the lifting task. The only difference is time and technique. The results will be the same.

Emergency Response Vehicles

The final component of rescue readiness is the readiness of the emergency response vehicles, including those transporting personnel and equipment to the scene of the accident and those transporting the injured patients to appropriate medical facilities. All of these vehicles and any specialty vehicles that may be requested must be ready to respond and function at the emergency scene.

Each vehicle must be in reliable condition and mechanically well maintained. All state-of-the-art safety features and equipment for crew members must be provided and used, including occupant seat belts, backup alarms, proper vehicle mirrors, emergency warning and lighting equipment, and enclosed riding positions. All portable equipment should be properly stowed on the vehicle and secured in a safe position. There are few things more discouraging than trying to cope with a rescue vehicle where the compartments seem to be designed around the principle of "self-unloading" tools. There is no need to look for tools within the compartment after you open the doors — they are all at your feet.

All available emergency warning lights, audible warning devices, and two-way mobile or portable radios should be in working order. For rescue scene safety, vehicle lights designed for illuminating the scene should be adequate in number and ready for immediate service. Portable handlights should be available for use by crew members working at the accident scene. Preconnecting equipment, particularly rescue tools and appliances that have many connections or components, is highly recommended. Any work that can be done before the incident response allows the crew members the opportunity to act more quickly and efficiently with fewer errors resulting. Examples include medical personnel carrying longboards with the necessary straps attached and in position and air or hydraulic-powered rescue equipment carried with the hoses already connected together.

ACCIDENT STAGE

The second stage in the life cycle is one that emergency service personnel have no control over: the *accident* stage. It begins when one or more vehicles is involved in an accident in which someone is injured or killed. The actual collision, with all its death and injury, generally lasts 1 second or less.

Forces generated during the impact move the structural components of the vehicle to make normal entrance or exit from the vehicle impossible. When a door is jammed or a steering column crushed into an occupant, we routinely say that we have "people trapped." This simple phrase actually describes a very dynamic and complex situation that presents countless challenges for emergency service personnel. The collision may have taken just 1 second to occur, but the work for fire, rescue, and medical personnel will take considerably longer.

At the moment the accident occurs, the persons affected by the collision technically become victims and remain so until emergency service personnel first make contact, directly or indirectly, with them. Once responding emergency service personnel of the first agency to arrive on the scene assume responsibility for their care and safety, the injured or trapped victims of the accident become their patients.

Golden Hour Begins

The *golden hour* is an imaginary time frame within which serious trauma patients have the best chances of surviving their injuries if extricated from the damaged vehicle, transported to a medical facility, and delivered to a surgical team (Fig. 2-3). At a rescue scene, we can neither slow nor stop the ticking of this imaginary life or death clock. Although the golden hour (generally considered a maximum of 60 minutes) varies with the nature of the injury and the seriousness of the problem, the serious trauma patients' golden hour does not stop when they leave the accident scene, nor does it stop when they are delivered to a hospital emergency room. Their golden hour is complete only when they receive surgical intervention by a trained surgical team.

The rescue philosophy of "get them out any way you can" can no longer be our guide. We must make the most efficient use of our patient handling time at the accident scene, carefully considering each of our rescue and extrication activities and the time that it

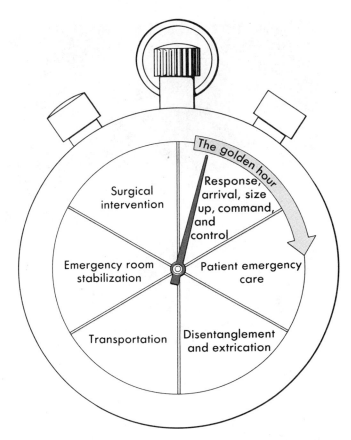

FIG. 2-3 The golden hour is an imaginary time frame within which a serious trauma patient has the best chances of surviving the injuries if extricated from the damaged automobile, transported to a medical facility, and delivered to a surgical team.

takes to accomplish. For most accidents, our actual vehicle rescue activities should take no more than 15 or 20 minutes. Ideally, patient transportation from the accident scene to the medical facility should take no longer than another 10 minutes. This leaves less than 30 minutes of the golden hour for emergency room stabilization work and delivery to the surgical team. All of our vehicle rescue activities should therefore be designed around the goal of a total of 20 minutes working time at the accident scene. There is no time to waste with a serious trauma patient. A life can literally be ticking away at the scene.

NOTIFICATION STAGE

The third step in the life cycle is the *notification* stage: rapid notification and activation of all appropriate emergency service agencies (Fig. 2-4). This stage usually begins when an accident is reported by

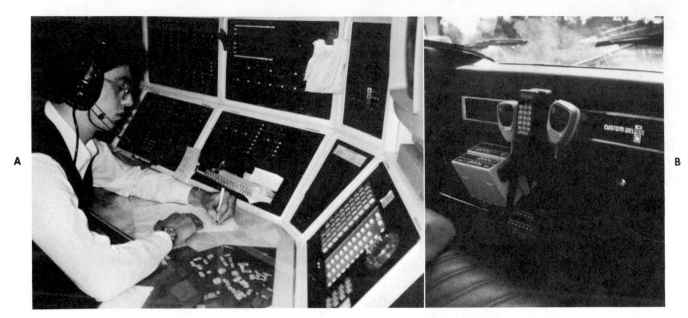

FIG. 2-4 **A,** The communication facility notifies all needed emergency service agencies. **B,** Field units, such as this fire department first response fire/rescue vehicle, have increased communications capability with installation of cellular telephone equipment.

telephone from the general public to telecommunications personnel who determine the nature and extent of the problem. Once the accident location, nature of the incident, and other basic factors are known, the appropriate agencies are rapidly alerted and dispatched to the incident. A protocol describing exactly which emergency service agencies to summon should already be in place in the community (Fig. 2-5). Its components should include a typical response to the various types of vehicle accidents and the roles for each responding agency to fulfill at the scene.

RESPONSE STAGE

In the *response* stage, various agencies respond to the incident based on the need determined during the notification stage. For example, when a call reports an automobile accident with no injuries, the appropriate law enforcement agency should be notified to respond. If, however, the initial call reports an accident with injuries, then a different level of response should be initiated. Any accident that produces injuries should prompt the notification and response of the appropriate law enforcement agency, emergency medical personnel, *and* a fire department engine company (pumper) with a crew of firefighters. Personal injury to vehicle occupants justifies the presence of a fire crew at the accident scene to establish and

preserve scene safety and to perform other important functions.

If the accident report indicates that occupants of any of the involved vehicles are or might be trapped, rescue company personnel and equipment should be added to the initial response assignment. When communications personnel have any doubt about needing the services of any specific agency, that agency should be notified to respond. It is easier to return a crew that is en route to the scene than to have a problem go uncontrolled while waiting for the unit's delayed arrival. Preplanned response assignments should be available for calls reporting situations that involve the presence of hazardous materials or multiple casualties because these incidents require the notification and dispatch of additional agencies initially.

Agencies that routinely work side by side at an accident benefit by developing assigned responsibilities for each agency to fulfill. The following example illustrates how standardized operating procedures and responsibilities can be established.

Recommended Agency Roles
LAW ENFORCEMENT PERSONNEL

• Investigate the accident to determine its cause and whether there are any violations of the law.

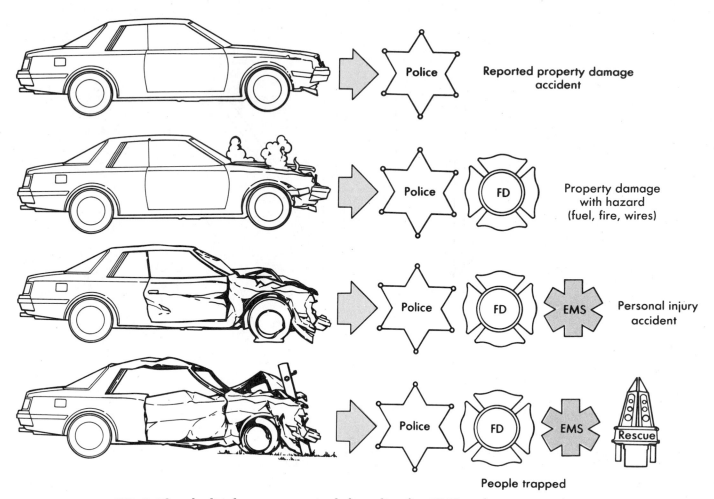

FIG. 2-5 Standardized response protocols for police, fire, EMS, and rescue agencies can be developed and implemented for a variety of vehicle emergencies.

- Establish and maintain crowd and traffic control measures at the incident scene.
- Make arrangements for any additional resources that may be required.
- Preserve the accident scene for accident reconstruction and investigation teams.

FIRE DEPARTMENT ENGINE COMPANIES

- Establish and maintain scene safety by control of safety hazards including but not limited to the following:
  - Extinguishing fires
  - Preventing fires
  - Handling spill or leak control
- Perform vehicle safety surveys including the following:
  - Energy-absorbing bumpers
  - Electrical system
  - Fuel and fuel system
  - Basic vehicle stabilization

- Assist law enforcement agencies in establishing and maintaining control of traffic and crowds in the immediate vicinity, if requested and assigned.
- Provide minimum of "first responder" level emergency medical service.
- Assist EMS personnel and rescue personnel as requested and assigned.
- Preserve accident scene for accident reconstruction and investigation teams.

EMERGENCY MEDICAL SERVICES

- Establish and maintain medical personnel/patient contact throughout incident.
- Evaluate condition of patients.
- Prioritize and administer necessary patient medical care.
- Assess need for disentanglement activities to free trapped patient.
- Advise rescue personnel of interior entrapment conditions as necessary.

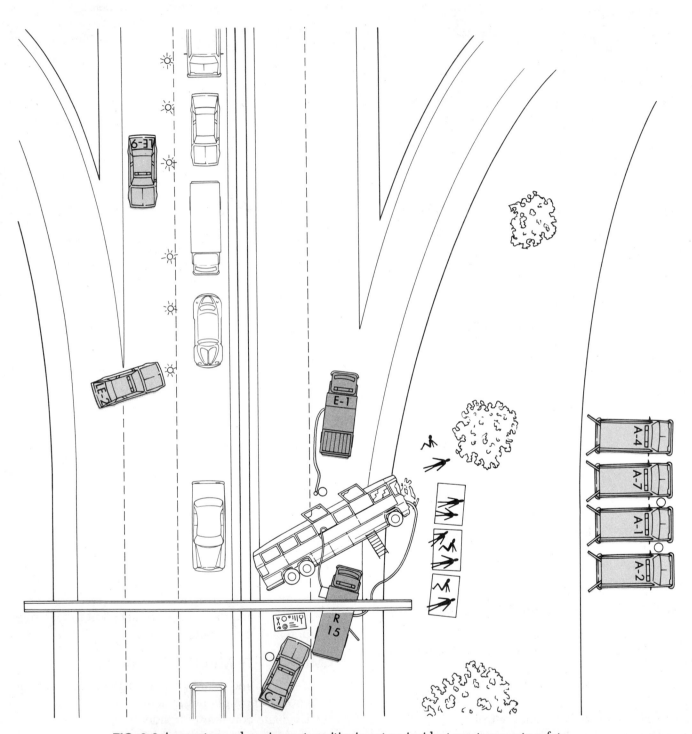

FIG. 2-6 Apparatus and equipment positioning at an incident must promote safety and allow for efficient and controlled operations.

- Properly package injuries and injured patients.
- Assist in extrication of patient from damaged vehicle.
- Transport patient to medical facility.

VEHICLE RESCUE AND EXTRICATION PERSONNEL

- Establish incident command.
- Perform vehicle stabilization.
- Provide initial and sustained patient access as necessary.
- Initiate disentanglement procedures as necessary.
- Assist EMS personnel as necessary.
- Implement necessary safety measures on damaged vehicles to prevent further injuries to patients or operating personnel.

Because the simultaneous arrival of law enforcement, fire, rescue, and medical crews rarely happens, each agency must be prepared to deal with the situation alone until additional crews arrive. When a particular response agency is absent from an accident scene, command personnel may have to assign personnel from one branch of service temporarily to fulfill some of the responsibilities of the other services. However, no member of any branch of service should become involved in another agency's realm of responsibility without the full knowledge, consent, and direction of command personnel. For example, if firefighters abandon their charged standby hoselines to direct traffic at an accident scene, the safety afforded by the standby lines is lost. In all cases, every action taken by every agency must reflect consideration for safety at all times.

ARRIVAL STAGE

As each responding unit arrives at either the accident scene or a predetermined staging area, the fifth stage, the *arrival* stage, of the life cycle begins. Although this stage is very short, it has a key role in the overall life cycle. Personnel arriving with each emergency service unit must execute several basic safety procedures. First, vehicles must be more than just parked — they must be positioned at the scene or at a staging area (Fig. 2-6). Without specific orders from command personnel already at the accident scene, standard operating procedures should call for positioning arriving apparatus to prevent the accident vehicles from being involved in a secondary collision. The accident vehicle must be effectively shielded from all approaching traffic in all directions.

When possible, emergency vehicles should be positioned uphill and upwind of the scene and at a safe distance (at least 100 feet) from the involved vehicles. This is especially important for rescue and engine company apparatus, which should be shielded from safety hazards such as fuel leaks or downed electrical wires. Positioning should also direct exhaust fumes away from patient treatment areas and damaged vehicles that are being worked on by personnel. Each vehicle operator is responsible for setting parking and emergency brakes in the "on" position. Larger vehicles, such as pumpers and rescue trucks, should also have their wheels chocked to keep them from moving unexpectedly.

SIZE-UP STAGE

While response vehicles and crews arrive and properly position at the accident scene, the *size-up* stage begins.

In the fire service, size up, a basic information-gathering activity, is the process of surveying and assessing the overall emergency scene. In vehicle rescue, three levels of size-up work need to be accomplished, each at a different point in time. First, there is *prearrival* or *response size up* (Fig. 2-7). This occurs during the

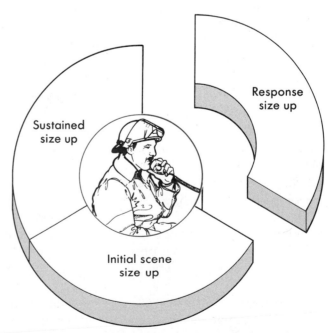

FIG. 2-7 Response size up occurs during the actual response of the emergency vehicles and personnel to the scene.

actual response of the emergency vehicles and personnel to the scene. Consider a dispatch call:

"Reported motor vehicle accident with people trapped....273 Castle Road at the corner of Pinnacle....time out 04:15 hours."

This dispatch gives responding personnel the basic information needed to anticipate events that have occurred and think about actions that may have to be taken on their arrival. The reported location in this case may indicate that the accident has occurred on a residential street, at a "T" intersection where serious accidents occur frequently. The fact that the call is being dispatched in the middle of the night is also significant because it indicates that safety for personnel, victims, and bystanders will be in jeopardy unless proper lighting of the scene becomes an early priority.

Among the important prearrival size-up factors for personnel to consider are the day of the week, the season of the year, the weather, the type of road or highway emergency response crews will be working on, typical traffic volumes, and response problems such as detours or trains blocking crossings. All of this size-up information is used by the command personnel to develop a clear picture of the overall rescue incident. By the time personnel are close enough to glimpse the actual accident scene, initial solutions to those anticipated problems should have begun to be formulated.

When emergency service personnel arrive at the accident scene, the prearrival size-up work now leads to *initial scene size-up* work. This scene survey, which lasts less than a minute, is one of the most crucial stages of the entire life cycle. Completing this quick and accurate analysis of the situation is a challenging and involved process. It lays the foundation for the rest of the activities that will take place at the scene. The information gathered during this size up confirms or verifies initial reported information and provides additional information to units still responding to the accident scene (Fig. 2-8).

Details of the size-up procedure are discussed in Chapter 4 in the context of the vehicle rescue incident command system, but it is important at this point to consider this stage in relation to the rest of the life cycle.

The supervising officer of an emergency crew begins the actual scene survey before exiting the emergency vehicle (while still in the fire apparatus, for example). The supervisor of the first-arriving emergency service vehicle, whether medical vehicle, rescue truck, or fire department pumper, makes a radio

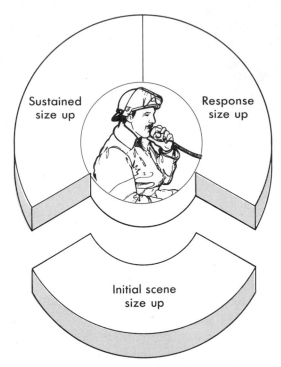

FIG. 2-8 Initial scene size-up work serves as the foundation for the rest of the activities that will take place at the scene.

report on the proper frequency, documenting arrival at the location and describing obvious points of information observed to that point. A simple, effective "report on conditions" for a medical unit that arrives first at the scene of our hypothetical collision on Pinnacle Road may include the following:

"Medic 30 to County, arriving Pinnacle Road just south of Castle....Two-car collision....A station wagon on its edge....We're investigating."

This message, recorded at the County Emergency Control center, documents the arrival of the first emergency service vehicle. If there is multiagency communication capabilities or the protocol to rebroadcast such information on the various channels, other responding units monitoring their radio frequency will receive additional information before their actual arrival at the scene.

The scene survey by the first-arriving crew continues until all basic and relevant information has been considered. A complete circle of the scene is generally required to assess the nature and degree of the emergency fully and initiate the necessary measures to handle the emergency.

Once this survey has been accomplished, a strategy developed, and specific evolutions begun, a more deliberate *sustained size up* can be initiated by the

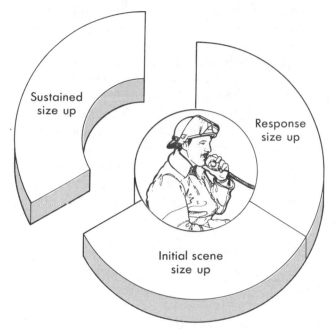

FIG. 2-9 Sustained size up allows command personnel to continue to make the proper strategic decisions.

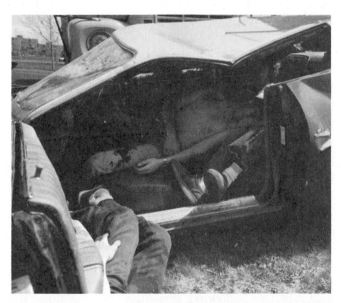

FIG. 2-10 The size of the emotional and psychological challenge to rescuers (as portrayed in this simulation school bus/automobile accident) may be overwhelming and may impair their ability to function at the emergency scene.

command officer. This size up defines a constant process of assessing all the activities that unfold during the entire span of the incident. Sustained size up for command personnel involves the constant balancing of what you have, what you need, and what you will

do. This process enables command personnel to continue to make proper decisions and to measure the success or failure of their decisions throughout the rescue process (Fig. 2-9).

Size up is an ideal term to describe the information-gathering work at an emergency scene because it refers to the "size" of the emergency, which is measured in several ways. First is its physical size: a lone auto that runs into a tree is one problem, while a 13-car chain reaction collision on a major expressway has a very different size. To an experienced supervisor, size up is also a measure of the physical and emotional challenges that the emergency presents. The sights and sounds that emanate from an accident scene sharply challenge the emotions of emergency service personnel and may be overwhelming to some individuals (Fig. 2-10). Consideration of this aspect of dealing with life and death is important to the success of operations at the emergency scene.

INCIDENT COMMAND STAGE

Although the seventh stage of the vehicle rescue life cycle — the *incident command* stage — is relatively new, progressive fire, rescue, and medical agencies are fully aware of the need to have supervisory persons on the scene to fulfill both command and safety functions. With the acceptance of incident command as a major function that must be accomplished during a rescue incident, we acknowledge that command, control, and safety supervision are vital to successful rescue operations. A specific individual must be in command of the incident at all times, especially when multiple agencies are involved.

The first important element of the incident command stage is establishment of command. Some agencies require that the first command person arriving at the scene of an emergency incident make a formal statement assuming command over the emergency service radio frequency; the supervisor of the first emergency unit states that the individual is "establishing command" at the scene, using the vehicle's radio number designation and identifying the incident scene by location or address.

As an example of this system, the person in charge of paramedic unit Medic 30, who arrived first at the accident scene discussed earlier, would transmit the following message:

"Medic 30 to County...arriving Pinnacle Road just south of Castle....Two-car collision....A station wagon on its edge....We're investigating. Medic 30 assuming *Pinnacle Road Command.*"

The command individual, known as the Incident Commander or IC, must be readily identifiable and available to personnel working at the scene. Whether designated by helmet color, the color of the protective coat or vest, or other identification markings, the IC must be easily recognized by all public and private agency personnel called on to assist at the accident scene. The officer's command post is the specific site selected by the IC to physically locate. (Recommendations concerning the location of a command post and its functions are discussed in detail in Chapter 4.)

The question of who is actually in charge at an accident scene can be answered by state legislation, local or regional operating procedures, or past tradition. Documented cases of physical confrontations between persons at an actual rescue scene arguing over who is in charge still haunt us. Command responsibility must not be left to chance or be determined by the personalities of the individuals involved. A unified command concept must be incorporated into a system that uses the talents and abilities of each emergency service agency to its best advantage. The responsibilities that rest with law enforcement, medical, fire, and vehicle rescue personnel should be decided well in advance of any actual accident and be based on what will yield the best overall operations. Once standardized procedures or protocols are in place and accepted by all emergency response personnel, the "who's in charge" controversy can be put to rest.

With initial scene size-up work complete, the commander identified, and the command post selected, it is time to develop the basic plan of action and the specific procedures to be followed. This information composes our rescue strategy and tactics. A strategy is a basic goal or a plan for action. The typical overall goal at an entrapment situation is to free trapped patients in the safest and most efficient manner and deliver them to the appropriate surgical team within a 60-minute time frame. Once the IC develops a strategy, what needs to be accomplished and how those goals or objectives can be met must be considered.

The methods employed to fulfill the objectives of the IC's strategy are the rescue tactics. Tactics at an entrapment incident include actual hazard control, scene stabilization, and patient care work. After the IC has developed a strategy and assigned the necessary tactics to be carried out, reports on the progress or lack of progress as events unfold must be received.

The results are analyzed, and new strategies or tactics developed. This assessment becomes the basis for the sustained incident size-up process.

Command personnel are responsible for establishing communications for the incident. The brief details of the initial on-scene radio report begin the process. Information on the nature of the situation, number of patients, need for additional resources, and progress reports are important parts of this communication process. The IC also ensures that face-to-face communication between personnel and agencies both on and off the scene takes place as necessary. The IC must know who is in charge of the assisting agencies at the scene and where they are located. Communication with that person or a delegate must be established to give and receive orders and direct activities between agencies.

It is extremely important for the IC to provide a timely progress report to the appropriate communications center to keep the communications center and other personnel and emergency service units advised of the situation. A major benefit to command personnel in transmitting this progress report on a regular basis is that they are forced to look objectively at their own operations and evaluate their progress.

It is vital that the size-up process continue for the life of the emergency. The good news and bad news must be accumulated and molded into a new or revised strategy as the incident continues. Command responsibilities are passed from first-arriving command personnel to those of higher authority when they arrive on the incident scene to ensure that the safety and efficiency of all personnel and activities are continually monitored.

Experienced senior-ranking command personnel do not automatically assume command as they arrive at the scene of an accident. To foster experience among junior officers, a street-wise commander may choose to simply advise and support the commanding junior officer, allowing this officer to continue to command and control the incident. The senior officer may choose to take command if there is a serious deterioration of conditions or if safety concerns dictate intervention.

A final word regarding the establishment of command: All ICs should do everything in their power to avoid "getting their hands dirty." Although the reality of today's minimum staffing levels often requires the IC to become a working member of the team, it is extremely difficult to fully command and control, develop safe operating procedures, and adequately supervise crews while involved in some intricate detail of the rescue. Officers must act as officers! When the IC or a crew leader becomes a "hands on" worker, the Incident Command System is weakened, efficiency is reduced, and overall safety is sacrificed.

SCENE SAFETY, STABILIZATION, AND SUPPORT STAGE

The eighth defined stage of the life cycle, which includes all hazard control operations is best remembered by its four key words: *scene safety, stabilization,* and *support.*

All safety hazards or potential hazards must be controlled as the incident is stabilized and necessary support activities initiated quickly and efficiently (Fig. 2-11). It is at this stage that assignments to *eliminate, control,* or *neutralize* existing hazards are made. The goal to remember is that once emergency service personnel arrive on the scene, things must get better.

The decision-making process for dealing with scene safety starts with consideration of safety hazards to people. Those who become first priority are the emergency service personnel themselves. *We do not and cannot trade lives for lives.* Emergency service personnel must not be committed into kamikaze rescues where their own lives are threatened. Although the very nature of our work involves risk, as professionals, we seek to minimize this risk (Fig. 2-12).

Our second priority is for those persons who are not yet involved in the incident. All residents, passing

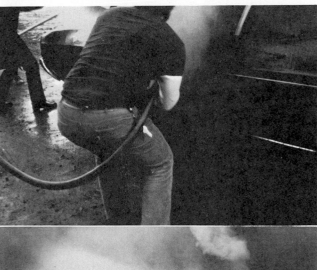

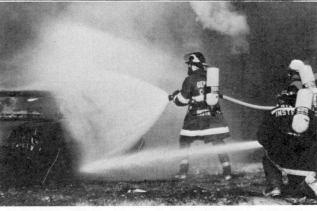

FIG. 2-12 **A,** This individual is not properly prepared or equipped for fire suppression and is at great risk of personal injury. Command personnel must not tolerate such unsafe acts at any time. **B,** These firefighters are properly equipped and following safe procedures as they handle this hazardous situation. Note full protective clothing with hoods, SCBA, and dual 100+ gpm handlines.

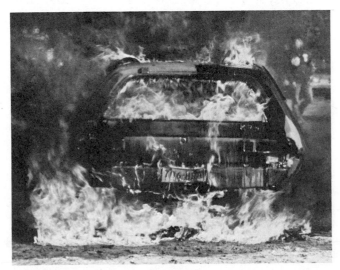

FIG. 2-11 All safety hazards must be stabilized as quickly and efficiently as possible.

motorists, and bystanders must continue to remain uninjured and uninvolved. It is these people, for example, who are considered when a large area evacuation at a hazardous material incident is initiated.

Our third priority is the safety of those already injured by the accident. Although they have the least chance of escape if a problem develops since their mobility is the most impaired, they must remain the last to be contacted if hazards at the scene prevent emergency crews from safely accessing them. It is crucial for the IC to face this reality; the safety of injured or trapped persons can only be ensured after the overall scene has been stabilized. The personal safety of fire, rescue, and medical personnel and control of the immediate vicinity must be ensured first.

An example of this priority system in action follows: At an accident where people are trapped, energized electrical service wires are found to have contacted

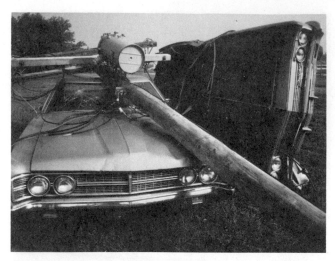

FIG. 2-13 Emergency response personnel must approach any accident involving downed electrical transmission lines with extreme caution. Electricity can be an invisible enemy with deadly potential.

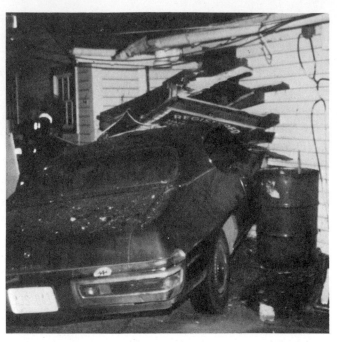

FIG. 2-14 Emergency personnel should note all potential hazards immediately. Remember scene safety, stabilization, and support activities should control hazards present or anticipated at emergency scene.

the damaged auto (Fig. 2-13). Emergency response personnel in this situation must cautiously approach the accident scene to avoid placing themselves in danger of electrocution. Bystanders gathered at the scene are immediately moved to a safe distance. When the safety of rescuers is ensured, attention then turns to citizens and lastly to those trapped in the wreckage. Failure of command personnel to consider the potential safety risks to rescue personnel and uninvolved citizens is negligence.

Control of scene hazards accompanies personnel safety considerations. Scene hazards that are obvious on arrival are referred to as "sight" hazards. Because they are usually easily detectable — a vehicle on fire, a large gasoline fuel spill, or energized electrical service wires arcing at an accident scene — they are generally serious in nature. "Intelligence" hazards, in contrast, are those hazards or conditions not readily visible or obvious, although they may be extremely deadly. Intelligence hazards require a rescuer's understanding of the potential that a situation can produce and an appreciation for what may only be perceived as a potential problem or hazard (Fig. 2-14). The ability to promptly recognize these potential hazards typifies an experienced emergency service professional. This understanding of and appreciation for potential problems is not only a skill but a discipline that must be studied and learned. It is a discipline that many people lack.

A damaged vehicle with batteries still intact, a loaded energy-absorbing bumper, or even a damaged

vehicle sitting on a level stretch of road possess safety hazards that silently await the rescue personnel. Other scene hazards include traffic control (Fig. 2-15, *A*), control of crowds at the scene, and downed electrical service wires. Crowd control includes control of "walking wounded" or uninjured vehicle occupants at a mass casualty incident (for example, when a bus vehicle is involved). Another crowd to control is emergency service personnel on the scene who are not presently being used (Fig. 2-15, *B*). These crew members should be considered as standby personnel and maintained in a central location at a safe distance from the work area. Control of our own emergency service personnel can be as simple as stretching a coil of rope around an accident scene and requiring all nonworking emergency service crew members to stand by outside the roped-off area.

One method of ensuring hazard detection and control is to have a fire department engine company dispatched automatically to the accident scene and to preassign hazard detection and control to the engine's firefighter crew. This "hazard group" knows in advance that their initial tasks include hazard detection along with initial scene stabilization. They arrive prepared to accomplish these assignments immediately and become our accident scene safety specialists.

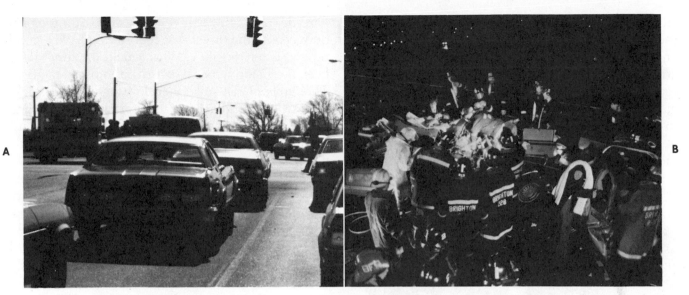

FIG. 2-15 A, Accidents cause traffic congestion. Traffic congestion causes accidents. **B,** Excessive numbers of fire, rescue, and medical personnel can be just as serious a problem as too few personnel. Crowd control includes control of our own "crowd" as well.

These crews develop their own standard operating procedures to ensure that basic safety and hazard control work is completed.

Stabilization of the involved vehicles must be accomplished at this early stage of the rescue. Every vehicle should be stabilized every time, whether it is found sitting on its tires on a paved roadway or perched precariously on its edge. It is a simple rule that we can all accept. (Detailed information of vehicle stabilization appears in Chapter 7.) When engine company personnel handle basic vehicle stabilization, medical and rescue personnel are able to concentrate on more involved tasks.

Support Activities

While safety hazards are being controlled, support activities to ensure continued safety for all persons on the rescue scene must be initiated. These actions are taken to assist or supplement the efforts that are taking place such as fire prevention, emergency scene lighting, and the staging of additional personnel and resources. Fire prevention support includes the deployment of portable fire extinguishers and minimum 100-gallon-per-minute fireflow handlines and may involve the deployment and maintenance of a blanket of an AFFF type of foam agent. Fire safety crews in full protective clothing should be standing by with this

equipment. One fire safety handline is required for each involved vehicle or each separate hazard area at the scene. The available water supply for the handlines and foam generation should be adequate to completely contain and control any fire or safety hazard that might possibly develop in a worst case scenario.

When a fire department dispatches a minipumper as the lone source of fire suppression, the relatively small quantities of water carried on this apparatus provide little more than a false sense of security. The limited water supply, usually 200 gallons, may control one small vehicle fire or contain a fire that is confined to one portion of the vehicle under ideal conditions. The small water supply leaves no room for error and no safety factor for operating personnel. If the fire involves a truck with combustible cargo or involves a large quantity of flammable fuel, the fire may not be extinguished or the fumes may not be properly dispersed. Lives may be lost. The assignment of full-size, Class A fire apparatus with water supplies of 750 gallons or more, capable of fire suppression and control with a good margin of safety, should be the rule for fire departments to follow.

A recent vehicle accident illustrated the importance of the prompt dispatching of appropriate fire apparatus. In this incident a loaded tractor-trailer truck crashed into a ditch alongside a remote section of an interstate highway, trapping the driver in the tractor's cab. A fire immediately broke out on the ground under the vehicle. When fire department personnel arrived with their pumper, they could hear the screams of the trapped driver. They used all 1000 gallons of water carried in their apparatus water tank to contain and control the fire that had by then spread to the vehicle and its cargo. The trapped driver, although burned over 55% of his body with second- and third-degree burns, was rescued alive. At a regional burn center, the driver was reported to have a good prognosis for recovery. What would the result have been if a minipumper had arrived to battle the fire? The limits of the small vehicle water supply might have sent that truck driver to his grave! It is foolish to risk the lives of everyone present at the scene just because the fire department likes to send the "little rig."

Lighting support work includes scene illumination, deployment of portable lighting units, and availability of handlights for use throughout the rescue scene (Fig. 2-16). Personnel support work includes having back-up or alternate crews as relief for rescue personnel subjected to physically demanding or psychologically stressful situations. Physically demanding work takes a heavy toll. An overworked rescuer works less efficiently and is prone to errors that may compromise everyone's safety. The physically drained individual becomes a "victim" of the incident and needs to be rehabilitated just as a patient needs medical care and attention. Psychological stress, a familiar hazard to all emergency service personnel, can also be reduced or prevented if relief personnel are available to replace those placed in physically or emotionally stressful situations.

Equipment support work at a vehicle accident includes EMS personnel setting up a tool-staging area,

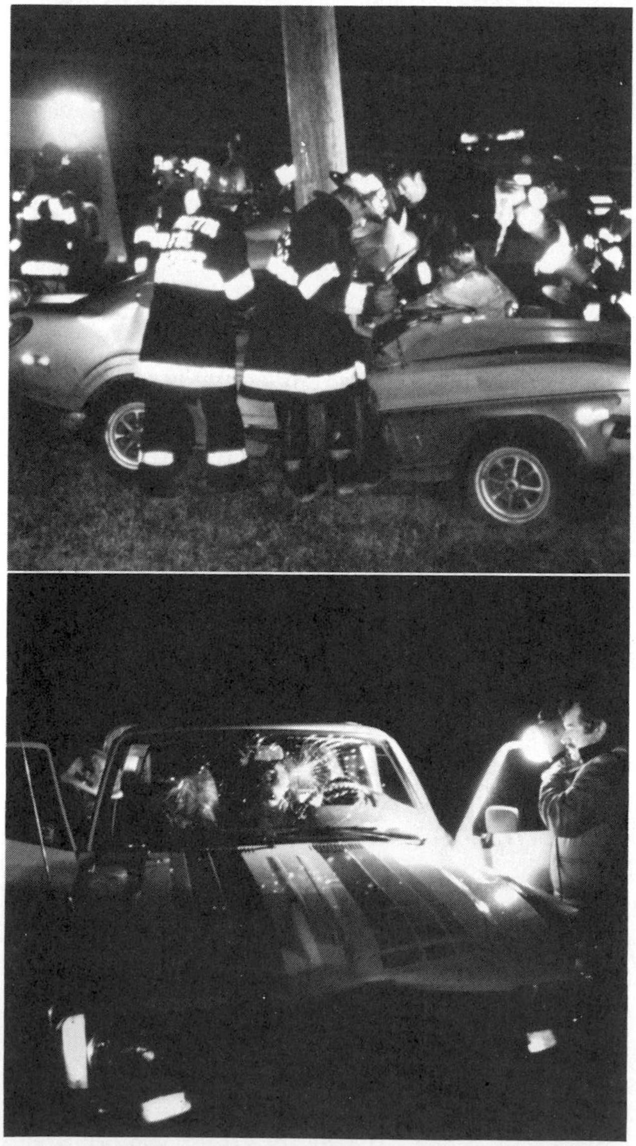

FIG. 2-16 A, Lighting is essential to safe and efficient rescue work. Examples of scene lighting include truck-mounted quartz flood lights, vehicle spotlights and headlights, portable Circle-D lights, and individual handlights. B, Every time you turn on a light at a nighttime emergency scene, scene safety is increased for all.

FIG. 2-17 A, Multicasualty incident supplies must include sufficient numbers of shortboards, longboards, and patient packaging equipment to meet the needs of patients in a school bus accident. New school buses can carry 84 to 101 students. B, Multicasualty disaster kit designed for storage at station and transport to emergency scene in ambulance when needed. C, Specialized rescue resources can include air cushion recovery units. Heavy loads can be lifted using relatively low air pressures. D, A utility company line truck can safely handle downed wire emergencies and is also equipped with hydraulic boom, winch, ladders, ropes, variety of hand tools, separate communications system, and trained crew. E, Specialized heavy-duty tow truck can be included within community's listing of outside resources available for emergency situations. This vehicle has 25-ton capacity split booms and a 30-ton capacity rear-mounted winch. Larger recovery vehicles, resembling portable cranes, have lifting capacities of up to 60 tons. F, Heavy Utility 27, operated by the Los Angeles City Fire Department, has heavy-duty tow truck booms and an on-board, high-capacity air compressor to power air-operated tools.

providing sufficient backup equipment for anticipated rescue assignments, readying fuel and funnels
for gas-powered units, and setting out compressed
air cylinders for air-powered rescue tools. Equipment support also includes rescuers' summoning
of mutual aid equipment or personnel from other
emergency service groups or outside agencies
(Fig. 2-17).

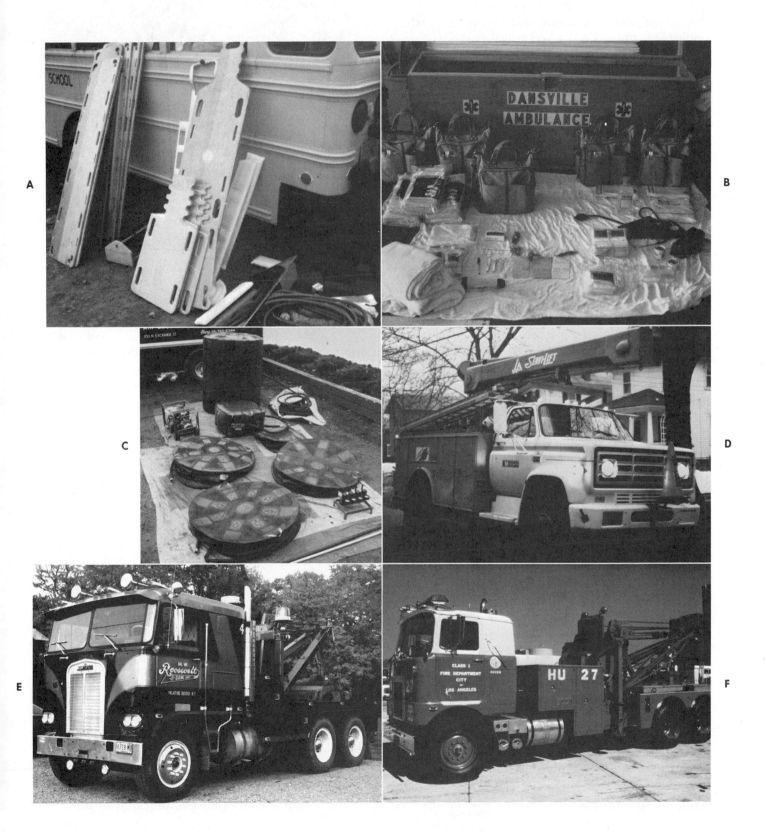

To be fully effective, scene safety, stabilization, and support must be a preplanned series of activities directed to control or correct existing or potential safety hazards. To gain control of the challenges at the accident scene, sufficient numbers of trained personnel, along with apparatus and rescue or medical equipment, must be readied to support the overall rescue effort fully.

PATIENT ACCESS STAGE

The chaos that greeted the first emergency service teams is by now being systematically molded into an organized system of operations. As the priority hazards are being dealt with and effectively controlled, other personnel begin the next step in our life cycle. At every accident where occupants are trapped in a vehicle, there must be an opening or pathway of sufficient size to enable qualified emergency medical personnel to make contact with each trapped patient. The process of making and using this pathway to reach those persons, our ninth life cycle stage, is the *patient access* stage.

Access to the injured persons, a very critical part of the overall rescue operation, is accomplished in several steps. First, because patients must be reached quickly to determine their status, *initial access procedures* are begun. This work must rapidly yield at least one pathway that will allow medical personnel to contact the patients. In some cases the collision has already provided initial access openings. These accident-generated openings include broken automobile windows and windshields or doors flung open during the crash. Some safety work, however, may need to be done to prepare the access opening for use. A broken side or rear window may need to have the remaining shards of glass removed or the bottom of the opening protected before anyone can reach or climb through to access the patient. Initial access involves using any available openings that exist in the vehicle yielding access to and contact with the occupants of the vehicle. Ideally, basic vehicle stabilization evolutions have been put in place before any attempts to access the interior of the vehicle.

If a damaged vehicle has no usable access openings (which is relatively rare in real-world situations), a *rescue-generated* access opening must be made (Fig. 2-18). A priority sequence has been developed for rescue personnel to use if no initial accident-generated openings exist. Initial access is first attempted by trying all doors, regardless of their exterior appear-

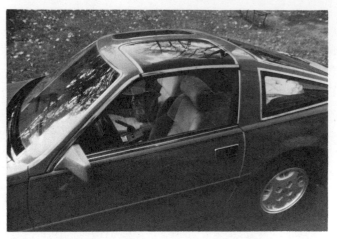

FIG. 2-18 Access should be gained within 30 seconds using the following priority sequence: (1) doors, (2) windows, (3) sunroof or T-top, and (4) windshield.

ance, to determine whether any door will open normally. Remember the instructions, "try before you pry." If no doors open manually or are obstructed, the tempered safety glass rear window, side windows, T-tops, or sunroofs are the next target. Their complete removal can quickly provide an effective access. Next, if access is still not possible, the removal of the vehicle's windshield is considered. With some practice, this can be done fairly quickly, although forcible removal produces large quantities of small slivers of broken glass. These salt and pepper glass slivers can cause additional injuries to unprotected patients trapped inside.

If necessary, each of these tasks can be done by one rescuer using simple tools. Initial access can thus be gained almost every time by using existing openings in the wrecked vehicle or using simple hand tools to make suitable openings.

When it is most effective, the process of gaining initial access takes no more than 60 seconds to accomplish. This does not mean that access to the patients should be provided within 60 seconds of the arrival of the emergency service crews, but that once initial size-up work has been accomplished and scene stabilization has made it safe to touch or work with the accident vehicles, access should be gained in the shortest practical period of time (Fig. 2-19).

Emergency service personnel may make the mistake at this point of not promptly accessing the injured. Medical teams that do not quickly gain access to the interior of the vehicle can miss a life-saving opportunity. The simple determination of a patent

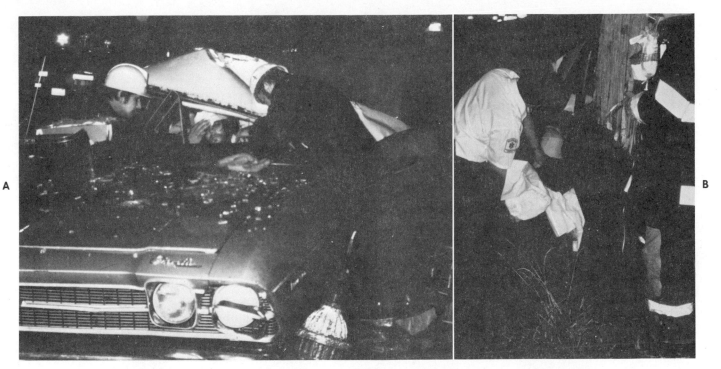

FIG. 2-19 A, Access should be gained as quickly as possible and is not necessarily the opening by which the patient will eventually be removed from vehicle. **B,** EMS work including patient stabilization should be accomplished before, during, and after the patient is extricated from the vehicle.

airway can save a patient's life. Patient access is therefore crucial during these initial operations; patients must be accessed quickly and safely so that their primary medical conditions can be ascertained. Waiting for heavy-duty rescue operations with sophisticated power rescue tools to be completed consumes precious seconds and delays immediate access to the injured, which can cost them their life. Remember, most initial access is accomplished by simply "reading" the damaged vehicle to discover its existing access openings or making usable openings with simple hand tools (Fig. 2-20).

Sustained access openings are openings that provide additional access to the overall patient area and are made after patients have been initially contacted and before more extensive work is done. Sustained access openings enable additional medical personnel to reach patients with the necessary equipment. A broken rear door window may have allowed one medic to enter the vehicle and access the injured persons initially. Continuing to "open up" the vehicle has many advantages and is an important responsibility of personnel once inside the damaged vehicle. Access to interior door locks, window cranks, and

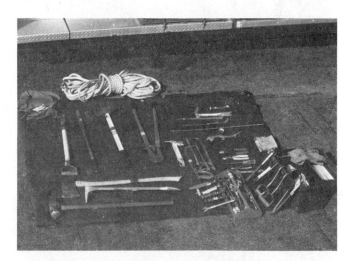

FIG. 2-20 Simple hand tools can provide intitial access to patients in most rescue situations. These tools are carried on a structural fire suppression engine that also responds to motor vehicle accidents.

door handles can aid in making further openings in the vehicle. When more openings are made, patient access becomes available, interior heat is vented during warm weather, and any fumes inside the vehicle are dispersed. Additional openings also improve communication between inside and outside rescue personnel and allow for more effective lighting of the interior areas.

Work done during the sustained access stage need not be very involved or require complex rescue activities. When pondering how to make sustained access openings or whether they are in fact necessary, the general rule for command personnel is "if in doubt, take it out." If those in charge believe that there is or may be a need for sustained openings, it is probably prudent to go ahead and order them to be made. For example, if an inside medic feels it would be beneficial to have additional doors or windows in a damaged vehicle opened or removed, the request should go to the person in charge of that operation and the evolution should be accomplished. If a rescuer suspects that a piece of metal may be in the way of a later evolution, it should be removed. One of the best examples of sustained access is roof removal (Fig. 2-21). Although a bit more involved than glass removal, this single

evolution can have the biggest and most profound positive influence on the outcome of the entire rescue and extrication process. If in doubt, take it out!

PATIENT EMERGENCY CARE AND TREATMENT STAGE

Once successful access to the patient or patients has been provided, emergency medical activities begin. The *patient care and treatment* stage continues longer than any of the other life cycle components. The medic/patient relationship is established when an injured or trapped person is contacted and the patient becomes the direct responsibility of emergency care providers. EMS personnel sort out injury severity if confronted with multiple numbers of injured patients. After this sorting or triage is accomplished, medical crew members initiate individual emergency medical care measures as appropriate and maintain and support each patient's medical needs throughout the

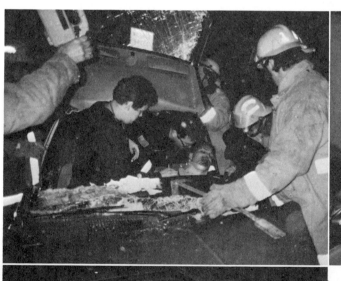

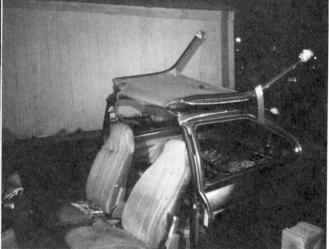

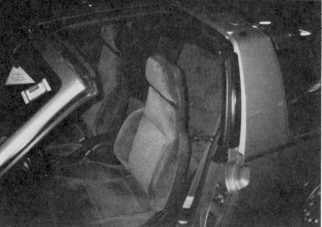

FIG. 2-21 **A,** Flip-top-box rescue evolution being performed to give sustained access to the trapped and injured driver. **B,** Exposed sharp glass and metal must be covered during extrication of patient to prevent further injury. Roof must also be secured in the flipped position. **C,** The sunroof panel has been removed as an example of increased patient access.

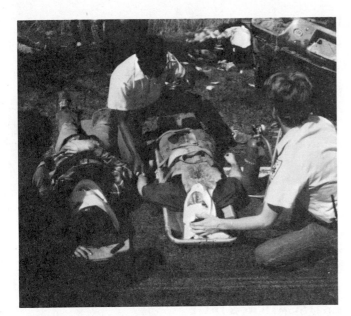

FIG. 2-22 Medical care measures are maintained throughout the entire period of contact with the injured patient. EMS crews must provide care for both physical and mental injuries to their patients.

remainder of the incident (Fig. 2-22). Patient emergency care and treatment ends for the emergency medical provider when the patient is transferred physically and legally to the medical facility or the patient is pronounced dead by a responsible medical authority. Medical care in the field must not stop once it has been started unless there is obvious death, a death pronouncement, or imminent threat to the life safety of the emergency care provider.

Emergency medical care responsibilities involve triage work, evaluating individual patient conditions, administering necessary care, and ensuring that patient handling neither causes further injuries nor aggravates existing injuries. This care evolves in several stages. During an initial patient assessment or survey, life-threatening injuries or conditions are recognized and corrected or stabilized. When further access becomes available, the patient receives continuing medical care, secondary surveys, and packaging. Patient packaging refers to two distinctly different actions — that of packaging the patient and that of dealing with individual injuries. Patient packaging includes immobilizing the head, neck, and spine to prevent further injuries complicated by spinal movement and the securing of a patient on a longboard for removal from the vehicle. Injury packaging might include immobilization of limb fractures to the extent practical within the confines of the wrecked vehicle.

Once packaged, the patient may be ready for removal from the automobile unless trapped in some manner. It is the responsibility of the inside-EMS personnel to ascertain whether and how the patient is trapped and what the patient's needs will entail as the rescue is accomplished. Inside-medical personnel must continually advise command personnel of the patient's medical condition, what entrapment problems exist, and what requirements the particular patient may have for removal. Suggestions about rescue work that might be indicated and reports on medical and rescue progress (or lack of it) must be relayed to the IC, who can make the most appropriate decisions on how to proceed.

Once EMS personnel have access to patients during the patient access stage, they take on an immense responsibility — for their well being and that of their patients. During the patient care and treatment stage, medical personnel must use all their skills and training to assess both injuries and entrapment problems. Inside-EMS personnel must develop the best means of treating the injured, providing the necessary care, and assisting in the process of removing the injured from the wreckage. It is a challenging assignment, both physically and emotionally. These important activities can only be accomplished when EMS personnel are adequately trained, sufficiently equipped, and protected from physical harm. (Recommended personal protection for EMS personnel is discussed in Chapter 3.)

DISENTANGLEMENT STAGE

One of the most crucial stages of the life cycle occurs as medical personnel attending the injured go into a holding action while those responsible for the necessary disentanglement work move into full swing. The actual unraveling of the vehicle, systematically moving or removing portions of the wreckage to make the patient readily removable, is the *disentanglement* stage (Fig. 2-23). The critical goal here is to not further injure the patient. The current definition of disentanglement means to remove the vehicle from the patient.

Disentanglement provides sufficient room within the vehicle's structure to permit medical personnel to provide proper medical care and patient packaging and release the injured patient from conditions that may have caused the entrapment. Disentanglement also provides the safest possible exit pathway for the packaged patient.

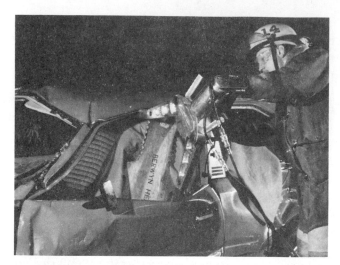

FIG. 2-23 Disentanglement: Remove the vehicle from the patient.

To accomplish these goals, rescue personnel must either distort the structure of the damaged vehicle back toward its original shape or take away the portions that block patient removal. This effort may take up most of the on-scene time. Case histories of tractor-trailer truck drivers being trapped in the wreckage of their overturned truck while medical and rescue personnel labor 5 hours or more are true. Fortunately, these long and difficult rescues are the exception rather than the rule.

The concept of the golden hour of life for the serious trauma patient allots only about 20 minutes for disentanglement work. At this point in the rescue process, vehicle stabilization, hazard control, and access work has been done. The difference between these efforts and what must still be accomplished to remove the patient is what the disentanglement stage addresses.

Disentanglement work is the science of putting energy back into the damaged vehicle structure in a manner that opposes the effect created by the dynamics of the original collision. It is the use of controlled and directed force to free a patient from what binds or obstructs the individual, permitting safe and efficient removal. Disentanglement may be simple or may constitute some of the most involved and difficult rescue work of the entire incident.

How the trapped patient is to be removed is determined by a series of ongoing decisions made by inside medical personnel attending the injured patient, the rescue officer in command of the disentanglement operation, and the IC, who assesses both exterior and interior activities. Exterior work, which generally paves the way for the interior operations, involves working with doors, roof and roof pillars, and the vehicle's glass. Interior work involves moving or removing items that are either crushed into or are in close proximity to the patient. Actual techniques are determined by the extent of entrapment and the nature of the patient's injuries and overall medical condition.

During disentanglement, inside EMS personnel must properly protect the patient from further injury. Rescue crew members working outside the vehicle must see that both patient and inside medic are protected or insulated from further injury resulting from the rescue work.

EXTRICATION STAGE

The process of physically removing the injured patient from the position within the wreckage is the *extrication* stage of the life cycle — removing the patient from the vehicle (Fig. 2-24). Several important activities must first take place. A two-part final assessment is made by the inside medic and the rescue

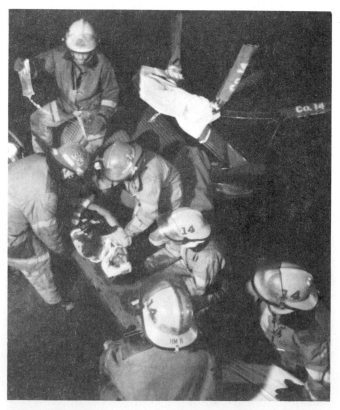

FIG. 2-24 Extrication: Remove the patient from the vehicle.

officer. They must determine whether the patient is ready for extrication by confirming that the patient is free of all obstructions and properly immobilized with patient packaging equipment and that the actual extrication pathway is adequate for patient removal. Inside medical personnel then conduct a final check of immobilization straps, survey the patient, and prepare for the activities that are about to take place. This assessment ensures that extrication will be carried out smoothly and safely. Medical and rescue personnel work together as the patient is properly moved onto a longboard device, secured, and moved from the wreckage. Actual patient handling is supervised and coordinated by attending medical personnel.

Once outside the confines of the wrecked vehicle, the patient and attending medic are located in an appropriate patient treatment area, generally the back of an ambulance. A specially designated patient treatment area may be established at incidents involving multiple casualties.

TRANSPORTATION STAGE

The process of moving the injured from the accident scene to the medical facility is the *transportation* stage of the life cycle. Transportation from the scene,

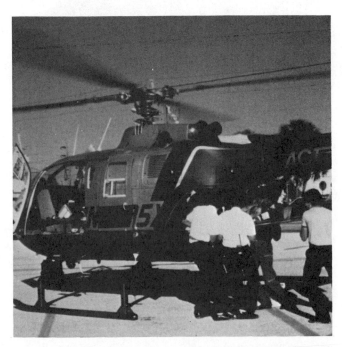

FIG. 2-25 Medical evacuation by helicopter is performed when patient injuries or other circumstances meet a predetermined set of criteria established by the emergency care providers. (Courtesy Bob Cross, Orlando, Fla.)

although generally by ambulance, might also be by fire department rescue vehicle, squad truck, or the specially designed pumper/medical units now available. Helicopters or fixed-wing aircraft, either publicly or privately owned, are also available in selected areas. The military term *Medevac,* an abbreviation of the words medical evacuation, is given to air transport used specifically when patient injuries or other circumstances meet a given set of criteria (Fig. 2-25). Other less common medical patient transportation methods include boats or snowmobiles.

During transportation, emergency medical personnel continue their sustained medical care. The patient, now on the medic's home turf, is further evaluated and treated appropriately. Communication with medical facilities can be established or continued. The emergency ends for noncritical trauma patients when medical personnel contact them and stabilize their conditions. For the severe trauma patient, survival even during the transportation phase may not be ensured until surgical intervention at the medical facility is achieved.

TERMINATION STAGE

For those left behind at the accident scene, once the final patient has been transported the emergency is over. The urgency of the rescue, so important in everyone's mind when there were people trapped, now diminishes. Vehicle rescue activities move into the final phase of the life cycle, the *termination* stage.

The incident is now being wrapped up as fire, rescue, and medical personnel wind down their involvement at the scene and return to their previous in-service status. The IC must assess whether the services of any agencies continue to be needed. If the accident scene has once again become a safe environment and the services of an emergency agency are no longer required, its personnel, equipment, and apparatus prepare for departure. Termination includes returning tools and equipment to vehicles for transporting back to quarters, proper servicing with fuel or other fluids (Fig. 2-26), and placement on the rescue vehicle. Fire suppression handlines and fire extinguishers deployed early in the incident are now returned to service. Other assisting agencies, such as the tow truck service, may enter the scene at this point and fulfill its legal responsibilities at the scene (Fig. 2-27). Tow agencies may have to do more than just move and secure damaged vehicles. In some states, tow agency operators are legally responsible for clear-

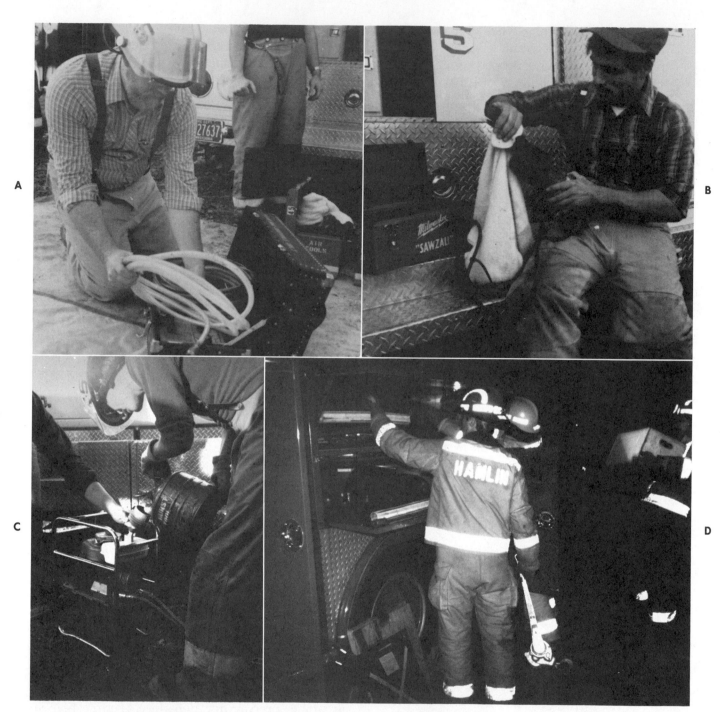

FIG. 2-26 Termination work for rescue personnel includes **A**, repacking, **B**, reblading, **C**, refueling, and **D**, returning equipment.

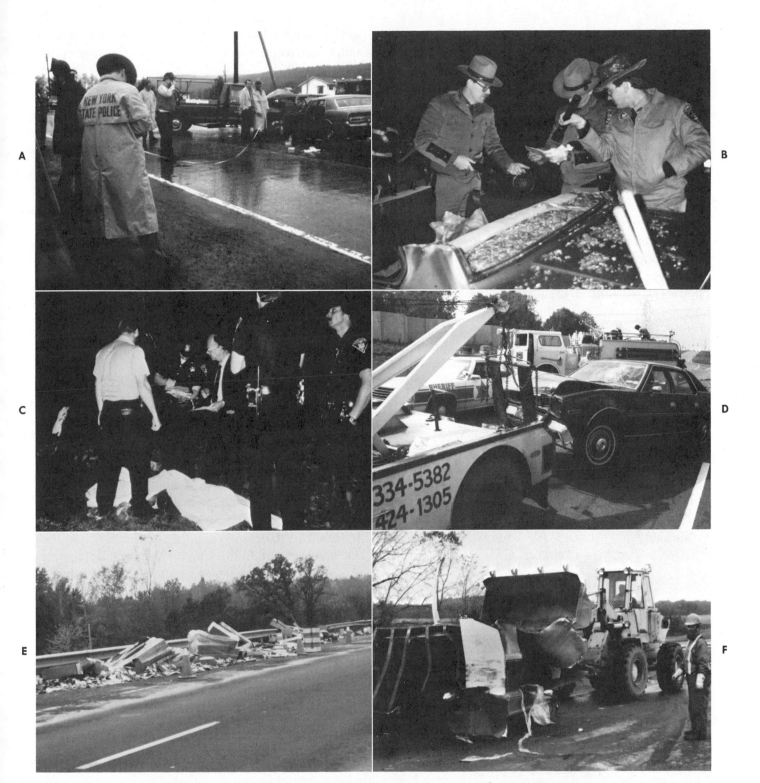

FIG. 2-27 Agencies fulfill their responsibilities at accident scene during termination stage. **A,** Police investigators document vehicle post-crash positions, **B,** account for accident victim's personal possessions, and **C,** assist the medical examiner's office with identification and documentation of traffic fatalities. **D,** Two agencies remove damaged vehicles, as standby handlines are reloaded by fire department engine company. **E,** A high-speed crash of two 18-wheelers on an expressway results in a tremendous amount of road debris requiring highway maintenance crews, **F,** to assist with the clean-up necessary to restore the flow of traffic.

ing the roadway of loose debris and foreign materials that would impede use of the road.

Once the scene itself has been cleared, medical, fire, and rescue personnel return to their quarters. In quarters, all tools and equipment used at the incident must be checked, accounted for, and readied for future service. During equipment cleanup, crew members can inspect the tools and equipment for loose or missing parts, breaks, or cracks. Clean equipment exemplifies team members who care about themselves, their public image, and those they strive to protect (Fig. 2-28).

During termination, necessary paperwork is done and a critique or evaluation of the rescue work may be conducted. This may include immediate discussion back at quarters and an organized critique session at a later date. Professional and progressive organizations critique themselves to better prepare for the future. After an emotionally draining incident, organized stress-debriefing sessions may be appropriate. In a small community, for example, when a well-known, life-long resident is killed in an accident, the emotional stresses can reach far beyond emergency service personnel. "Stressed-out" emergency service personnel must be recognized by their superiors and treated appropriately. If this occurs at the scene, they should be removed and attended to as soon as possible. Remember, it is not just the patient that we treat who can sustain scars for life. We must recognize both our abilities and our weaknesses. A rescue worker who "freezes" under stress at a future incident is likely to be

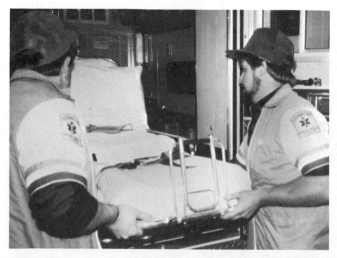

FIG. 2-28 Termination of one incident leads to readiness for the next. Emergency service personnel must always be at one step of the vehicle rescue life cycle.

a victim who has gone untreated because of our failure to recognize and deal with this aspect of human frailty.

It is important to remember that this final stage of the vehicle rescue life cycle leads directly into readiness for the next emergency. In reality, each emergency service team should always be at one stage of the vehicle rescue life cycle for it to function effectively as our guide to safe and efficient operations.

SUMMARY

A collision has occurred at a busy intersection in a metropolitan area. One vehicle has been hit broadside and pushed to the side of the intersection and now rests precariously on its driver's side. The driver, a 22-year-old woman, is unconscious and still seated in the driver's position. The second vehicle, a full-sized automobile, is across the street. Its two front-seat occupants are also injured.

The fire department pumper crew arrives ahead of the rescue truck and ambulance responding from a different station. First-arriving firefighters are overwhelmed by the emotion of the accident, and without the knowledge of their officer, two firefighters go to the driver's door window of the overturned vehicle, locate the injured driver, and yank her out the broken window until she is lying on the street. The woman survives the accident but is later found to be paralyzed for life. Did this result from the accident or from the so-called rescue? In this true story, essential stages of the life cycle were never completed. The injured patient paid a tragic price for our incompetence.

At a different time and place, a one-vehicle collision occurs on a rainy weekday morning. The overweight driver of a small compact automobile loses control of his vehicle and runs head-on into a large utility pole. The front end of the car, still in contact with the pole, is severely damaged. The driver has his legs and knees wedged into the dashboard and his face bloodied by the injuries he has sustained. The collision has jammed the doors of the compact shut. Steam emanates from under the buckled hood as rush hour traffic snarls and a large crowd begins to gather. The first emergency crews arrive.

The command officer, a fire department lieutenant, immediately assumes command and quickly orders basic traffic and crowd control procedures initiated. Hazards of the power pole and the vehicle are accounted for and controlled as the vehicle is quickly stabilized. Medical personnel reach the injured driver through a window opening prepared by the rescue crew. The patient is assessed, receives medical care, and is then immobilized. The patient and the medical crew member inside are protected, shortboards are placed inside the front doors, and the doors are opened and widened. Almost simultaneously, another rescue team sets up to move the steering wheel and column, along with the dash. Once disentangled, the patient is gently moved to a longboard and transported to a waiting ambulance. All this is accomplished within 12 minutes of the arrival of the first emergency service crew. One week later the driver of the automobile, now on crutches, hobbles into the local fire station to say thanks for a job well done.

Both these accidents actually occurred as described.

In the first scenario, important steps were omitted, severely compromising the health and safety of the rescuers and the injured patients. In the second accident, emergency service personnel followed correct procedure. Their professionalism yielded a viable patient who was extricated in an impressively short time with all safety precautions given full consideration.

Which team do you want to be a member of? The difference is simply the commitment of both officers and crew members to follow a systematic procedure at each and every accident. The difference is a commitment to believe in the vehicle rescue life cycle, the system that defines the delicate balance of medical, fire, safety, and rescue efforts necessary for safe and successful vehicle rescue operations.

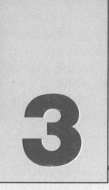

Vehicle Rescue Safety

OBJECTIVES

At the end of this chapter, you will be able to:

• List and describe the three major categories of emergency service personnel hazards related to vehicle accidents.

• Define the safety concerns associated with each major hazard area.

• Understand the effects of each specific safety concern or hazard on emergency scene activities.

• List and describe procedures or specific methods necessary to deal with a given safety hazard to prevent injury or death.

A tractor-trailer has overturned on an expressway. Medical, law enforcement, and fire department personnel arrive on the scene. One occupant of the truck has been ejected a short distance from the damaged cab. The driver is dangling from the wreckage. Should the medical crew immediately rush over to the victim lying on the ground and provide medical care? Should the rescue team immediately begin work to disentangle the driver from the wreckage of what was once the cab of the truck? Should traffic be diverted around the scene or stopped completely? How far back should crowd control be maintained?

These decisions are typical of those that must be made quickly under less than ideal conditions at an emergency scene. A correct decision minimizes the danger posed to emergency service personnel, the public, and the patient. One incorrect decision, on the other hand, can lead to injury or death for all. The overturned truck in this instance may contain dangerous products that will injure or kill those who come in contact with them, or it may suddenly ignite in a massive fuel fire. The truck may be perched percariously and suddenly shift or collapse onto unsuspecting emergency personnel.

As soon as emergency service personnel arrive, all activities must be directed at improving the safety of the accident scene. This chapter focuses on the basic safety precautions that must be considered if successful vehicle rescue operations and the safety of all persons are to be ensured. Emergency service personnel are being injured and killed in preventable situations. We are often our own worst enemies. The following pages identify the causes of many of these injuries and deaths and discuss ways to develop procedures to prevent their occurrence at future operations.

HAZARDS

Any situation with the potential to do harm is a hazard. All accident-scene hazards fall into one of three general categories. *Environmental hazards* are weather related. They include extremes of heat, cold, wet, dry, and darkness that threaten crew and patient safety and must be dealt with properly at an emergency scene.

Incident scene hazards relate directly to the specific incident scene and include control of crowds, traffic, the danger of downed electrical wires, the presence of hazardous materials, even the very location of an emergency. A vehicle perched precariously on the edge of a bridge railing or one that has crashed into a structure causing a partial building collapse are examples of scene hazards requiring special safety activities early in the incident.

The final category is extremely important and includes the primary hazards that most often confront emergency service personnel. *Vehicle hazards*, those directly related to the vehicle itself, include fuel, electrical system, cargo, stability of the vehicle, sharp glass and metal, hot antifreeze, engine oil, and battery acid.

The first step in increasing safety and survival for emergency service personnel is to make each individual acutely aware of the real and potential safety problems to be found at an accident scene.

Emergency Response Safety

A 60-year-old volunteer firefighter suffered fatal head injuries when he was thrown from the back step of a pumper that was involved in a collision. The pumper with its crew of eight was responding to an automatic fire alarm with warning lights on and siren operating. As the pumper proceeded through a residential area of the fire district, it collided with a van at a cross street. The out-of-control pumper then skidded, turned 180 degrees, and pushed the van into and around a utility pole. The firefighter died 19 days later.

In Houston, Texas, a 32-year-old career firefighter died of injuries sustained during a fall from a pumper responding to an automobile accident and fire. He had been standing in the jump seat area. As the driver/operator approached the accident scene and slowed the apparatus, the firefighter apparently lost his balance and fell to the pavement. He was wearing full protective clothing, but his helmet reportedly came off on impact. He died of a skull fracture and broken neck.

These reports from the files of the National Fire Protection Association (NFPA), a major center for the collection and analysis of U.S. fire and safety data, identify important trends in injuries and deaths to emergency service personnel. According to the NFPA, in 1988, accidents to emergency service personnel responding to or returning from emergency scenes claimed the lives of 5 career firefighters and 32 volunteer fire service personnel, accounting for almost one third of the year's total; an estimated 5080 U.S. firefighters were injured while responding to or returning from emergency incidents (Fig. 3-1). From 1979 through 1988, 334 firefighters died while responding to or returning from emergencies and other incidents. This total includes 235 fatalities while actually responding to alarms and 159 fatalities while operating emergency or privately owned vehicles.

These deaths and injuries are needless and, in most cases, readily preventable. If the process of driving or being a passenger in an emergency vehicle is the common thread among these accidents, safe vehicle operation must become the focus of an intensive effort to improve the safety of our personnel.

Analyzing accident reports for emergency vehicles clarifies our knowledge of problem areas in vehicle response. For example, 318 motor vehicle accidents involving ambulances in New York State were reported in a single year, killing one person and injuring 419 others. Most of these accidents occurred during daylight hours, while the weather was clear and the roadway dry; only 20% occurred during rain or snow or under conditions of darkness. Most also occurred on straight and level sections of municipal streets, and nearly half at traffic control devices while the ambulance was proceeding straight ahead. The most common contributing factor found by the statisticians

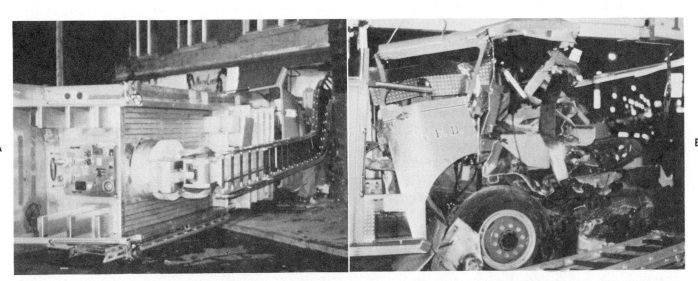

A

B

FIG. 3-1 A, This 22-ton fire apparatus swerved during emergency response to avoid a pedestrian and rolled over into a building. Officer and driver received serious injuries resulting in one permanent disability. **B,** Fire apparatus after removal from building. Note massive destruction of jump seat area of vehicle. (Courtesy Judy Galloway, Syracuse, NY.)

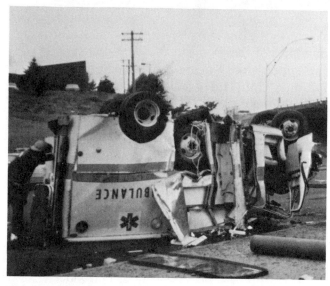

FIG. 3-2 Statistics from several states indicate that the majority of ambulance accidents during emergency response occur during daylight hours on clear, level roads.

was human error. This accident scenario has remained essentially unchanged in New York State for the last 7 years (Fig. 3-2).

Motor vehicle accidents involving fire apparatus and police vehicles also fit this pattern. Accident summary information from Virginia reports that over a 3-year period, the state's 7000-plus emergency vehicles had an accident rate three times that of ordinary motor vehicles. It is clear that these problem areas are common to emergency service providers throughout the country.

TRUE EMERGENCY

The first step in reducing needless injuries and deaths is to change our personal attitudes toward emergency vehicle driving and operation. We cannot "blow them out of the way" or assume that all motorists will yield to our emergency vehicles. To respond to each and every emergency at top speed, with lights flashing and siren blaring, reflects total disregard for the safety of both crew members and the general public. This attitude puts the driver in a game of Russian roulette, a game that cannot be won. Each emergency vehicle operator must accept responsibility for a safe and efficient emergency response.

Emergency service personnel must understand the definition of a "true emergency." As defined by the U.S. Department of Transportation Emergency

Vehicle Operator's Course, a true emergency is any situation in which there is a high probability of death or significant injury to an individual or group of individuals or a significant loss of property, which can be reduced by the actions of an emergency service. This definition has gained legal acceptance nationwide. How many of our lights and siren responses really fit this court-tested definition? If two emergency vehicles travel a total distance of 10 miles on an expressway, one vehicle traveling at the posted speed and the other vehicle exceeding the posted speed by 5 mph, the faster driver would arrive only 54 seconds ahead of the slower and safer one. If you, as the driver of the speeding vehicle, were involved in a response accident, could you justify your operating procedures in court before a jury? Following the same reasoning, protocols should be developed that encourage or even mandate that emergency warning lights and sirens *not* be used for responses to training sessions, parades, or routine runs to cover or fill in at a neighboring station.

Many years ago, the California State Highway Patrol forbade the use of sirens and warning lights by emergency vehicles traveling on the thousands of miles of that state's expressways. The consensus is that the lights and sirens actually disrupt the traffic flow patterns and produce fear and confusion on the part of the motoring public.

Emergency medical personnel should also consider transporting stabilized patients to medical facilities under nonemergency conditions. Given the current state-of-the-art in emergency medical care, the true emergency for patients is often over when trained and equipped emergency care providers arrive at the scene. Patients receive controlled care and their condition generally stabilizes. In the case of collision trauma patients in life-threatening and rapidly deteriorating conditions, however, swift transportation is justified. This includes conditions of uncontrolled internal bleeding, traumatic asphyxia, acute respiratory distress, complicated childbirth, congestive heart failure, drug or poison ingestion, anaphylactic shock, diabetic coma, or hypothermia. Fortunately, calls of this nature account for a small percentage of total EMS calls.

Even transporting a heart attack (AMI) patient or performing CPR on a patient during transport may not justify a rapid, high-speed run to the hospital. Medical care providers know from personal experience that manual CPR cannot be performed effectively at vehicle speeds much above 30 mph. Regardless of the condition of the patient in the care of any medical crew, a primary EMS responsibility remains a safe response to the incident and a safe transport to the medical facility.

Intersections

Because intersections are the most frequent crash site for responding emergency service vehicles, there is a clear need to design and implement operating procedures that require operators of emergency vehicles to come to a complete or momentary stop at all traffic control devices such as yield signs, red lights, and stop signs. Electronic systems now available give responding emergency vehicles the capability of controlling traffic signals. When the fire department in Syracuse, New York, equipped their emergency vehicles with such a system, the accident rate for fire vehicles fell dramatically.

Standard operating procedures must also be established for situations when two emergency vehicles approach the same intersection from different directions. Mandatory radio communications between vehicles approaching an intersection are possible when common radio frequencies exist. The emergency vehicle that must turn at the intersection must yield to the vehicle that will continue straight through the intersection.

Some emergency service personnel have the mistaken idea that police escorts and multiple emergency vehicle responses in bumper-to-bumper fashion are safe. When vehicles follow each other too closely, drivers have little or no time to act or react to rapidly changing response conditions. Citizens in private vehicles may clearly hear and see one emergency vehicle, allow it to pass, and then blindly pull into the path of other oncoming emergency vehicles. Unless they are unavoidable, there should be no multiple vehicle responses in convoy fashion. Adequate spacing between vehicles must be maintained so that each vehicle is observed and reacted to as an individual response unit. Escorting of emergency vehicles, particularly ambulance units by police department vehicles, also presents a high degree of risk. Unless the emergency vehicle driver and crew officer are unfamiliar with the incident location or some other justifiable situation exists, police escorts of emergency vehicles should be avoided as unsafe.

Response safety can be increased when all responding emergency vehicles confirm the exact location of the incident. Confusion among crew members (for example, whether the emergency incident is at 112

Down Street or 112 Brown Street) increases the chance of emergency vehicle response accidents. Responding vehicles may be caught unaware when a misinformed crew makes an erratic turn onto Brown Street when everyone else expected them to continue another four blocks to the correct location on Down Street.

When emergency vehicle operators (EVOs) know the expected response route for their vehicle and those of other responding crews, the response to the scene is smoother for all personnel. Vehicle operators can listen for the radio response acknowledgments of other responding vehicles whenever common radio channels are used. If multiple vehicles are dispatched to a given location, the sequence of these responses alerts other crews to the possible vehicle arrival sequence at the scene. To avoid an accident with another vehicle, the driver and crew officer must anticipate the actions of the vehicle ahead, the one behind, and those approaching at intersections. Crew officers and drivers must remain constantly aware that other drivers may not hear their sirens or see their emergency warning devices. Extra precautions must be taken when approaching traffic in or near intersections. Operators must expect the unexpected and drive defensively.

RIDING POSITIONS

Each emergency vehicle operator and supervising crew officer must be held responsible for the safe and efficient operation of their vehicle. The responsibility should be placed directly on the operator to check and confirm that all personnel riding in or on the emergency vehicle are fully dressed in appropriate protective clothing and are seated and belted before the vehicle begins its response from quarters.

Riding positions on emergency vehicles must be controlled. Crew members in jumpseats and enclosed riding positions must be required to be seated with their seat belt restraint devices properly used. In the case of an accident, jumpseats, or "buckets" as they are sometimes called, offer more protection to fire service personnel who must ride in exterior positions than to those riding the rear step of the apparatus. Current trends in American fire apparatus design were brought about by changes in nationally accepted minimum apparatus standards, and they require provisions for all responding personnel to be located inside enclosed and protected positions on the emergency vehicle.

BACKING UP

Accidents that occur when the emergency vehicle is backed up are also preventable. Vehicles should be placed in positions or locations that do not require backing up to reduce accident potentials and should have audible warning devices to warn those near the vehicle when backing is unavoidable. Large-size or long-length vehicles should have special convex back-up mirrors or the newer rearview television cameras and monitors installed to allow vision along the back of the vehicle. A policy should also be in place that mandates the positioning of an assistant near the rear of the vehicle to assist during backing maneuvers.

Staging of Personnel, Equipment, and Apparatus

At the scene of the emergency, *staging* responding emergency vehicles and crews away from the actual work area gives on-scene personnel a safer and less crowded working environment. Later-arriving emergency vehicles should automatically be positioned the equivalent of a city block from the nearest edge of the incident scene. Crews and vehicles that stage at this minimum distance are readily available for assignment at the scene, relocation, or return to service as necessary.

APPROACHING THE INCIDENT SCENE

Arriving crews must learn to expect the unexpected from those already on the accident scene. Emergency personnel are busy scanning the accident and moving back and forth to assess the situation and plan their initial actions. Later-arriving vehicles and crews must allow for this preoccupation with the scene and proceed into the immediate area with great caution. A firefighter intent on donning self-contained breathing apparatus to combat a vehicle fire could accidentally step into the path of an arriving fire vehicle, or an excited citizen could suddenly run into the path of an arriving ambulance. Personnel on the scene may also attempt to guide later-arriving vehicles and crews with hand signals that may be misunderstood, increasing the potential for accidents.

SAFE SCENE POSITIONING

There are lessons to be learned from the tragic death of a 31-year-old career firefighter in Birmingham, Alabama, who was struck and killed by a passing car while working at the scene of an accident. He was wearing proper firefighting protective clothing and standing next to his fire apparatus while assistance was being rendered to accident victims. An oncoming car veered around a police vehicle and into the highway median, narrowly missing the fire apparatus and running him down before he had time to react. He suffered multiple trauma injuries that proved fatal. The car's driver was found guilty of manslaughter and driving under the influence of alcohol. According to NFPA records, 11 firefighters were struck and killed by vehicles at emergency scenes. Assistant Fire Chief Jim Yvorra of Berwyn Heights, Maryland (to whom this book is dedicated) was one of 139 firefighters to die in 1988. He was struck and killed at an accident scene by a passing vehicle. From 1979 to 1988, firefighters struck at or near emergency scenes were most often operating at traffic accidents or vehicle fires. Most fatalities occurred after dark or under conditions of poor visibility.

One initial measure that can be taken to minimize these unfortunate occurrences is the proper positioning of our emergency vehicles to shield and protect the accident scene. Dangers posed by approaching or oncoming traffic must be eliminated to prevent secondary collisions. Proper vehicle positioning involves more than just stopping where convenient. Emergency vehicles must be properly *positioned* on the emergency scene, which includes placing them in the safest and most advantageous location to minimize exposure of emergency service personnel to oncoming traffic.

Positioning is influenced by many factors, some of which can be controlled. The actual arrival sequence, for example, may dictate positioning, with first on the scene generally meaning closest to the action area. This can be good or bad. Other vehicle-positioning factors include the function of each vehicle and its crew and standard operating procedures that dictate positioning or placement. It is important to recognize and anticipate potential hazards and their strike zones.

Under normal circumstances and if possible, the initial emergency vehicle to arrive at the accident scene should be properly positioned on the *approach* side of the accident in the same lane of traffic as the involved vehicles and between oncoming traffic and the accident. In this position, the emergency vehicle's lights warn approaching traffic of the presence of an incident ahead, and the vehicle acts as a physical barrier between the accident scene work area and approaching traffic. When the accident is located in the same lane or lanes of traffic as those being used by the arriving emergency vehicle, approach-side positioning also enables the vehicle operator and crew officer to survey the scene from inside their vehicle. If the response is at night, the crew can use the headlights and vehicle-mounted spotlights for initial scene illumination. Additional units should properly stage away from the incident on their own approach side and await the initial scene size-up report and additional orders from the first-arriving vehicle officer commanding the incident at this point.

If accident vehicles are blocking lanes of traffic and causing a backup, emergency vehicles may be forced into the opposite lane of traffic because it provides the only access to the accident scene. Whenever an emergency vehicle must be positioned in a lane of traffic facing the normal flow of traffic, extreme caution should be exercised. Under these circumstances, emergency vehicle operators should consider turning off the headlights so that drivers of oncoming vehicles are not blinded.

When traffic control requires bringing traffic to a full stop in both directions on a street or highway, command officers may direct emergency vehicles to position to block off an open lane of traffic. This positioning greatly increases exposure of the vehicle and its crew to secondary collisions. Although positioning emergency vehicles in off-roadway locations provides protection for the vehicles, it may deprive personnel operating on the scene of needed protection.

Additional emergency vehicles positioning at the scene may find locations on the *departure* side of the accident the most beneficial. Positioning beyond the scene enables later-arriving crew members to view three sides of the accident scene as they pass by and allows them to leave the scene when necessary without being parked in.

When no obvious or unusual hazards are present, no emergency vehicle arriving at the accident scene should be positioned closer than 100 feet from the nearest vehicle involved in the accident. This spacing provides a minimum safe working area around the accident vehicles and diverts exhaust fumes from the emergency vehicles away from the work area. If one or more vehicles involved in the accident are burning, this distance should be increased. A 100-foot distance is a minimum recommendation, and it should be increased whenever there are doubts about the safety and stability of an accident scene. The 100-foot distance is intended to minimize the exposure of operating personnel and the emergency vehicle to hazards such as an exploded bumper. EVOs should be keenly aware of the fact that when an energy-absorbing bumper launches itself, it is likely to travel a fairly straight path. This is why crews must avoid approaching burning vehicles from either the front or the rear. Positioning or working within this strike zone puts the apparatus and its crew in grave danger of being struck by the unguided bumper if it shoots off the burning vehicle.

A minimum clear area of 2000 feet should be maintained initially if a hazardous material is or may be involved in the incident. This would include the presence of any pressurized storage cylinders or toxic, reactive, or explosive materials. This minimum distance may increase to 3000 feet or more in all directions depending on the nature of the incident.

In most situations it is also best to position emergency vehicles uphill and upwind of the accident scene, if possible, to avoid hazard areas. If a vehicle is leaking gasoline, the fumes typically travel downhill and downwind to low terrain areas such as sewer drains, ditches, and gullies. Because they must be evacuated and have all sources of potential ignition near them isolated, these low-lying areas should be avoided when choosing a position for emergency response vehicles. Safe vehicle positioning at an accident involving a utility company power pole requires vehicles and crews to avoid any area under overhanging transmission lines and near power transformers, which could short out. Command personnel must quickly ascertain the stability of the overhead wires, the damaged pole, adjacent power poles, and adjoining spans of transmission wires.

In all situations, if the operator or crew officer is in doubt as to how much space to put between the accident scene and the nearest emergency vehicle, a rule of excess should prevail. *If in doubt, stay back for safety's sake.* It is far easier and safer to move the vehicle forward than it is to be forced to rapidly back it up or abandon it entirely should an unanticipated, life-threatening situation develop.

Vehicles on Fire

March 10, 1984, is a day that no firefighter in Travis County, Texas, near Austin, will ever forget. On that day, Assistant Chief Marvin Ridgeway suffered fatal injuries when a burning pickup truck's fuel tank exploded, catching him in a massive fireball. Chief

Ridgeway, who was standing about 20 feet from the burning truck, wore a golf shirt, jeans, and sneakers, with only his fire department helmet on for protection. He had left his wet protective clothing at home that day to dry on his patio. His clothing ignited and burned as he was engulfed in flames; he died 10 days later.

Other incidents involving emergency service personnel have been so plagued with things going wrong that they sound like fabricated "tall tales." Such is the case with a documented incident that occurred in 1974 near St. Louis, Missouri. It began when a driver lost control and his car overturned, coming to rest on its roof on the roadway. Gasoline from the vehicle spilled and ignited. The lone occupant, trapped inside the burning vehicle, was screaming and trying to escape as help arrived.

The first-arriving emergency service personnel included a crew from the fire department with a pumper and several police officers. The firefighters stretched a small-diameter booster line from the pumper and battled to extinguish the fire. As the flames subsided, personnel shut the hose down, but they could still hear the trapped occupant screaming.

In an effort to free the trapped person quickly, the firefighters and the police, joined by some citizens who had stopped at the fire, lined up on the passenger side of the vehicle and began to roll the vehicle back over onto its wheels, pushing it by hand. As this makeshift effort was underway, gasoline from the fuel tank again spilled out onto the hot blacktop, instantly reigniting the fuel vapors. The people who were attempting to push the vehicle over were engulfed in an inferno. The car fire was extinguished for a second time. The decision was then made to free the person without rolling the car off its roof. The severely burned person was eventually removed from the vehicle alive but succumbed to his burn injuries 3 days later.

VEHICLE FIRE HAZARDS

A vehicle fire is a serious safety threat. In the Missouri incident, the second fire should have been prevented. That fire, caused by the rolling of the automobile, resulted entirely from wrong decisions made at the emergency scene. The goal of all motor vehicle incident responses is to make the overall situation better and safer. In times of excitement or stress, actions may be undertaken that are neither appropriate nor correct. When this happens, it is usually

because those at the scene have become victims themselves, caught up in the emotion of the moment.

In the 1970s, the Insurance Institute for Highway Safety, an independent nonprofit scientific and educational organization, conducted vehicle-to-vehicle crash tests to assess the problem of automobile accidents and fire. The Institute crashed six new automobiles at a moderate 35 mph into the rear ends of six other new autos. In each case the fuel system of the stationary target vehicle ruptured, spilling a considerable amount of gasoline from the tank or its adjacent fuel system components. In one test, spontaneous ignition of the spilled fuel occurred at a crash speed of 38.8 mph. (Analysis of the accident data revealed that lethal quantities of burning gasoline were injected into the passenger compartment, surrounding the test mannequin in the driver's seat with flames in one third of a second from the moment of the rear impact while the crash was still underway.)

A burning vehicle can be considered a "time-bomb" of potential disaster whose "fuse" has been lighted before the arrival of emergency personnel. Initial actions at a fire incident must therefore be directed toward snuffing out this fuse.

A burning passenger automobile, the most common type of vehicle fire encountered, presents a host of real and potential hazards. Pressurized containers found throughout the vehicle may overheat and explode. The hydraulic piston units of the energy-absorbing bumper systems located on each bumper, the vehicle strut suspension units, and the increasingly common hydraulic-pressurized lifting cylinders for the hatchback, tailgate, hood, or trunk are all potential hazards.

The hollow metal drive shaft of an automobile can fail under heat exposure, as can inflated rubber tires. The tires will first burn for a brief period, then rupture explosively, increasing the intensity of the fire in the vicinity of the tire and up to a distance of 3 to 4 feet out from the vehicle as the frame of the automobile instantly drops closer to the roadway. If the wheels are split rims, heat exposure can cause a violent failure of the entire wheel assembly. In this instance, portions of the metal rim can rocket a great distance, causing fatal injuries to anyone in their path.

The fuel-evaporation emission control system of a typical automobile consists of a metal or plastic fuel tank, a vapor-holding canister, various connecting lines, and a filler cap provided for a sealed fuel system. When this system is exposed to rapid heat build-up, the sudden and unexpected release of pressure

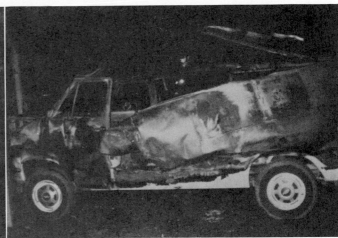

A

B

C

FIG. 3-3 A, Fire of electrical origin in dashboard resulted in leak of pure oxygen in this van containing a mobile oxygen refilling station. Resulting explosion blew side door off vehicle and bowed roof structure. **B,** Driver side of van after fire suppression. Note side body panel separation and incinerated forward roof section. **C,** Interior view reveals oxygen storage cylinders involved in fire and explosion.

can present a serious safety problem.

Another hazard area of a burning vehicle is the trunk or cargo storage area. Items carried in these areas, like aerosol cans, gasoline cans, or pressurized propane cylinders for backyard cooking grills can become explosion hazards (Fig. 3-3).

The issue of toxicity is also an important concern at a burning vehicle incident. Materials composing the interior seats, cushions, or vinyl trim generate toxic gases that can injure or kill unprotected emergency personnel (Fig. 3-4). Fiberglass or plastic body panel and trim materials, such as the Pontiac Fiero's Enduraflex, decompose and release hazardous by-products of combustion, including hydrogen cyanide. The toxins are carried away by the plume of smoke rising from the fire. Proper self-contained breathing apparatus must be used during fire suppression and overhaul situations. The growing threat posed by toxic hazards may also justify mandating that emergency medical personnel have access to and be properly trained in the use of this apparatus.

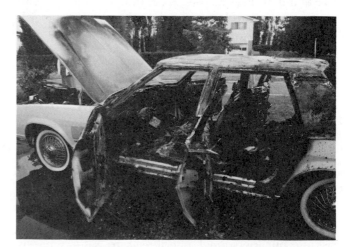

FIG. 3-4 Total burnout of full-size automobile demonstrates the large amount of combustible materials present on vehicles.

FIG. 3-5 A, Firefighters await arrival of engine company to scene of burning Volkswagen van. **B,** Delayed arrival of apparatus causes firefighters to move in with portable fire extinguishers. Vehicle suddenly undergoes flashover as captured in this dramatic photo. Note rubber-mounted rear window exploding from vehicle at the tongue of the flames and fireball visible in rear window moving toward front of vehicle. (Courtesy Tompkins County, NY, Fire Service.)

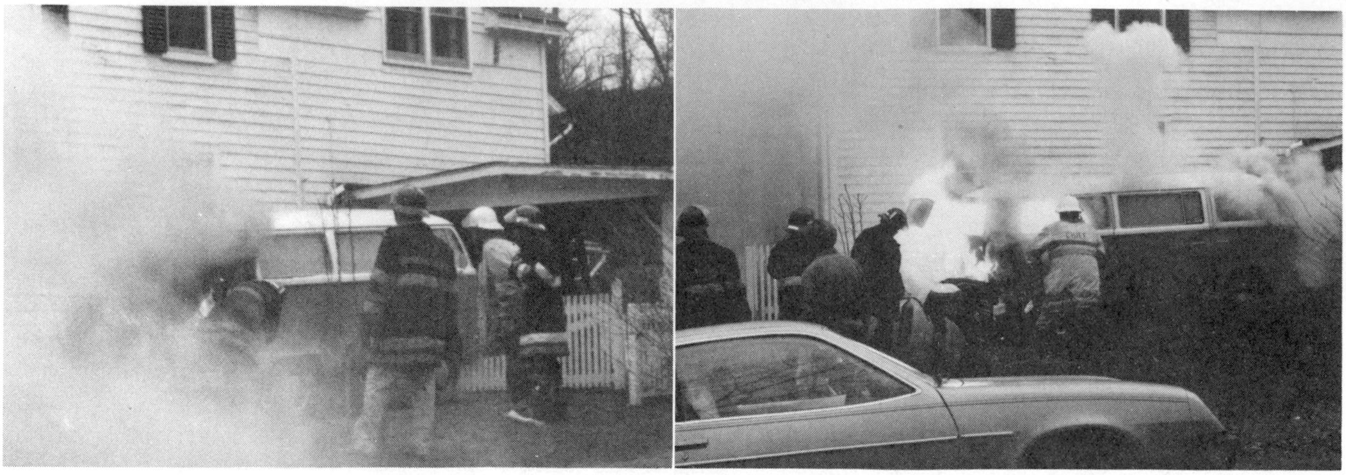

Firefighters may also encounter the phenomenon known as flashover, which is the heating of combustible components to the point where the contents of a vehicle ignite spontaneously. A small fire, barely visible through huge amounts of thick brown and black smoke, can suddenly become a raging inferno when flashover occurs. Firefighting crews must be ready for a sudden increase in the intensity of a vehicle fire at any time (Fig. 3-5). A seemingly small fire can cause unprepared personnel to lower their guard, making them extremely vulnerable to injury.

RESULT OF FIRE

Today's typical automobile construction materials are extremely fragile and easily destroyed by the slightest exposure to fire. Realistically, when firefighters observe visible open flame on a vehicle, it is likely that the car has already been damaged beyond what is practical to repair. Open flame is a true signal of the "death" of a modern-day auto. Emergency service personnel must reevaluate aggressive commitments to all-out vehicle fire attacks. We may be risking our personnel needlessly to save what is already beyond saving.

As with all emergency operations, hazard recognition is the foundation of successful vehicle firefighting. All actions must be directed toward being safe and protected at all times. All firefighters must believe that until the last flicker of flame is gone and everything

has cooled down, the vehicle has the potential to explode with deadly force at any time, and they must proceed as though it is about to do so. Only with this attitude can firefighters give the burning vehicle the respect it deserves.

The vehicle fire attack handline should have the capability of flowing a minimum of 100 gallons of water per minute. The flow of a 1¾-inch handline, for example, provides safety to the crew on the line and makes for a quick and efficient fire knockdown. Firefighters must be fully protected with approved protective clothing and self-contained breathing apparatus, which provides the necessary respiratory protection. Remember, if there is a fire of sufficient magnitude burning in a vehicle, that vehicle is usually considered "dead on arrival." It will be "written off" by the insurance company for its salvage value. The safety of the firefighting crew members must therefore be paramount. To risk exposure to the fire and its products of combustion would be suicidal; it is an attitude that cannot be tolerated.

As the fire attack gets underway, consideration should be given to chocking the front and back of one wheel of the burned vehicle when safe to do so. This procedure is intended to minimize the chance of vehicle movement along the ground.

One member of the fire attack crew should have simple forcible-entry tools during fire combat. With a tool such as a Halligan type of pry bar readily avail-

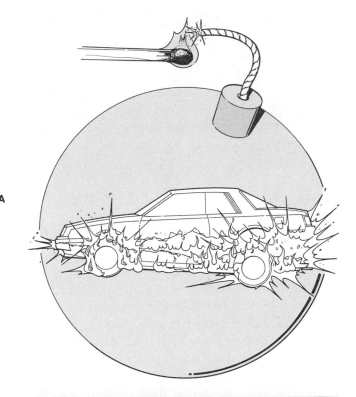

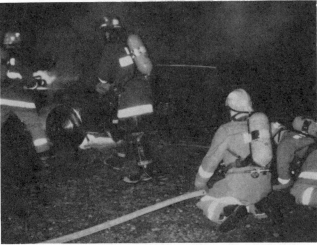

FIG. 3-6 A, Burning vehicles must be considered time bombs whose lit fuse is burning toward disaster. All activities must be directed to quickly and safely snuffing out potential explosion hazards. **B,** A cooling spray of water on the undercarriage, the "safety sweep," can buy valuable time for firefighters as they suppress the vehicle fire.

able, the crew can immediately vent automobile windows, move hot metal, or hold or prop hoods or trunk lids in the open position.

Members of the firefighting crew must direct their actions toward *getting the upper hand on the lower*

foot. This reminds them that nearly all immediate explosion hazards on a burning vehicle are found within the lower 12 inches of the automobile, somewhere between the front bumper and the rear bumper (Fig. 3-6). It is critical that the firefighting crew take the time at this point to "buy a life insurance policy" by applying a few seconds of cooling water spray along the undercarriage area. After this initial cooling sweep, the fire attack line can be moved into proper position to combat the body of fire.

The electrical power of an automobile that has been involved in a fire should be shut off. As soon as the fire has been extinguished, the negative battery cables could be disconnected or cut if the battery is still intact and capable of developing an electrical charge. Personnel must be wary of melted battery casings that expose the acid still contained within the cells.

NEED FOR STANDBY PROTECTION

Most safety actions that a firefighting crew initiates at an automobile accident are preventive in nature. Standby handlines or fire extinguishers are readied in anticipation of problems. Prevention work is not just standing by; prevention is an active process, not a reactive one.

The fire hazards on a vehicle, its quantity of dangerous fuel, and the many sources of ignition potential at an automobile accident have led progressive emergency service organizations to mandate that a fire department engine company be dispatched automatically to an accident serious enough to result in personal injury to the occupants. (For recommended vehicle and emergency crew responses, see Chapter 2.) If an ambulance is needed at the scene, those present also need the safety and security provided by a standby engine company. It must be remembered that a typical ambulance has only a small, dry chemical fire extinguisher in its inventory. It is much too late to use this extinguisher once the automobile has erupted into an inferno. Pumper crews would rather respond immediately and stand by than arrive at a tragedy caused by something their presence could have prevented in the first place.

Vehicle Fuel Leak and Spill

Leaks and spills of vehicle fuels present serious safety problems. Fuel leaking from any component of the fuel system can cause a small spill or cover a large area of the accident scene. The first and most impor-

COMMON PROPERTIES OF GASOLINE

Weight: 5-6 lb per gallon
Vapor density: 2.5 to 4, with 3.4 average
Flashpoint: –45° F
Ignition temperature: 495° F to 918° F
Explosive limit: 1.3% to 7.4%
Flame propagation in vapor/air mixture: 15 ft/second
Vapor travel: 400 ft downgrade on calm day
Energy of explosion: 1 gallon properly vaporized has
    explosive force of 88 sticks of dynamite

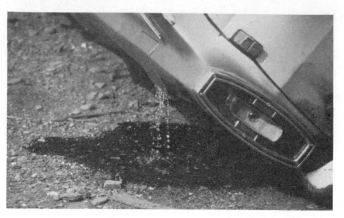

FIG. 3-7 The source of a fuel leak must be located and dealt with quickly and safely.

tant safety procedure for emergency service personnel to undertake at an accident with a fuel leak or spill is hazard recognition. The best and most reliable information about the presence of a fuel leak or spill must come from the scene survey conducted by emergency service personnel.

Fuel hazard safety work therefore begins with a size-up survey. Fuel contained within the tank or cylinder that is not leaking is relatively safe unless the container is damaged or the vehicle moved. When there is no apparent leak, precautions are still taken in anticipation of a problem that may develop. If a fuel leak is observed, the next step is to identify the nature of the fuel. Although the most common vehicle fuel is unleaded gasoline, the presence of diesel fuel or an alternate fuel such as propane, butane, or natural gas is a possibility.

Gasoline, the most common automobile fuel, has some important characteristics that all emergency service personnel must know (see box). Certain properties of gasoline influence preventive safety actions that are taken at an accident.

If a leak is detected, its source must be located. The leak can originate from the actual tank or container, any of the fuel lines, the filler neck, or the fuel cap (Fig. 3-7). An estimate of the quantity of gasoline or diesel fuel spilled is important. The amount of the present spill plus any additional amounts anticipated to continue to leak may be enough to require that outside agencies (such as environmental conservation personnel) be notified.

Crews must begin to deploy the safety handlines and fire extinguishers as appropriate. The standby 100 gallon-per-minute handline must be properly positioned in a "cut off" position. If a fire develops, the firefighter at the nozzle must have the capability of driving the fire and products of combustion away

from the patients, medics, and rescue personnel. The same standby line may be employed to divert existing fumes and vapors away from personnel and sources of ignition. The vapors of hydrocarbon fuels, particularly gasoline, act as an anesthetic to humans. As they displace oxygen, the oxygen levels necessary to sustain life are lowered, rendering the victim unconscious. Death can result from this oxygen deprivation.

Fire crews on these standby lines must don full personal protective equipment including Nomex firefighting hoods and leather-palmed gloves. Many progressive engine company officers also require their personnel on standby hoseline duty to wear their breathing apparatus units and have the facemask available for immediate donning. It must be remembered that if a fire erupts, these safety people must successfully combat the flames and need maximum protection to fulfill this assignment. The positioning of multipurpose, dry chemical fire extinguishers is a quick way to get at least a minimum level of protection to an immediate hazard. Personnel can be assigned to fire extinguishers while protective handlines are being stretched and readied for service.

At this early stage of the incident, crowd and traffic control should be initiated with the first emphasis being for those downwind of the spill. Quick crowd control also minimizes ignition sources presented by spectators lighting smoking material with a match or lighter. The supervising officer may also assign personnel to the task of eliminating potential sources of ignition. This safety work may include shutting off the ignition switches of damaged vehicles, although the internal arcs caused by shutting or closing an electrical switch have ignited flammable vapors at accident scenes. Other safety work includes rendering elec-

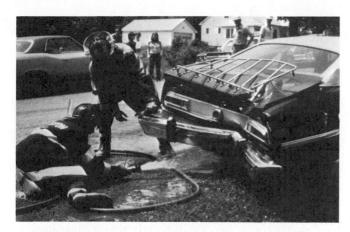

FIG. 3-8 A "flush job" or "wash down" represents an unsafe action under most circumstances. Note firefighters inside bumper strike zone and water spray pushing gasoline liquid and vapors closer to patients, rescuers, and vehicle ignition sources.

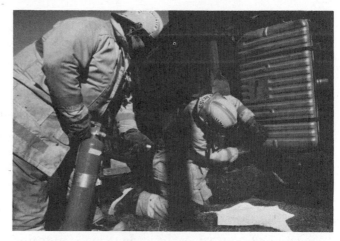

FIG. 3-9 Utility company type sealant material stops leak of gasoline, as absorbent pad contains spill and protective fire extinguisher is readied.

trical systems safe, checking the integrity and location of catalytic converters, and monitoring the use of highway road flares.

It is unsafe to flush a spill of gasoline fuel into the sewers or to the side of a road. The fuel floats on top of the water and simply spreads out, making a larger potential hazard area (Fig. 3-8). Crews should not fill a fuel tank with water in hopes of "inerting" the hazard of the fuel in the tank. Not only does this action not reduce the hazard potential, it can cause further problems with the liquid fuel and the fuel vapors. The intentional puncturing of a fuel tank — opening it up in the mistaken belief that such action will reduce its explosion potential — is another practice that should be discontinued.

Action taken to control a fuel leak should be done with caution. Gasoline in contact with exposed skin removes natural oils and fats. Continued exposure can yield skin rashes and other irritations. Direct contact with a liquid fuel can also saturate the protective clothing worn by personnel, causing it to act as a wick if exposed to ignition. Vapors given off by the fuel can also become trapped inside protective clothing.

The many specific techniques that can control a fuel leak include plugging, capping, clamping, removing the fuel supply, and shutting off the fuel source. Some of these actions, like shutting off a valve on a natural gas fuel cylinder or tightening the fuel fill cap on an automobile, do not require tools, while others require simple tools or equipment. A golf tee may be all that is needed to stop the leak in a vehicle fuel line that has been broken open. A wooden, cone-shaped plug may

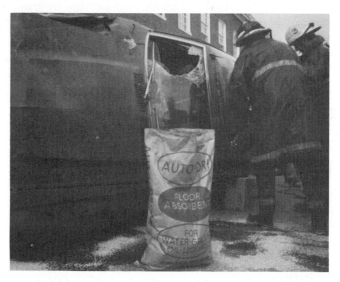

FIG. 3-10 Absorbent materials can contain spills of engine oil, antifreeze, transmission fluid, and motor fuels. Granular absorbent material can also provide traction under slippery ice or snow conditions.

seal the leak in a gasoline tank. A putty type of sealant material may be used to plug a tear in a tank (Fig. 3-9). In most instances, simple tools or techniques will either stop the leak or reduce it to a more manageable problem.

Every effort should be made to contain external liquid fuel spillage by placing containers or trays under a leak. The quick deployment of absorbent granular material (similar to cat litter in appearance) can minimize the spill area by containing the material within absorbent dikes (Fig. 3-10). Agents can be employed to cover liquid fuel spills. Deploying and maintaining aqueous film-forming foam (AFFF) over a spillage of fuel is an extremely effective means of providing safety at a spill scene. It is vital that fire service personnel realize that AFFF does *not* neutralize the spilled fuel. AFFF simply forms a film that acts to minimize vapor escape and ignition of the fuel. Special inerting agents are commercially available that reportedly neutralize the flammability of hydrocarbon fuel.

Emergency service personnel should see that spilled fuel and any contaminated dirt or absorbent material are properly disposed. The assistance of private waste management companies, hazardous material teams, and government agencies specializing in hazardous material cleanup work may be necessary. Procedures for dealing with contaminated materials should be adopted in advance of any local incident.

Portable internal combustion engines used by emergency service personnel must be monitored. These engines, necessary for powering rescue tools, supplying electrical power at the scene, or for scene illumination, must not be placed in locations where flammable vapors are present. The diesel engine of an emergency vehicle parked in a flammable gasoline vapor cloud, for example, will "run away" with itself, burning the vapors taken into the engine until the engine actually self-destructs.

Leaking vehicle fuels have the potential to cause tremendous death and destruction. An incident involving a leak of any type of fuel is potentially deadly and demands the utmost respect from emergency service personnel. Actions taken to minimize the safety hazards of a fuel leak must be quick and correct.

Vehicle Electrical System Safety

The major safety hazard associated with the electrical system is the electrical current, which operates the starter, fires the engine, and allows the electrically powered accessories to operate. Accessories such as the starter, electric fan, or supplemental restraint system can still function without the engine running. Crew members can also receive shocks from the electrical system, have an electrical spark ignite vapors, or have the battery explode violently. It is crucial that emergency personnel shut off the ignition switch of the damaged vehicle as quickly as possible and work to take away the electrical power to the vehicle.

A vehicle's electrical system can be both friend and enemy to emergency service workers. Decisions on how to control electrical system hazards can only be made at the scene on a case-by-case basis. It is safest and most effective if power from the battery is disconnected at the battery post or cut at the ground cable (see Chapter 1).

DOWNED WIRES

Electricity is transmitted through transmission and distribution wires up to the size of a half dollar in diameter. These wires routinely carry up to 19,900 volts of current in residential neighborhoods, with higher currents moving through major distribution lines. Amperage is the measure of flow of current through an object — the wire in the case of power lines. This amperage is the killing factor in electrical shock. The voltage is only important in that it determines how much amperage or current will flow through a given body of resistance.

As little as $1/10$ amp of current flowing through the human body can be fatal; some authorities set this figure as low as $1/20$ amp. A person contacting a 19,900-volt line down at an accident could have a current of 19 amps flowing through to ground. This is 190 times the amperage needed to kill. Wires containing common household 120-volt or 220-volt service also have sufficient amperage to be fatal to humans.

In electrocution cases, the current flows by means of the shortest and most direct pathway to reach ground. The parts of the body through which the current flows as it grounds itself can be severely damaged. If a person is standing in water, which serves to reduce the resistance to ground and allows more current to pass, the resistance to ground when contact is made with a 19,900-volt line can increase to 130 amps or more. The potential effects of electrical current on the body include the following:

- 1 ma (milliamperes of current) causes no sensation and is not felt.
- 2 to 8 ma causes sensation of shock but is not painful. Individual can release contact at will because muscular control is not lost.
- 8 to 15 ma causes painful shock. Individual can let go at will. Control is not lost.
- 15 to 20 ma causes painful shock. Control of adjacent muscles is lost.
- 20 to 70 ma causes painful shock. Severe muscular contractions with extremely difficult breathing occur.
- 100 to 200 ma causes painful shock and ventricular fibrillation of the heart.

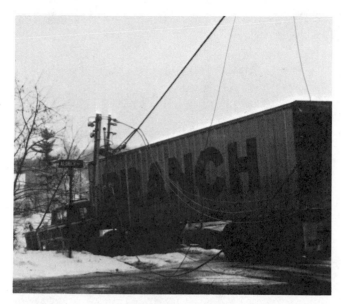

FIG. 3-11 Downed electrical wires along with broken or damaged poles and transformers represent safety hazards that must be recognized immediately at the accident scene.

- 200 ma or more causes severe burns and muscle contractions so severe that chest muscular reaction clamps the heart and stops it for the duration of the shock.

It may not be possible by simply looking at a person to determine whether electrocution has occurred. The patient may show no visible signs of electrocution if, for example, they had stepped into energized water.

If there is a possibility that energized wires are down or a power pole has been damaged, personnel initially should not get close to the scene (Fig. 3-11). All crew members must remain in and on their emergency vehicles until the area is determined to be safe and all other responding personnel notified immediately. Personnel should proceed as though all power wires are energized. When trying to determine exactly which lines may be down, the officer and crew members can scan the adjacent power pole and compare it with the damaged pole. They must also remember that transmission wire has memory — it will tend to return to its spooled state by recoiling when broken, which can cause the wire to move into contact with a person standing nearby.

After confirming that power poles are damaged or lines are down at the accident scene, emergency service personnel must notify the local utility company immediately. The services of these electrical professionals should be requested and the general nature of the emergency described to enable the utility company to determine the situation's priority needs. Emergency service personnel then continue to control the scene, treating all wires as energized. No rescuer should touch an involved vehicle until it is determined that the vehicle and the ground around it are not energized and will not become energized (Fig. 3-12).

Victims or accident vehicles should be approached by personnel moving in "duck walk" style — walking while slowly sliding their feet side by side. This waddling movement may allow the rescuer to detect electrical current that is flowing through the ground. As the distance closes between the rescuer and the charged wire, resistance forces change in the ground. Referred to as *ground gradient*, this invisible force field runs outward in all directions from the electrical source. If these force fields were visible, they would resemble waves from the splash of a rock thrown into a pond. The closer to the electrical source, the greater the amount of current that can flow through the ground and enter the body through one leg and discharge through the other. A tingling sensation in the feet, as if the toes have gone to sleep, tells the rescuer that the wire is "hot." Going any closer to the energized source would be dangerous, placing the rescuer at risk of injury. The ground gradient strike zone at this particular time in this particular incident has been identified.

Current may be transmitted through objects other than the ground. Special precautions must be taken when rescuers suspect that nearby steel highway guide rails, metal fences, telephone lines, even cable television transmission wires have been contacted by a downed transmission wire. The wire can readily energize everything it comes in contact with, extending the electrical strike zone great distances. The Niagara Mohawk Power Company, headquartered in Syracuse, New York, conducts a training school specifically designed for emergency service personnel. The program's instructors relate the story of a telephone repairman electrocuted 15 miles from the scene of a car accident. His death occurred when broken wires at the automobile accident scene contacted the same telephone lines on a nearby utility company pole. The phone lines transmitted the fatal electrical current to the lineman.

Personnel must maintain adequate clearance around all sides of the electrical strike zone. Traffic and crowd control measures must be enforced. Communication between all emergency service per-

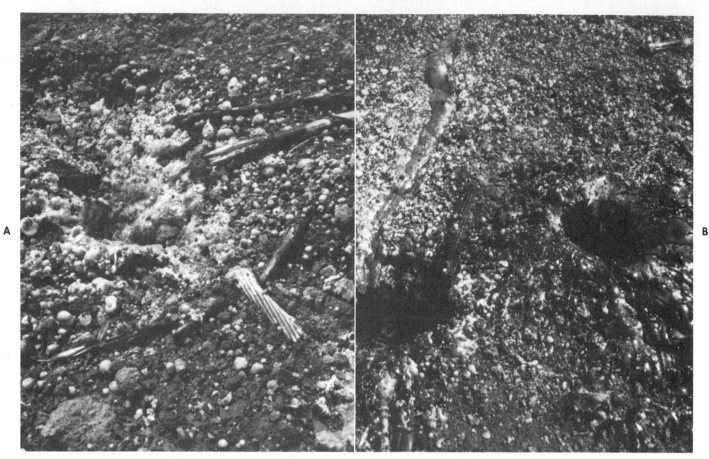

FIG. 3-12 A, Downed wire with sufficient amperage caused sandy soil to turn to glass. Note bare wire is approximately the diameter of a person's thumb. **B,** Original position of downed 34,000-volt power line is still evident in farmer's cornfield.

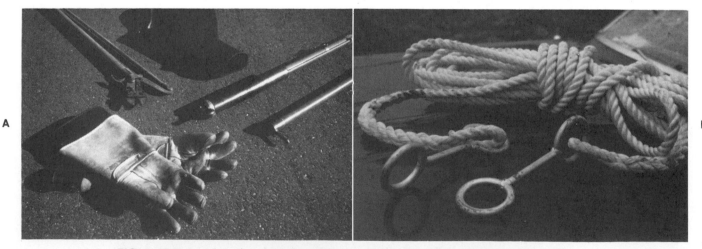

FIG. 3-13 Examples of tools and protective equipment used by professional utility company personnel when dealing with energized wires include, **A,** linesman's gloves, cutters, clampstick, and **B,** synthetic rope with weighted metal ring ends.

sonnel must make everyone fully aware of the danger and the exact location of the strike zone. If broken wires are sparking and flipping around, some crews may attempt to secure the broken end by placing a heavy weight such as a rolled up length of fire hose near the end to control its whipping action. The danger of this procedure is that those trying to anchor the free end may be contacted by the wire or electrocuted by the ground gradient current. Before any attempts to move or secure a wild wire are undertaken, supervising officer personnel should assess the risks of carrying out this assignment (Fig. 3-13).

Personnel should resist the temptation to move a downed wire, particularly when the wire is not moving, arcing, or showing any signs of being energized. Remember, *do not* touch or move the wire, even if it appears dead. Downed wires must never be trusted! They can be quick and silent killers.

When occupants are inside an electrically energized vehicle, quick action must be taken to ensure their safety. Immediate visual and verbal contact with the occupants should be established and maintained, even if those inside do not acknowledge the communication or are unconscious. Loud shouting or the use of a bullhorn or public address system on the emergency vehicle may be necessary. These accident victims should be convinced to "wait it out" inside the vehicle if at all possible. Their best chance of survival lies in waiting for the electricity to be shut off. In order for those inside the vehicle to feel secure, they must always be able to see a concerned rescuer paying attention to them. If they look around and see no one, they may feel abandoned, panic, and attempt to get out of their predicament.

Because of the higher carbon content in the rubber, steel-belted radial tires can burst into flame spontaneously from high amperage flowing through them. This presents an immediate danger for those inside the vehicle. Engine company personnel may be instructed to discharge water from a high-volume fog stream onto the fire in an effort to control or contain it. Evacuation of an energized automobile should be preceded by careful and complete instructions to the occupant. They should be instructed to slowly open a window or door and *jump and roll* in a direction *away* from the downed wire. This gets the person clear of the energized source before contact is established with the ground. If the victim touches the vehicle and the ground simultaneously, they will complete an electrical circuit with their bodies and be electrocuted.

If the occupant is determined to get out of the energized vehicle and cannot be dissuaded, emergency service personnel have no choice other than to provide them with the jump and roll instructions and assist them as necessary. Once a person has successfully escaped from the vehicle, they should be "captured." They may, in their state of shock and excitement, attempt to return to the vehicle to reach others or retrieve a personal belonging. Monitor the activities of anyone in these circumstances. Do not give them the opportunity to make a fatal mistake.

As we have seen, electrical hazards are not to be taken lightly. The utmost care must be taken if safe operations at an emergency scene are to be ensured. As a general rule, an electrical wire should never be moved unless there is a clear indication that a life will be lost if it is not. The preferred action is to secure the services of professional utility company personnel. Do not attempt a rescue unless you have been trained by these professionals to do so and have the necessary equipment and personnel.

Traffic Control Safety

Emergency service personnel working at highway scenes are killed every year. These deaths have a common bond: in each case effective traffic control was not accomplished. Traffic problems cause traffic accidents. Traffic accidents cause traffic problems.

Prompt traffic control reduces traffic problems at the scene of an emergency and prevents secondary collisions. Although crowd and traffic control are considered a basic police agency function, lack of control — of the crowd or the traffic — seriously affects the safety of all concerned. Traffic control must be an integral part of our hazard control activities and is necessary even when personnel are limited in number. Under minimum staffing situations, personnel on the emergency scene must learn to use their vehicles as initial traffic control devices.

Warning of traffic approaching an accident scene must be established to be appropriate for prevailing conditions such as traffic speed and volume, local terrain, accident location, weather, and the type of highway. In the absence of law enforcement personnel, it is vital that at least one responsible emergency service crew member be assigned to basic traffic and crowd control. On high-volume, high-speed expressways the dedication of one crew member as a traffic scout is urgently needed. This person faces oncoming traffic and acts as the "eyes in the back of the head" for other crew members. While other working personnel are intently concentrating on the action at the scene, the traffic scout concentrates strictly on the actions or reactions of approaching traffic. Should a problem motorist appear — one apparently oblivious to accident traffic control efforts — the scout warns fellow workers. Having someone dedicated to covering your rear can be a lifesaver!

As traffic is alerted and controlled, motorists should be advised of actions to take with their vehicles. Traffic should be kept moving if possible. Immediate localized traffic detours that move approaching traffic around the accident scene are recommended. If traffic is detoured and kept far enough away from the action area, motorists are less likely to stop and cause traffic congestion at the scene. What is to be avoided is the complete stopping of traffic, especially for any extended period. If traffic is stopped completely on high-volume interstate highways and expressways, traffic snarls can occur in all directions at the rate of one mile for each minute that traffic is not moving. After five minutes of total shutdown, the possibility of getting additional emergency service units into or out of the immediate accident area becomes extremely difficult and time consuming and may be even impossible (Fig. 3-14). Once allowed to stop, motorists may let their curiosity get the best of them. They may park on the shoulder of the road or just abandon their vehicle where it is to go to the action they see ahead. This adds to traffic congestion and increases the size of the

crowd that must be controlled. A detour around the accident area minimizes traffic congestion and maximizes scene protection. If the driving lane is blocked, it may be safe to move traffic along open lanes or the shoulder.

Notification of approaching traffic can be done by various means. Initially, vehicle emergency warning lights provide notification of a hazard ahead. Operators of emergency vehicles must realize that during night incidents, particularly on two-lane highways, the headlights of their emergency vehicle may totally blind approaching vehicles and personnel as they look toward the accident scene. Certain vehicles on the accident scene may be requested to use low-beam headlights or even parking lights alone to minimize this problem. Red-burning highway road flares, a generally accepted means of warning of a traffic impediment, are inherently dangerous at an accident scene. Flares can ignite combustible materials or flammable vapors within their flammable range. The residue that spits from a burning flare can cause significant injury to unprotected hands or eyes. Personnel using flares for traffic control should be sure that the flare is all that is going to ignite and that the flare itself is the only thing present that is going to get burned (Fig. 3-15).

Individual flare spacing should start at the closest edge of the accident scene and continue toward approaching traffic at 15-foot intervals. If an individual's walking pace is 3 feet in length, another general rule for estimating the length of the line of flares is "twice the posted speed in paces." A 35 mph speed limit roadway would require flares to be placed up to

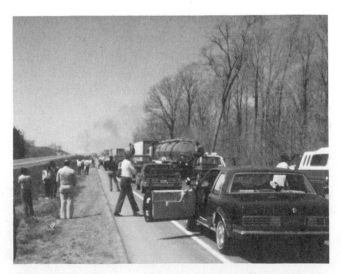

FIG. 3-14 Traffic stopped on expressway due to vehicle fire. Note motorists on far left documenting their presence by taking pictures with car fire in background.

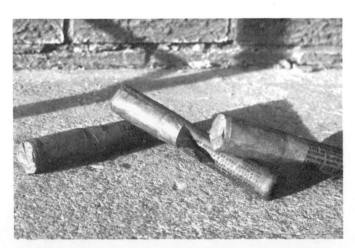

FIG. 3-15 Use of flares in stacked arrangement to notify approaching traffic of hazard ahead. Bottom flare burns down and in doing so ignites flare above it.

70 paces from each side of the accident scene, or approximately 210 feet. On a highway where traffic may be expected to be traveling between 55 and 65 mph, this line of flares should continue for at least 300 feet, the length of a football field from goal line to goal line. If the accident has occurred on a hill or at a curve in the roadway, flares should be placed to adequately warn approaching traffic on the other side of the hill or curve. If in doubt, continue to light flares. They must both direct the flow of oncoming traffic and provide some degree of safety to operating personnel.

Personnel may also warn and direct oncoming traffic with portable flashlights or portable strobe type of warning lights. It must be remembered that these devices only warn the fully alert and responsible motorist. At no time should any traffic control measure be blindly relied upon as the sole means of traffic control.

Emergency Scene Security

Although protecting the personal belongings of the accident victims is primarily a police function, all medical and rescue personnel should assist in this task. Debris found at the accident scene, personal belongings, even vehicle skid marks play important roles in the accident reconstruction and investigative work that follows a serious accident. To the rescuer or firefighter, material on the highway may look like junk and open beer bottles in a vehicle may seem insignificant. Yet these items may well be the key to understanding an injured person's condition or the circumstances that caused the accident itself.

Emergency service personnel should also be trained to protect their own rescue and medical supplies, tools, and equipment. This may mean assigning personnel to the emergency vehicle to act as "babysitters," ensuring that equipment removed from the vehicle or tool staging area is used by authorized persons. Medics who fail to provide security for their valuable EMS equipment and medical drug supplies run the risk of having these items lost to theft.

Engine company and rescue vehicle operators should remain in close proximity to their vehicles to provide security for the apparatus and protect tools and equipment against theft or loss. These operators additionally become valuable communications links between the scene and other units or the communications center. They should also be required to establish a rescue tool staging area in an appropriate location

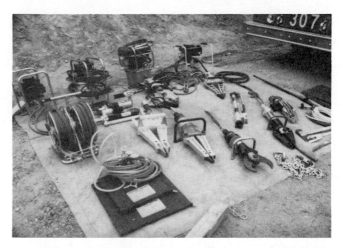

FIG. 3-16 Example of staging area at vehicle rescue training session. Note use of tarp and positioning near rescue vehicle.

near the apparatus by placing a large salvage cover or tarp on the ground. Rescue tools and equipment, as well as additional medical supplies, can then be placed in this staging area (Fig. 3-16).

When the vehicle operator is located between the vehicle and the staging area, anyone assigned to get an item from the tarp or the vehicle has a knowledgeable guide to help locate the tool and keep track of its movement. The apparatus operator can also inspect returned equipment, restore it to service, and maintain a current inventory of equipment as it is replaced on the vehicle.

The operator of a vehicle with an electrical power plant and scene lighting equipment should also be assigned to deploy electrical power and lighting to the accident scene.

Scene Lighting

Effective scene lighting greatly increases the safety of operating personnel and patients. Every time you turn on a light, you increase scene safety. Emergency scene lighting has value during both night and day operations and should adequately illuminate all work areas without becoming a hindrance to operations. Lighting efforts begin with portable handlights and flashlights and are supplemented by portable lights powered off electric generators and by vehicle-mounted floodlight units.

Placement of lights at the scene should provide for complete coverage of the incident. Deep, dark shadows should be eliminated. When lights are too few in number or are placed incorrectly, hazards may not be visible. Failing to see downed electric wires at an accident scene — usually black wires on a rainy, dark night — can be a fatal shortcoming. Proper lighting aids in gathering important information. During daytime operations, lighting can be used to illuminate shadow areas surrounding a vehicle. Work under or inside a vehicle (examining a trunk area for example) can be done more effectively when lighting fills in the shadows.

Lighting can also become a problem at an emergency scene. Incorrectly used headlights, spotlights, and portable floodlights can temporarily blind workers or those approaching the accident scene, hampering operations. Lighting of a scene should be well rounded — placed behind and above the workers to minimize the chances of light shining directly into their faces. The goal of scene lighting is to provide effective illumination of the entire accident scene.

Portable and fixed lighting should be both adequate in number and readily available. Team leaders and group or division commanders should be required to ensure that each crew has proper lighting at each area. There is no justification for ever operating at a rescue incident in the dark!

Crowd Control

Emergency service personnel learn early in their careers that a crowd of spectators can appear out of thin air, gather in the blink of an eye, and quickly get as close as possible unless definite control measures are established. Crowds at an accident scene are liable to restrict the activities of the working personnel, make inappropriate comments about the accident, introduce ignition sources as they light cigarettes, confiscate personal belongings, and destroy accident evidence. Spectators can quickly become patients if caught too close to a safety hazard. Protection for the crowd is best accomplished by *distance*, the single most important aspect of effective crowd control.

Although control of crowds is basically a police function, emergency service personnel must determine how far away to keep spectators and, if assigned by their officer, assist police personnel in carrying out this function. The crowd should not determine where it stands, what it hears, and what it sees. Methods of crowd control vary with the situation. Generally, a strong law enforcement presence on the scene provides effective enforcement of crowd control measures. Emergency service personnel may quickly

establish crowd control by deploying physical barriers such as ropes or plastic crowd control barrier tape. Barriers can be formed by having emergency personnel stand side by side or temporarily hold up tarps as shields. The shielding technique is also effective during removal of burned or decapitated bodies or whenever the privacy of a patient must be ensured.

Crowd control is a top safety priority in the early stages of an emergency and is critical to the prevention of further injuries. It is the responsibility of all personnel to see to it that these vital control measures are established. If in doubt about crowd safety, back people up!

Hazardous Material Safety

A hazardous material spill proved serious to the first-arriving police officers at an overturned tractor-trailer truck on the New York State Thruway just before Christmas in 1981. The rollover caused the truck to come to rest in the ditch along the shoulder of the road. The driver escaped. The first 2 state police officers to arrive at the scene treated the incident as just another routine winter truck accident on a cold dark night. Totally unaware of the danger, the troopers, eventually joined by 10 other law enforcement officers, continued to work in and around the damaged truck. One officer contacted a liquid that was leaking from the truck's trailer, stepping in it and getting it on his uniform. When he went inside his vehicle to use the radio, things started to happen. In the heated automobile, the liquid warmed up and gave off toxic gases. The trooper suddenly became ill, as did 6 of the 12 police officers on the scene.

The officers had unwittingly exposed themselves to the poisonous chemical toluene di-isocyanate. Symptoms of eye, throat, and lung irritation developed quickly. Two of the most seriously injured troopers received permanent disabilities and have since retired. It is that quick and that easy to go from being a rescuer to being a victim. With hazardous materials accidents, you may not get a second chance.

Emergency service personnel must not attempt a victim rescue at an accident involving hazardous materials unless the nature of the hazard has been properly identified, the rescuer is trained to deal with the material involved, the needed equipment is available, and there are enough personnel present to ensure a safe operation. Personnel cannot operate safely when conditions are unstable or unpredictable (Fig. 3-17). Command personnel must consider the impact

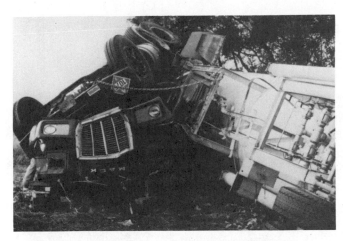

FIG. 3-17 Fatal LP-gas transport truck accident portrays the real-world possibilities of hazardous materials at vehicle rescue incidents. Scene was approached only after determining it was safe to do so. We do not trade lives for lives!

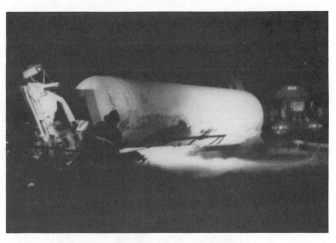

FIG. 3-18 Super cold (cryogenic) liquid nitrogen leaking from damaged truck can have detrimental effect on rescue equipment and be harmful to operating personnel. Off-loading was required before driver's body could be recovered.

of a hazardous material on the emergency personnel and their equipment. Internal combustion engines used at the emergency scene need oxygen in their incoming air to function, just as humans do. If a hazardous material has created an oxygen-deficient atmosphere, these engines cannot function and rescuers and accident victims can suffocate. If rescue personnel must operate in positive-pressure, self-contained breathing apparatus units to survive, the unprotected victim may already have died of suffocation. A leaking liquified compressed gas with its chilling sub-zero temperatures can deteriorate hydraulic rescue hoses or solidify hydraulic fluids. Caustic or corrosive chemicals that come in contact with rescue equipment can put the units out of service by destroying vital rubber or neoprene components (Fig. 3-18).

Experienced command personnel learn to accept the fact that they cannot accurately predict the sequence of events that can unfold at a hazardous material incident, despite extensive training and education in this specialty field. Hazardous material training does equip them for early detection and recognizing the potential for a dangerous or hazardous situation to develop. But even specialty teams trained in hazardous material abatement procedures do not commit their personnel or resources until the material has been identified, decontamination procedures are in place, and resources are adequate.

Identification of the suspected material is the all-important first step at an incident. Knowing the identity of the product is vital and determines the procedures that will be used. Possible sources of information include the vehicle operator or owner, shipping papers, invoices, bill of lading documents carried in the vehicle, vehicle warning placards, and package labels. Emergency service personnel can use binoculars to survey the accident scene and search for vehicle identification markings at a safe distance from the hazardous material. It is important to remember that identification numbers or shipping papers may be incorrect or inaccurate at the time of the accident; they should be treated as valuable but not totally reliable (Fig. 3-19).

When little or nothing is known about a product, an evacuation and standby operation is recommended. At major incidents, first-arriving units may be fully committed to evacuation activities. This should continue as reliable hazardous material information is received. Emergency service personnel confronting a hazardous material incident need educated help quickly. Reference material such as the U.S. Department of Transportation's *Emergency Response Guidebook* can assist in formulating initial strategic decisions and should be consulted. They are, however, only designed to guide on-scene personnel through the first 10 minutes or so of the incident. The accuracy of some

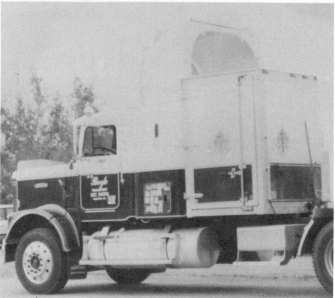

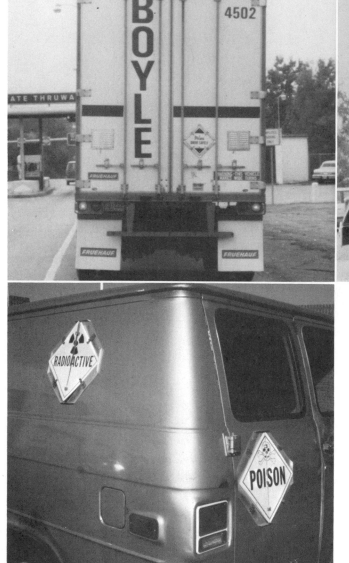

FIG. 3-19 Vehicle placards are not always reliable. **A,** Placarding is not visible as personnel approach rear of truck trailer. **B,** It becomes evident that vehicle may contain explosive Class A hazardous materials. **C,** This van's owner proudly displays the "Poison" and "Radioactive" placards as a novelty. Other than the front bucket seats, the van is empty.

information in the book has also been disputed (see box on p. 91). More definitive information can be obtained by telephoning the National Response Center (NRC) or the Chemical Transportation Emergency Center (CHEMTREC). Operated by the Chemical Manufacturers Association and located in Washington, D.C., CHEMTREC operates a 24-hour-a-day, toll-free hotline at 1-800-424-9300. Given such information as the DOT identification number, name of the chemical involved, or the product name of the hazardous material, a CHEMTREC operator can provide additional product information and recommendations for emergency personnel.

Personnel calling CHEMTREC or the NRC should not hang up or disconnect the established lines of communication with the center. Operators will cut off the communication when they feel it is appropriate to do so.

DOT EMERGENCY RESPONSE GUIDEBOOK

The IAFF Department of Occupational Health and Safety wants you to be aware that the 1987 *Emergency Response Guidebook*, which has recently been published by the U.S. Dept. of Transportation, contains erroneous information that could jeopardize your safety and health.

The IAFF is currently conducting an investigation to determine the extent of inaccurate information contained in the 1987 guidebook. The IAFF membership will be kept informed of the findings. Listed below are some of the initial concerns raised by the guidebook.

The IAFF is extremely concerned about the misleading information provided by DOT on the protection offered by structural fire fighting protective clothing. The definition utilized by DOT states that it can be used as "protection to restrict inhalation of, ingestion of, or skin contact with hazardous vapors, liquids and solids." In many of its emergency action guides, DOT states that "Self-contained breathing apparatus (SCBA) and structural fire fighter's protective clothing will provide limited protection."

STRUCTURAL CLOTHING AT HAZARD INCIDENT

Please be advised that firefighter protective clothing is designed to protect firefighters against adverse environmental conditions during structural fire fighting. It is not designed for use as proximity, approach or entry clothing or for protection from chemical, radiological, or biological agents. The labeling requirements of NFPA 1971: *Standard on Protective Clothing for Structural Fire Fighting* warn: "DO NOT USE FOR PROXIMITY OR FIRE ENTRY APPLICATIONS OR FOR PROTECTION FROM CHEMICAL, RADIOLOGICAL OR BIOLOGICAL AGENTS."

The DOT implication in the guidebook that such limited exposure may be achieved without any health risks is erroneous. The fact is that your structural fire-fighting protective clothing has never been tested to withstand even limited exposure. While under practical conditions, limited exposure to hazardous materials may be unavoidable, it should be understood that such practices could lead to acute or chronic health effects.

CONTACT NRC

In a direct slap in the face, DOT has prominently added emphasis to the importance of contacting CHEMTREC in the new guidebook. The IAFF had urged DOT to list the National Response Center (NRC) at 1-800-424-8802 as the primary emergency response number. The IAFF has adopted a resolution requesting all IAFF affiliates to demand that their fire departments immediately use NRC instead of CHEMTREC. A call to CHEMTREC does not fulfill any statutory or regulatory reporting requirement of the federal government. CHEMTREC is operated by the Chemical Manufacturers Association.

The NRC streamlines the federal response mechanism by providing a single, continuously staffed location that receives and refers for action and/or investigation all reports of environmental, etiological, and biological incidents throughout the United States. After receiving a report, the NRC immediately relays the information to a predesignated Federal On-Scene Coordinator (OSC). Generally, the Environmental Protection Agency responds to inland zone incidents. The NRC also notifies other federal agencies and officials as appropriate. The OSC contacts the company or party responsible for the incident to ensure that proper action is being taken to minimize impact and cleanup of the spill. The NRC also offers extensive computer capabilities, including systems to identify unknown chemicals, determine the trajectory of a spill, and other information vital to emergency response.

Within its guidebook, DOT recommends the use of water spray or fog for dealing with flammable gas or vapor mixtures. This is basically the same DOT recommendation found in its 1984 guidebook. This recommendation is in direct opposition to the warning issued by the National Institute for Occupational Safety and Health in 1985. NIOSH warned:

Fire Departments and teams responding to incidents involving flammable gas or vapor mixtures are cautioned that the use of water spray (fog) streams to prevent ignition or control flame propagation may be extremely dangerous:

- Significant fires or explosions can occur despite the use of water spray. Under certain conditions, the use of water spray may in fact increase the severity of such fires and explosions.
- It is unlikely that handheld hose streams can produce a water spray with sufficiently small droplet size and uniformly high water concentrations to render inert a flammable atmosphere.
- The use of water spray cannot be relied upon to quench a fire in a flammable atmosphere.

Another area of concern to the IAFF is the lack of any warnings about long-term health hazards. The health hazards cited by DOT pertain to acute effects only. DOT refuses to put information in the guidebook about long-term health effects of exposure to hazardous materials.

The guidebook has been criticized for inaccurate information by the National Transportation Safety Board after its investigation of the hazardous materials incident in Somerville, Massachusetts. A new report by NTSB surrounding the incident in Miamisburg, Ohio, found that DOT has yet to take the necessary corrective action.

The IAFF urges all fire departments to take extreme caution when utilizing the *1987 Emergency Response Guidebook*. The IAFF recommends seeking other sources of information and contacting the NRC during any hazardous materials incident.

Modified from IAFF International Fire Fighter: DOT emergency response guidebook: use with caution, IAFF 71:11, 1988.

Emergency service personnel should give the following information to CHEMTREC or NRC:

- Your name and callback number
- Nature and location of problem
- Quantity of hazardous material involved
- Type of material involved (gas, liquid, chemical)
- Current state of material (leaking, burning)
- Time frame of incident
- Other hazardous materials involved
- Population affected
- ID number of product
- Specific name of material
- Shipper or manufacturer
- Type of container (on railcar, truck, open storage, housed storage)
- Carrier's name and name of consignee
- Local conditions, including weather

While the information-gathering and incident decision-making processes continue, command of the incident must be established. The services of varied support groups will be required at a major incident once definite plans for dealing with the hazard have been formulated. As soon as possible, additional fire service and rescue resources, specialized hazardous material emergency response teams, and other appropriate outside agencies should be notified and requested to respond.

The nature of the hazardous material involved may necessitate evacuation of the area. Everyone — emergency service personnel and the general public — must remain in a safe area. As a safety zone is established, controls must be in place to ensure that unauthorized people remain outside the danger area. Emergency service personnel must remain uphill and upwind of the incident. A sudden windshift or the downwash from the rotating blades of a helicopter, for example, may change the evacuation area for those too close to the incident.

Different hazardous material problems require different evacuation distances, ranging from several hundred feet to several thousand feet depending on the material, the quantity involved, and the nature of the emergency. An important strategic consideration in this decision is the location of the most intense exposure area. The immediate life-threatening area to be evacuated might be downhill or downwind, for example. Unless otherwise specified, the recommended minimum distance for evacuation safety is 2000 feet in all directions. Specific information and guidance are available from resources such as the NRC, CHEMTREC, or hazardous material reference books.

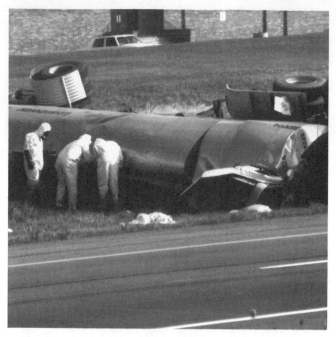

FIG. 3-20 Hazardous material emergency response team members work in encapsulating suits to contain and control leak of hazardous liquid industrial waste.

Incoming emergency units must be staged uphill and upwind of the incident. These crews should only be committed as needed and those entering the dangerous hot zone should be limited in number and strictly controlled. Dispatch protocols for hazardous materials incidents should provide first-responding units with immediate access to wind speed and wind direction. This information should be broadcast on all radio channels for all agencies involved to facilitate strategic decisions early in the incident.

Specialty response teams may be able to confine and control the hazardous material once all safety provisions are in place (Fig. 3-20). At this point, rescue or body recovery operations can take place if needed, with crews taking care to avoid contamination of personnel, patients, equipment, and vehicles. Explicit procedures for decontaminating people and equipment must be understood by all personnel.

TRANSPORTATION ACCIDENTS INVOLVING RADIATION HAZARDS

Radioactive materials are routinely transported by the military, trucking firms, common carriers like the United Parcel Service and Federal Express, and the U.S. Postal Service. When transportation accidents involve radioactive materials, emergency service personnel should limit their actions to what they are trained to do.

Three major types of ionizing radiation may be encountered at an accident. Ionizing radiation is dangerous because it can alter the cells of the human body. Alpha radiation, the first type, is emitted from a low energy source and can be stopped by a single sheet of paper, a few inches of air space, or a layer of light clothing. The second type, beta radiation, is emitted from sources at higher energy levels; effective shields include clothing, a layer of glass, or thin metal sheeting. The most serious problem with exposure to beta radiation is its possible introduction into the body by inhalation, ingestion, or contact with open wounds. Once inside the body, the radiation can last for prolonged periods of time and cause serious consequences.

The most harmful type of ionizing radiation, invisible gamma radiation, penetrates the human body. Gamma rays can only be detected with specialized detection equipment. The few effective shielding materials include heavy lead or concrete.

Radiation amounts received at any given accident depend on three important factors: the length of *time* the person is exposed, the *distance* the person is from the radiation source, and the *shielding* between the individual and the source.

There are two basic types of radiation transportation accidents. In a "clean" radiation accident, victims have been exposed to a radiation source and are thus irradiated. As patients, these people present no danger to emergency service personnel. In the more dangerous "dirty" radiation accident, victims have been both exposed and contaminated by radioactive particles in and on their bodies. In this instance, packages may be scattered about and radioactive containers may be found broken or leaking as the accident scene itself becomes physically contaminated with radioactive materials. Decontamination of victims, rescuers, equipment, and vehicles must take place in dirty radiation accidents. Personnel must remember that irradiated patients present no hazard to rescuers, but contaminated patients do.

There are two important priorities for personnel arriving at a radiation accident. The first is recognizing the presence of radiation, a skill that can be developed through training. Vehicle and container placards or package labels all identify the presence of radioactive material (Fig. 3-21). Training in determining radiation potential is available through hazardous material training programs.

Once the presence of radioactive materials has been confirmed, the second priority is establishing and maintaining scene safety. Protecting those who are not involved or exposed is critical. Evacuation of immediate and surrounding areas may be necessary. Well-meaning citizens can be totally unaware that they are exposing themselves and others to radiation hazards. Personnel responding to actual or suspected radiation transportation accidents must institute all appropriate safety measures, including ensuring safety for themselves. This can be done by maintaining correct evacuation distances, using available shielding such as buildings or terrain features such as hills, and positioning uphill and upwind from the incident.

Procedures for handling radiation accidents are similar to those for accidents involving other hazardous material. Prompt requests for information and technical assistance are again necessary as responding personnel carry out the required procedures on the emergency scene to the level they are trained to accomplish safely. If you do not know what you are doing, you should not be doing it. That is common sense. *This is no time for on-the-job training.*

Medical personnel should be prepared to provide care for either irradiated or contaminated patients. Protective clothing must be available to medical crew members, and they must know how to use it. Systematic rotation of medical crew members should be considered to limit the radiation dose received by any one individual as life-saving medical work is carried out. Working in cooperation with local hospitals, medical personnel must know in advance how, when, and where radiation-contaminated patients should be transported.

Rescue teams must have appropriate personal protection in place and approach victims from an uphill and upwind location if possible. Patients should be removed from the vehicle or accident area as quickly as possible even if this must be done before complete emergency medical care is instituted. Time is critical in radiation exposure incidents — so are distance and shielding. It may be feasible to shield the radiation from the victim rather than the other way around. Concrete, bricks, or dirt of sufficient thickness may help to reduce the radiation emitted from the accident.

In efforts to limit the contaminated area, the patients, the rescuers, and any of their equipment should be moved to a secure area, monitored, and decontaminated as necessary. Further decontamination procedures may be instituted by personnel at the receiving medical facility.

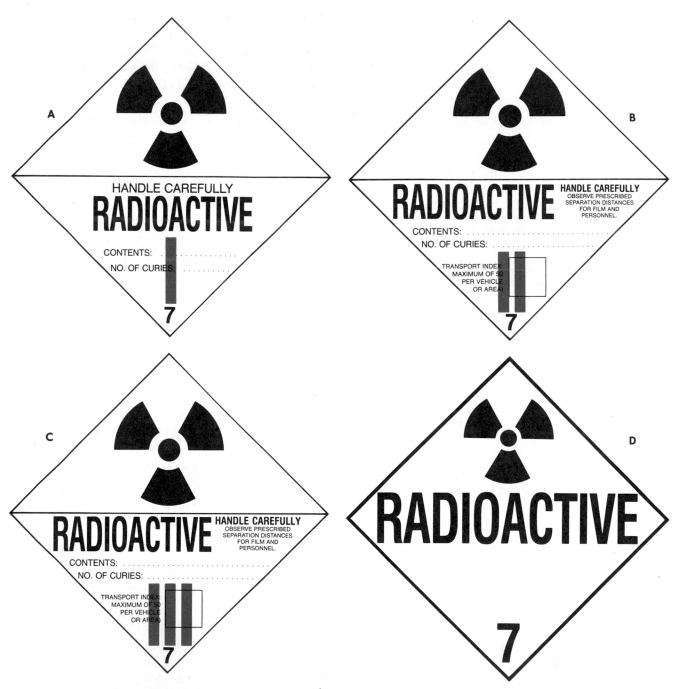

FIG. 3-21 A, Class I packages (marked with this label) emit 0.5 millirem (mrem) of radiation per hour. At a distance of 3 feet from the surface of the package, personnel will not receive any radiation. **B,** Class II packages (marked with this label) emit 5 mrem of radiation per hour. At a distance of 3 feet from the surface of the package, personnel will be exposed to 1 mrem. **C,** Class III packages (marked with this label) emit up to 10 mrem of radiation per hour. Any transport vehicle containing any quantity of Class III radioactive materials must also display **D,** a radioactive materials placard.

Radioactive material, like other hazardous cargo, presents the potential for the unthinking "hero" to die young. All personnel must learn to quickly recognize the presence of radiation at an accident and develop a personal and professional respect for its lethal consequences.

Patient Safety at the Accident Scene

Safety for the accident victim is an important concern for all emergency service personnel. Just how important this protection can be is illustrated by an incident involving a bus loaded with handicapped adults that was struck by a tractor-trailer truck. The first-arriving emergency worker, the assistant chief of the protecting fire department, found that most of the driver's side of the bus had ripped open on impact, trapping people inside. The truck, which burst into flames on impact, had come to rest alongside the bus, trapping the driver inside the burning cab. Flames crested high into the sky as smoke and heat from the fire impinged upon the bus and its trapped and injured occupants.

While responding, the first-due pumper received the chief's initial size-up report of the fire condition and was given specific orders for the engine crew to attack the fire as the top priority. Even in this difficult situation, when faced with the largest multiple casualty incident of his life, the chief remained aware of the importance of controlling the immediate life-threatening problems at the accident scene. Physical safety can become a top priority at an accident scene. It may be prudent to remove the hazard from the victims, as was done in this case, rather than try to remove the victims from the hazard.

O.B. Streeper, president of the Emergency Squad Training Institute and a pioneer instructor in the early days of vehicle rescue training, reported that at one time 27% of all persons trapped in vehicles were further injured by the actions of the emergency crews working to rescue them. Disregard for the physical safety of rescuers and accident victims can continue to produce statistics that are unacceptable in our field of service.

Concerns for the safety of injured patients at a vehicle accident fall into one of two categories. Patients must be protected from further physical injury by efforts to ensure their *physical safety*. The second category is less well understood and often neglected but equally important: the patient's *mental safety* must also be ensured.

Safety concerns for the patient's physical well-being begin when emergency service personnel first arrive at the scene. Initial efforts include protection of the entire scene, particularly the patient's vehicle. If people are near the damaged vehicle or injured persons are trapped inside, proper positioning of the emergency vehicles protects them from secondary collisions. Protection for the damaged vehicles also includes proper vehicle stabilization and hazard control. Supervising officers who quickly detail personnel to stabilize all accident vehicles and efficiently control scene hazards fulfill an important role in ensuring patient safety. Officer size up and the establishment of command are similarly positive steps that improve safety for both patients and workers.

Efforts to account for all occupants of all vehicles are very important. At an accident involving a Chevrolet Corvette that had hit a power pole, emergency service personnel found the driver inside the vehicle, trapped in the driver's seat area. The passenger's seat, however, was empty. That side of the vehicle—the impact side—had totally disintegrated on impact. Because of the possibility of an ejected occupant, efforts to search the immediate accident scene were ordered. No additional patients were located; the driver was later found to have been the lone occupant of the vehicle at the time of the collision. It is interesting to note, however, that the searchers discovered debris from the fiberglass-bodied vehicle more than 700 feet from the point of impact.

Unfortunately, patients also need protection from the emergency service workers themselves and the work that they perform. It seems ironic, but in any given incident the greatest threat to an injured patient's survival can be the mishandling they receive while in the care of emergency workers. The rescue tools themselves, even when used correctly, present hazards. The very presence of hydraulic fluid under pressure can be hazardous to any unprotected person near the equipment. The intense noise and vibrations produced by an air chisel or an air gun rescue tool cutting through metal on the damaged vehicle can cause great distress without ever touching the patient. Falling objects, glass fragments, and bare metal edges are other rescue hazards that can cause injuries unless proper precautions are taken.

Physical protection for victims inside a vehicle and for medical crew members who must remain inside may be provided in several ways. The simplest but not the most effective means is the use of a cover. A firefighter's protective coat should not be used as it

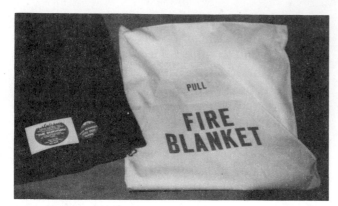

FIG. 3-22 Fire-resistive wool fire blanket serves as one example of ensuring patient physical protection from broken glass and sharp metal.

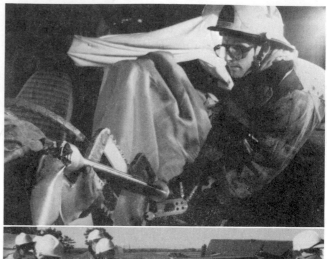

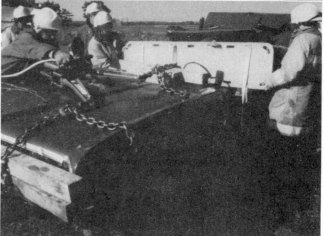

FIG. 3-23 A, Wood shortboard demonstrates insulation of patient as power ram is used to move dash and fire-wall structure. **B,** Longboard being used to demonstrate insulation of patient trapped by wheel and column. Note placement of rescue tool operator on passenger side of vehicle to increase operator safety.

covers very little of a person's body, and rescuers who valiantly offer their coat to the patient are left with a reduced level of personal protection themselves. It is not heroic to offer your coat to a victim, it is stupid.

The most common soft protective coverings are typically cloth blankets made of a fire-resistive, non-combustible material such as 100% wool, an aluminized material, Nomex, or PBI synthetic fabrics. Disposable yellow paper and plastic blankets are also used at accident scenes to protect the patient from further harm (Fig. 3-22). Although the cloth or paper blanket will keep loose dirt and glass granules off an injured patient, it affords very little protection against injury from a heavy rescue tool, razorlike slivers of glass, or exposed, sharp metal edges. Protecting a patient with only a "soft" blanket cover is one half of the necessary patient protection effort.

Additional protection should be provided by employing wooden shortboards or longboards to "insulate" the patients. A conscious effort to always place one of these wooden boards between the work that is being done and anyone under the protective blanket should always be made (Fig. 3-23). The addition of the ¾-inch thick layer of wood between the hazard and the person significantly improves the safety of those inside a wrecked vehicle. These boards must be held firmly to prevent their contacting the patient during the rescue evolution.

Other safety equipment available for the physical protection of the patient and inside personnel include tarps, covers, split fire hose, safety goggles or glasses, and hearing protectors (Fig. 3-24).

When protection from the noise of rescue tools and rescue operations is provided, patients should be told what they are going to hear and why they are being protected. Ear protectors should be placed over the ears of inside medical personnel and injured patients before a high-noise-level tool is used.

Physical safety for the patient cannot be stressed enough. For example, when personnel are gaining initial access or sustained access to the interior, the first glass that should be broken is the piece that is farthest from the injured patient. The remaining side door window glass should then be rolled down and broken inside the door cavity, minimizing the amount of broken glass near the patient and confining the broken glass to a smaller area.

Physical safety becomes particularly important under conditions of high heat, extreme cold, rain, or wind. Though these weather conditions cannot be

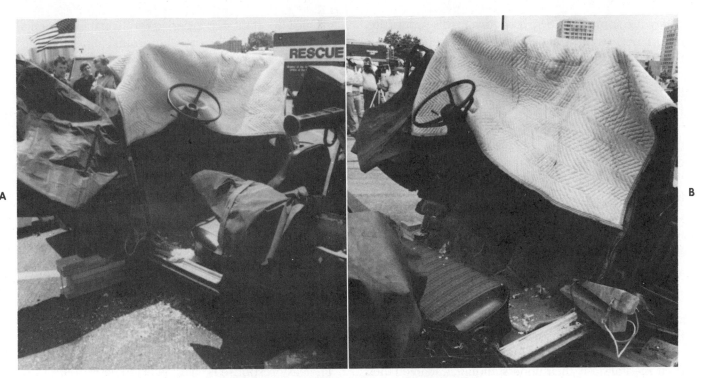

FIG. 3-24 **A,** and **B,** Use of furniture covers from household moving companies along with heavy-duty canvas tarps and old fire hose protect patient and rescuers alike from potential contact with sharp glass and metal.

mastered, they must be addressed. During rain or snow conditions, a temporary shelter made by rigging large fire department salvage covers over the automobile may keep workers and those inside adequately protected. Conditions of high heat pose special problems for patients and rescuers. Emergency personnel should consider how long they could sit in a vehicle with all the windows rolled up on a hot, sunny day. Temperatures inside a closed vehicle on a sunny day can exceed 135° F in a relatively short time, compromising the safety and well-being of those inside.

When faced with these conditions, rescuers must ventilate the vehicle by either natural or artificial means. Natural ventilation includes opening doors and windows quickly. Artificial ventilation can be accomplished by having fire department personnel set up a ventilating fan like those used at structure fire situations. The smoke ejector fan is first placed on a tarp to minimize loose dirt and dust that may blow around during its operation. When placed on the roadway outside the vehicle, the fan moves fresh air into and through the vehicle and removes dangerous smoke or fumes that have accumulated inside.

Cold weather conditions also require special pro-

cedures. Warm blankets help to maintain body warmth, as do blankets or fire service salvage cover tarps that shield the inside of the vehicle from cold winds. Portable quartz heater units, such as those used by local utility company or phone company crews during cold weather, can provide safe, efficient heat to a selected area inside a damaged automobile. Portable floodlights from an emergency lighting plant can provide both light and a degree of warmth. Instant Hot Packs, wrapped in towels, can maintain patient warmth. Medical personnel trained in ALS procedures can also use them to warm IV solutions before they are administered. Because extremes of hot or cold also affect the work of the medical and rescue personnel, rotation of working personnel is vital to everyone's safety.

Unnecessary body movement is another critical area of patient physical safety. Movement that damages an injured person's spine can compromise survivability by interrupting the basic functions necessary to sustain life. For emergency medical crews rendering care to those within a damaged vehicle, the accepted standard operating procedure is to immobilize the patient *as found* while inside the vehicle.

There are some specific exceptions to this procedure, but in most circumstances, it is best for patients when there is minimal movement of both the damaged vehicle and themselves until effective patient immobilization and packaging have been accomplished. Patients should receive necessary medical care, injury immobilization, and packaging before being extricated. Under routine circumstances, failure to accomplish basic immobilization procedures signals that an emergency service team either lacks proper training or mistakenly believes that immobilization is only important if the patient is complaining of pain or injury to the neck or back.

Mental Safety at the Accident Scene

The second major category of patient safety to consider is the individual's mental safety. Injured persons suffer both physical and mental injuries. What the patients see or hear at an accident scene can affect their mental state, their understanding, and even their memories of the event. Mental injuries could continue to occur long after the initial collision if unpleasant events were experienced during the rescue process. Common signs and symptoms of mental injuries include crying and other expressions of grief, paranoia, emotional distress, and various debilitating psychological disorders.

Rescuers routinely protect accident victims from further physical injury at an accident scene by using soft and hard insulation devices such as blankets and wood shortboards. Consideration for the injured persons' mental state must also accompany this physical protection. Injuries can occur here that are just as harmful and just as tragic as any physical injury could ever be. Consider two drivers of vehicles involved in a collision. The first driver sustains only minor cuts and abrasions and is being treated in the back of an ambulance unit by a medic. Imagine if you can, the horror of this individual when the second driver, who is critically injured, is extricated and placed in the same ambulance for transport. This avoidable scenario shows a lack of awareness of the mental injuries that affect all accident victims.

Protecting patients against mental injuries is a challenging assignment. It takes considerable effort on the part of medical and rescue personnel to consider the consequences of everything seen, said, or done in the presence of an injured patient. It is vital that all emergency responders remember that hearing is the last sense to go as patients lapse into unconsciousness.

One important step in caring for the patient's mental anguish is to establish early communication. It begins as medics compile patient history and assessment information and must continue throughout the entire rescue. The first medic to reach the patient may say something as simple yet effective as "Hello, I'm John…I'm with the fire department." This can be followed by brief questions to determine the extent of injuries and explanations of what is going to happen. "I have to put this collar around you," John may continue, "to help prevent any injury to your neck or your back…. This will only take a moment."

Inside medics responsible for the patients should be honest with their comments. Explanations should be brief, basic, and believable accounts of conditions as they exist. One of the most common questions asked by an injured person is "Am I going to be all right?" This question shows that the patient is aware of the predicament and has enough trust or confidence in you as the attending medic to respect your answer. The easy response is "Yes, everything is going to be just fine now… just relax and we'll get you out of here in no time." This may work for some patients, but it may turn others against you — they know they are hurt, and they are concerned. A more positive and reassuring answer that acknowledges that they are injured but advises them that everything possible is being done for them by trained and competent people is more appropriate.

It is an unwritten rule that emergency service personnel must say that they know nothing about the condition of anyone else in the car with the patient. When asked, "My wife, is she going to be all right?" the medic may already know that the woman in question has been crushed under the vehicle and is beyond help. Nonetheless, the reply is that the medic does not know how she is doing but that someone is caring for her. Personnel communicating with the patients must also contend that they know nothing of whose fault the accident was. The questioner might be the injured driver, so intoxicated that the individual can hardly talk, who perhaps caused the accident. The professionalism of the attending emergency workers must never falter to the extent of agreeing or disagreeing with the person about the cause of the accident. State openly that you do not know and change the subject.

A patient once contacted should not be deserted. The contact person can be rotated, but communication should never be lost, even for a moment. A feeling of confidence and trust must develop between the

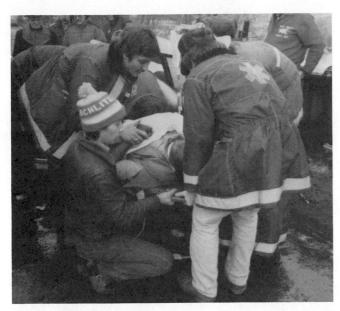

FIG. 3-25 EMS personnel maintain continual contact with injured patient from initial assessment throughout entire patient care process. Individual care provider may change, but the continuity of care to the patient remains constant.

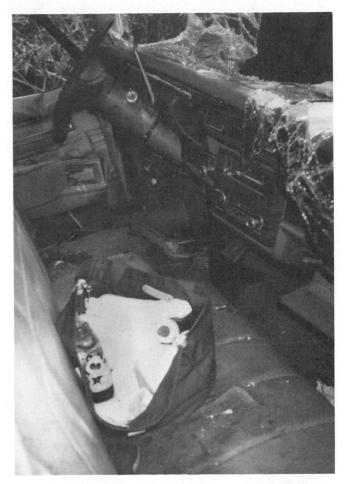

FIG. 3-26 Patient's personal property should be retrieved and secured by appropriate authority. Note presence of diaper bag and baby supplies may indicate presence of a possible undiscovered child passenger.

medic and the injured patient (Fig. 3-25). Patients should be protected as much as possible from what they see and hear taking place outside the vehicle. Protection from unpleasant sights can be accomplished by shielding or covering. It must be remembered, however, that when you cover patients with a protective blanket taking away their sight, you intensify their remaining senses. They can no longer see what is happening around them, but they still have their sense of hearing, smell, and touch. They may intensely focus their energies on what is being said around them. Comments between rescue personnel, such as "It doesn't look like that guy over there is going to make it," can be very harmful for the emotional well-being of other patients. In addition, a complaining patient can unnerve an entire crowd of people, sending them into a panic. The "screamer" makes it hard on everyone. The screamers and complainers should be talked to and reasoned with to get them to quiet down and relax.

Rescue and medical personnel should also use care in describing or naming certain rescue tools and techniques. Regardless of what the manufacturer has chosen as a brand name or model name for the tool, the name may be inappropriate when used in front of a patient who is unfamiliar with the concepts of vehicle rescue. Picture a conscious person trapped in a wrecked vehicle. One leg is pinned, causing great

pain. Other rescue work has taken place, and for the patient, it seems as if the incident has lasted for hours. Suddenly a rescuer's head pops inside the vehicle and tells the patient to relax, saying, "We're just going to use our cutter now, and we'll have you free." To the patient, a cutter may be a special tool that amputates legs! Reasoning that rescuers have given up on the leg and in desperation are going to saw it off to get the person out of the wreck can throw the patient into a total panic. Similar emergency scene terms such as *Jaws* or *blowing a door* also conjure up thoughts that can completely demoralize an otherwise stable patient. Be careful what you say, what you do, and what you allow the patient to experience. Always be aware of the patient's mental and physical state.

Another way to protect the patients' mental state is to protect their personal property (Fig. 3-26). Items they value should be accounted for, retrieved, and possibly sent with them to the medical facility. Whether it is a child's teddy bear, a man's glasses, or a woman's purse, it is valuable to the owner and can be a great source of comfort. Respect the patient's needs and treat the patient as you would wish to be treated if you or a member of your family were in distress.

Emergency Personnel Safety

One of the most common causes of injury to emergency service personnel operating at vehicle emergencies is the lack of proper protective clothing and equipment. Even when there is ample personal protective equipment available, it may not be used correctly. Fire and rescue personnel may wear their boots but fail to pull them up fully. They may place safety goggles around the brim of their helmet yet fail to put them on during rescue operations or leave their gloves in their turnout coat pockets as they operate equipment. They may wear a helmet backwards or fail to buckle up their protective coat.

Some personal protective equipment may also be wrong for the nature of the hazard. Outdated protective clothing, such as the orange-colored plastic gloves still being sold to fire service personnel, no longer conform to nationally accepted minimum standards and represent inadequate and unsafe personal protection.

Each individual's personal protective "envelope"

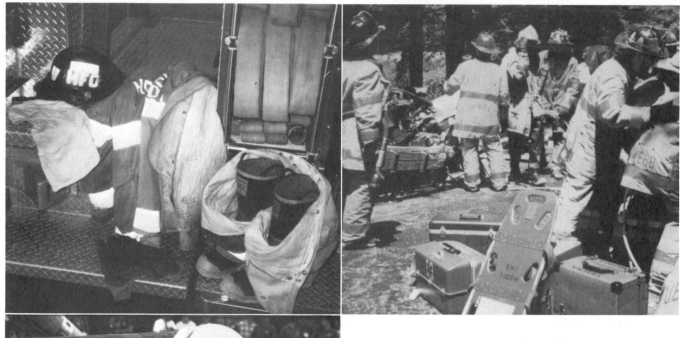

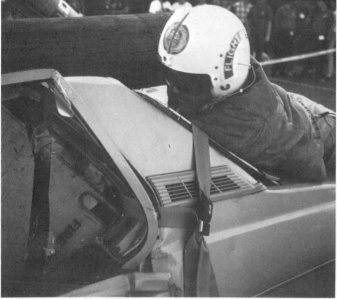

FIG. 3-27 **A,** Recommended personal protective envelope for vehicle rescue crews includes fire boot or work boot with steel toe and sole, upper and lower body protective clothing (turnout coat and bunker pants), fire-resistive hood, leather-palmed gloves, and approved helmet. Recommended but not shown are safety glasses and firefighter accountability identification tag. **B,** Standard operating procedures requiring use of protective clothing at rescue incident promotes greatest degree of safety for personnel. **C,** Pilot's helmet provides for head and eye protection.

must include several important components (Fig. 3-27). Personal head protection protects against falling and flying objects (impact-resistant suspension systems are designed into the helmet structure) and shields the head from radiant heat in a fire situation. Acceptable types of head protection for vehicle rescue situations include fire department protective helmets, industrial hard hats, police riot style of head gear, and motorcycle helmets. Inside medics working within damaged vehicles, who tend to remove their helmet when it is needed the most, can benefit from use of hard hats or motorcycle helmets, which protect the head but are less likely to be an obstruction in confined work areas. These helmets require the wearer to use acceptable eye protection. Any helmet, regardless of the style or type, must be worn and worn properly to provide its intended protection.

Eye and face protection must be provided by approved safety goggles or safety glasses with side shields. The standard fire service helmet-mounted 4-inch or 6-inch flip-down safety visor provides inadequate protection at an accident scene when used alone. Only safety goggles or glasses provide the necessary eye and side protection severely lacking with the flip-down shield. The best combination is simultaneous use of the eyeshield and the goggles or glasses. Face and neck protection is provided by wearing the structural firefighting type of fire-resistive hoods.

The fire-resistive material used in the construction of structural firefighting coats provides upper torso protection from fire, heat, and the abrasion hazards commonly present at an accident scene. The turnout coat is also an excellent means of identification at both day and night operations. Its disadvantages are its bulk and retention of body heat. Although emergency service coats consisting of a single shell of fire-resistive material that offer some of the benefits of the full coat are being marketed, they may give the wearer a false sense of security. The bright-colored nylon "team jackets" commonly worn by members of an ambulance corps or fire department offer inadequate personal protection under all emergency situations (Fig. 3-28).

Lower-body protection for personnel operating at an accident is best provided by the use of approved fire department structural firefighting pants. These "bunker pants" are specifically designed to protect the wearer as much as possible from various hazards that will be encountered (Fig. 3-29). Personal foot protec-

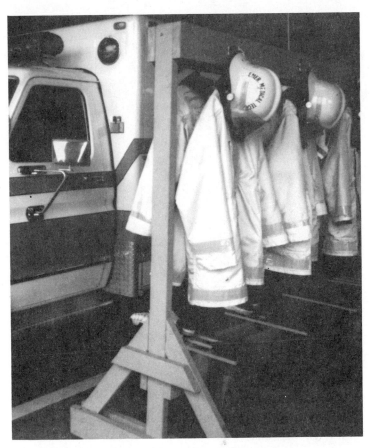

FIG. 3-28 Example of fire-resistive protective clothing, fire boots, and approved helmets used by EMS crews for operations at vehicle rescue incidents. Identification of personnel is also enhanced by use of safety gear.

tion must keep feet dry and warm and protect them from punctures or falling objects to the soles, toes, shins, and arches. This level of protection is provided by the standard fire service structural firefighting boots with steel toe, steel insole, and steel shin guard. Boots, commonly called ¾-*length day boots,* leave an exposed body area between top of the boot and bottom of the protective coat. These rubber boots *do not* offer insulation from the transmission of electricity. If these day boots are worn by personnel operating at an incident, long-legged pants must be worn underneath and the boots pulled completely up (Fig. 3-30).

Emergency service personnel may also wear approved high-top work boots for foot protection. This is particularly common among fire service personnel on the West Coast. These boots do protect the foot, are less bulky to wear, and provide increased mobility and good ankle support. When used as foot protec-

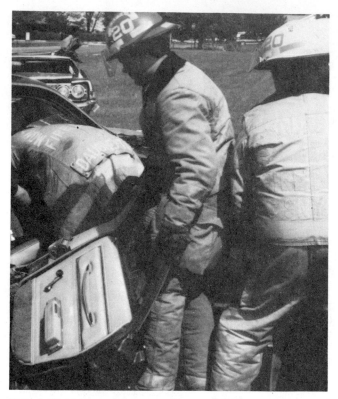

FIG. 3-29 Fullest protection of the rescuer's lower body is best afforded by use of short work boot and structural firefighting bunker pants.

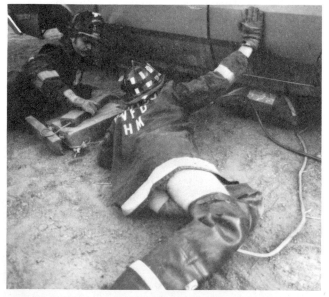

FIG. 3-30 Shortcomings of fire department "day boots" are evident as rescuer works at this rescue evolution.

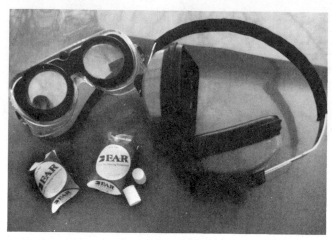

FIG. 3-31 Examples of hearing protection for patients, EMS, and rescue personnel include foam rubber ear plugs and industrial ear muffs. Eye protection includes safety glasses or goggles designed to resist fogging during unpredictable weather situations of heat or cold.

tion, these boots must have a steel toe and insole and be completely laced and zipped.

Hand protection for rescue personnel must include a glove that is lightweight enough to allow for grip and control and be maneuverable enough to allow the user some degree of dexterity. The glove must provide abrasion resistance, protect the wrist area, and have a leather palm for puncture and cut resistance. As has been noted, plastic-coated gloves are unacceptable for accident scene use.

The hearing protection necessary for any patient, EMS provider, tool operator, or apparatus operator exposed to unusually high levels of noise at the accident scene can be provided by approved industrial hearing protection devices. Standard industrial ear protectors placed over the head, although effective for noise abatement, cannot be worn with a separate helmet. Hearing protection of this type must be integrated into the helmet or hard hat. Industrial foam rubber ear plugs may also provide adequate hearing protection (Fig. 3-31).

INFECTIOUS DISEASE PROTECTION

Emergency medical concerns call for protecting emergency workers against infectious diseases such as AIDS or hepatitis. Personal protection includes disposable coveralls and paper face masks, latex rubber gloves, pocket masks, and airway devices (Fig. 3-32). The intent is to eliminate contact between the rescuer and a patient's blood, body fluids, or excreta. When

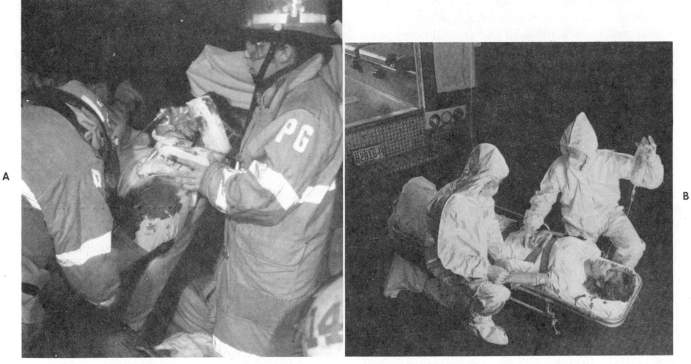

FIG. 3-32 A, Medical crew members use latex rubber gloves and proper eye protection in conjunction with full body protection at an accident scene. **B,** Equipment designed to minimize rescuer contact with patient's body fluids includes airways, pocket masks, latex rubber gloves, and disposable full body coveralls with head, face, eye, and foot protection. (Courtesy Mar Mac Manufacturing, McBee, SC.)

basic safety precautions are undertaken at all incidents, the risk of exposure to infectious disease at the emergency scene is reduced. State or local health departments and medical facilities can be contacted for specific information. Exposure to patients with incurable infectious diseases has become an important reality for us all, at any time and in any place.

UNSAFE PROCEDURES: PAYING THE PRICE

Hazards underestimated or not considered by those on the scene can lead to injuries and deaths. Ignorance coupled with inadequate mental preparation is a dangerous combination. A casual attitude on the part of emergency personnel allows them to become their own worst enemies. Tunnel vision, that fatalistic approach to emergency operations, can yield many dangerous surprises too late into the operation.

Injury to an emergency service crew member places an extra burden on remaining crew members. Just one injured crew member may require a one- or two-member escort to medical aid, where one or two additional emergency service people may be needed to render medical assistance. As treatment is being rendered, other members may find it difficult to concentrate on completing the necessary tasks. When personnel are limited in number, the care rendered to the original patient may be reduced while the additional "victim" is cared for. The patient's well-being may thus be threatened by the very people who were summoned to help.

Emergency service personnel have a responsibility to themselves and their co-workers to always wear protective equipment sufficient to meet the hazards of the work environment. Individual crew members must learn not to work beyond their limitations of knowledge, equipment capability, physical ability, and endurance. When personnel overextend themselves or their equipment, safety margins are reduced. The maximum effective working time for any worker at an incident is determined in part by individual ability and endurance. Under normal situations, barring extremes of heat, cold, or psychological stress, personnel should be expected to operate effectively for a maximum of 20 minutes. When they are exposed to heavy physical exertion or weather extremes, their effective operating time can be reduced by 50% to a maximum of 10 minutes. After this period of time, they should receive on-scene rehabilitation to allow them to regain their physical and mental composure and replace essential body fluids. It is harder to regain your ability to function effectively once you have become totally exhausted than it is when you are relieved while still functional. Recovery time is quicker and results are better with frequent crew rotations. Rotating operating personnel is vital to ensure individual health and personal safety.

When operating rescue equipment, crew members must know the function of the equipment, be able to use the equipment or tool properly, and be fully aware of its limitations. All risks associated with the operation of each tool must be considered and anticipated. For example, crews working with air bag or air cushion rescue equipment are well aware that the bag or cushion can slip out from under an object being lifted if the load shifts unexpectedly or the bag is placed in an improper position. This equipment is also vulnerable to exposure to heat or chemicals and can be punctured. Basic knowledge and understanding of such rescue equipment can be gained through quality training programs and reaffirmed by the real-world experiences of rescue personnel. To be as safe as possible, rescue personnel must also have good common sense, good mechanical aptitude, and the physical strength to properly apply tools and equipment.

Each organization must be responsible for providing personnel with the best and most appropriate personal protective equipment available. We cannot expect workers to be safe unless protective equipment is provided and its use mandated. Moreover, the proper tool must be used in the proper manner, for the proper job, and by appropriately protected emergency personnel.

SAFETY OFFICER

Preventing injuries and deaths among emergency service personnel begins with awareness of the fact that responsibility for safe practices and procedures ultimately lies with the administrative and management staff of each organization. When management assumes basic responsibility for safety, a viable safety-oriented training program for the organization can be developed, properly administered, and evaluated.

At the heart of this safety issue is the need for effective command. Leaders must be present at the emergency scene, and they must act to fulfill their command responsibilities. If safe operations are to take place at a vehicle emergency, the leadership present must truly believe in the "Safety First" rule.

As a means of establishing an organization's safety program, the position of *safety officer* should be created and supported by management. The individual or individuals serving as safety officer or safety unit must be experienced personnel who have a good understanding of the nature of the work. They must fully understand the kinds of emergencies that may be encountered and know the various activities that must take place at any given incident. Safety personnel must have the training and background to recognize real and potential hazards and be proficient in the techniques necessary to control them (Fig. 3-33). They should be trained in educational techniques so that they can conduct safety-oriented training programs within their organization. Emergency vehicle operation and incident command and control, as well as specific practices and procedures, must be within their instructional capabilities. They must be able to present state-of-the-art methods of accomplishing each and every given task that give emergency service personnel safety top priority. Members of the organization must truly believe that safety *is* the most important goal of each and every operation.

Training that emphasizes the correct and *safe* way to accomplish a given assignment is vital to a good safety program. The willingness to accept new ideas and develop new methods for confronting job hazards will reap great benefits by creating safe attitudes among emergency service personnel. Old ideas die hard. Tradition still rules in many areas of the work we are called to do. An organization that is safety oriented is eager and willing to accept input and flexible enough to progress to a safer, more efficient style of operation. Each organization takes on its own personality. The personality should reflect open-mindedness and the desire to be safe.

To further improve the health and safety of emergency service personnel, many career and volunteer fire departments are adopting physical fitness training programs. When members participate in maintenance-oriented physical fitness activities, the physical strength and agility, endurance, and mental alertness required for the proper and efficient performance of duty can be ensured. Effective results have even been obtained from programs conducted on a voluntary basis in which individuals control the pace of their own conditioning.

Finally, if on-the-job injuries and deaths for emergency providers are to be reduced, the leaders of each organization *must* set the correct example for all to see

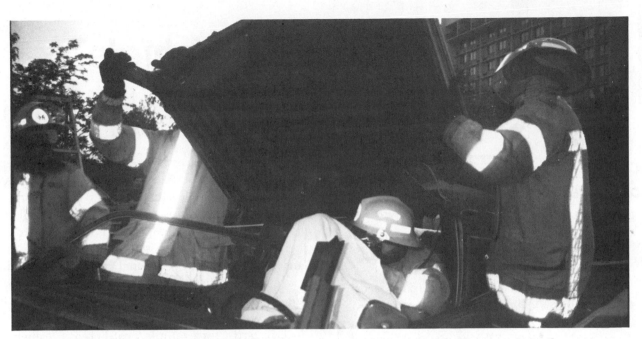

FIG. 3-33 Safety officer will require that flipped roof be secured and exposed metal cut areas be taped or tarped.

and follow. Leaders must show that they are safety believers in everything they say and do. The famous "do as I say, not as I do" philosophy can seriously undermine efforts to improve safety within an organization. It is a sad thing to hear stories of vehicle rescue instructors injured during training programs because of their own careless disregard for safety. The time has come for those in each rescue-oriented organization and those who serve as vehicle rescue instructors to set an example for all to follow. New crew members always remember their first impressions, particularly if they look up to and respect the senior person in their group or their first training instructor. That person, in the role of image-maker and trendsetter, must assume the responsibility to truly "do as I say, and as I do!"

SUMMARY

If emergency personnel truly have a desire to serve, they must first have a desire to serve safely. Personnel of any emergency service agency must be fully aware of environmental, incident scene, and vehicle safety hazards. Safety is a state of mind, something that must be practiced in training and on the streets. Safety must be a priority in everything we do, with our own safety and that of our brother and sister rescuers always at the top of the list. It is not heroic to wade through a pool of spilled gasoline to pull a victim out of a vehicle — it is stupid. It is not brave to work with rescue equipment at a serious auto accident clad only in T-shirt, jeans, and sneakers — it is foolish. It is not professional to be injured responding to, working at, or returning from an emergency incident — it is suicidal. If you want to be brave, heroic, and professional, be *safe*. The rest will follow.

4

Commanding Vehicle Rescue Incidents

OBJECTIVES

At the end of this chapter, you will be able to:

• Accurately outline the positions of the Incident Command System structure in graphic form.

• Understand procedures necessary to reduce the rescue reflex time upon arrival of emergency service personnel.

• Accurately describe and understand the meaning and function of the terms strategy and tactics.

• Accurately describe and fully explain the correct procedures for establishing command at an incident scene.

• Explain the actions and responsibilities necessary to fulfill any position of the Incident Command System.

• Accurately describe the three types of motor vehicle accident incident profiles.

• Accurately describe the three category areas of assessment information at an incident scene.

The world we live and work in is constantly changing. As emergency service providers, however, we remain creatures of habit. In the field of vehicle rescue, we tend to inherit our practices and procedures from past generations, accepting the reasoning, "If it worked 20 years ago, why shouldn't it work now?" These old habits limit our effectiveness in commanding and controlling the scene of a vehicular incident.

This chapter focuses on the actions that the individual in command of the incident must take in order to meet the basic objectives of the life cycle discussed in Chapter 2.

A period of confusion confronts emergency service personnel as they arrive at an accident scene. Effective actions are sometimes delayed until this brief chaotic period passes. A goal of all emergency agencies on the scene is to initiate actions that have a positive effect on the situation and will bring order to the confusion as soon as it is safe and practical. It takes a brief moment to comprehend what is unfolding before our eyes. The elapsed time between the initial arrival of emergency personnel and the point at which effective activities are begun is defined as our *reflex time*. This reflex time must be kept as brief as possible so that we waste no time after our arrival. Fire or fuel leak hazards, for example, can intensify quickly as time ticks away on the serious trauma patient's golden hour clock of survival.

In our efforts to get fire, rescue, and medical operations underway, our safety concerns must be kept in perspective. The person in charge of the overall incident must therefore quickly survey the scene and develop a plan to organize, command, and control the various agency personnel who are or will be beginning operations. The organizational tool that should be used for commanding and controlling a vehicle rescue incident is the *Incident Command System* (ICS). This proven system both minimizes the early confusion at an incident and reduces incident reflex time to a minimum.

The ICS originated in the early 1970s in California. Developed and instituted by Firescope (Firefighters of Southern California Organized for Potential Emergencies), it was designed primarily for the management of large wildland fires. The National Fire Academy Model Incident Command System presented here, which evolved from this wildland fire experience, has been specifically adapted to motor vehicle accident rescue situations. The ICS enables the person in charge to take available size-up information effectively, draw upon prior training and experience, and develop the correct incident objectives for emergency crews. An action-centered command structure gives those managing the emergency the means to achieve maximum results from their personnel, improve overall operational efficiency, and ensure that safety considerations are in place.

The ICS structure is established from the top down (Fig. 4-1). The responsibility to begin controlling and mitigating the emergency is placed with the initial person in charge, the Incident Commander (IC). The system expands in modular fashion based on the size, complexity, and challenges of the particular incident. It is like a toolbox. A wide range of system components or "tools" are available within the system, but only those needed to accomplish effective command and control are used. A minor accident, a simple ICS.

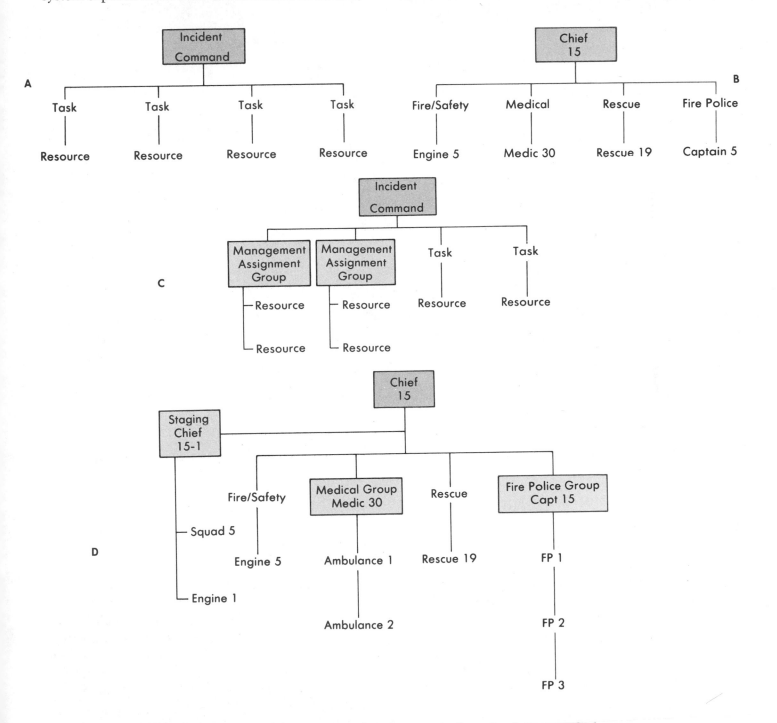

FIG. 4-1 A, Charting the assignment of single resources for a simple motor vehicle accident. **B,** Example of ICS unit assignments for a simple motor vehicle accident. **C,** Charting the staffing of management assignments at a more involved working rescue incident. **D,** Example of unit assignments for a working rescue incident.

Continued.

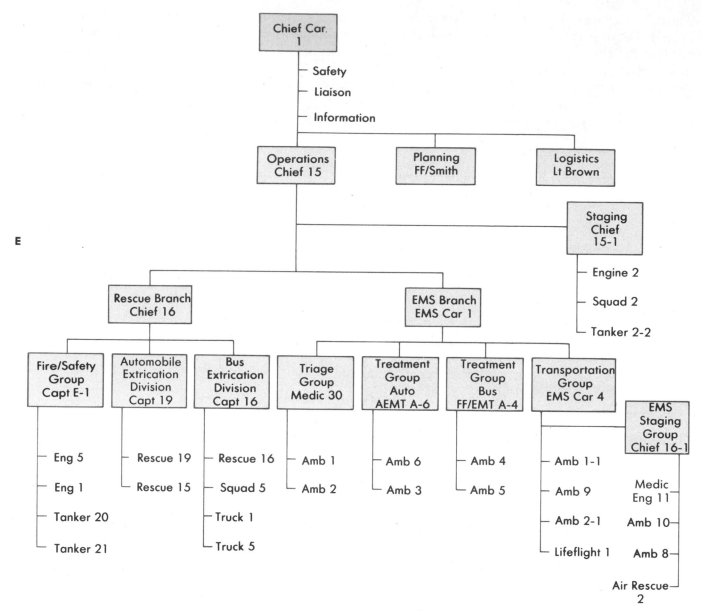

FIG. 4-1, cont'd E, Example of ICS structure for a major rescue incident with a multiple number of patients.

A more complex and challenging accident means the addition of more components. Depending on the need and available personnel, any or all ICS components can be put in place. The ICS should be used *at all incidents,* regardless of their size or complexity. Practice on the small ones makes for efficient operations at the "big one" where the system is truly essential.

Although vehicle accidents need proper ICS management just as much as fire or other emergencies do, emergency service personnel tend to let accident scenes remain unorganized, sometimes chaotic events because they usually involve only a few people or emergency vehicles. People can die because of this attitude.

The ICS works only when an individual fully accepts command responsibility and has the ability to put the system into operation. Someone *must* be in charge of the entire incident from first arrival to termination of the emergency. Later-arriving personnel must find a management system in place and functioning when they arrive. Effective command established from the very earliest moments yields the greatest success and highest level of safety to operating personnel.

Many problems are eliminated when first-arriving personnel establish command and control of the incident. The senior person on the ambulance unit, the officer arriving with the engine company, or the first police officer on the scene can establish initial command, gather critical size-up information, and begin to develop the necessary strategies.

The model ICS designates levels of responsibility in a geographic area by the formation of *divisions* and in specific functional areas by the formation of *groups* (Fig. 4-1, *C* and 4-1, *D*). Because accidents are generally of a smaller scale than fire incidents, our system normally uses only three or four divisions. (Examples of divisions are outlined in the sample ICS organizational chart). Engine companies, truck or ladder companies, rescue or squad companies, and other specialized crews are usually deployed as *single resources* within the ICS. A single resource crew has a specified number of personnel (three to seven) and an identified leader. Each single resource crew leader reports directly to the next higher supervisory level within the ICS. At motor vehicle accidents the use of a crew is the most common method of resource management.

Divisions or groups assist in maintaining the "span of control" in which each officer supervises a reasonable number of individuals. An essential element of a successful ICS is the maintenance of a span of control of five to seven individuals per supervisor, with five as the optimal number. An incident is thereby reduced to manageable proportions through the delegation of responsibility and authority to group or division supervisors. When there are more objectives to be met, more personnel to supervise, or when the incident covers a large geographic area, the IC can further delegate authority to subordinates by the formation of *branches*. A branch is a level between divisions or groups and the IC. A branch and its officer are responsible for implementing actions appropriate to the assignment.

As incidents increase in complexity or size, such as in a multicasualty incident or a rescue covering a large geographic area, the IC may need to delegate major functional responsibility to maintain an effective workload and span of control by establishing an Operations branch.

Operations' function is headed by an operations chief — commonly designated by radio as *Operations* — who supervises the branches, each of which has a command officer. Branch, division, or group officers,

as supervisors, should be experienced personnel with good fire, rescue, and medical backgrounds. Good choices for these officers include fire department company officers or senior personnel.

One successful way to designate an Operations officer is to have the first-arriving command individual move from the IC role when relieved by either a higher ranking officer or a more qualified individual to become the operations officer. This person, already familiar with the incident, can readily assume that position. Once an individual is assigned to supervise a division or sector, that individual assumes that position's title and is contacted by the radio designation of *extrication, medical,* or *operations.*

All supervisory officers must account for operating personnel assigned to them and monitor their activities to see that safe operating procedures are followed. All operating personnel communicate either face-to-face or by radio with the assigned division, group, branch, or crew officer. This officer then reports to the IC or the Operations chief, depending on the command structure.

The Operations' functions and all established branches, divisions, and groups are controlled by the IC either directly or through the chain of command. At most accident situations the IC can effectively serve as overall supervisor. Required crews, groups, and divisions to be established for a vehicle accident include those for law enforcement, fire safety, extrication, staging, treatment, and transportation. Any of these might include all the personnel, equipment, and apparatus of a fire department engine, rescue company, or medical crew. At a vehicle accident, often only one or two individuals fulfill the responsibilities of a particular group or crew.

As the vehicle rescue incident unfolds, the IC may request additional resources. The crews need to be assigned, but the IC may not immediately know where, when, and how to use the resources most effectively. The simplest solution is to assign all arriving companies to report to staging, a specified area where apparatus and personnel are assembled. Companies in staging are ready for immediate deployment, and their status is controlled by the staging officer.

Traditionally, individual crews have been given specific tasks but have had *no* management responsibilities. This is not the best method to follow. The ICS thus shifts more responsibility to all members of each crew as a single unit resource. To take maximum advantage of the ICS organizational structure, any leader or officer of an arriving crew may be called to become a command officer. Rescue, fire, medical, and police personnel must therefore be aware of the correct procedures to follow when they need to assume command of a portion of the incident. Accordingly, remaining crew members must be capable of functioning on their own while their officer or crew chief handles command duties.

This may sound like one IC and eight division officers are needed to extricate one trapped driver from a car, but this is not the case. It must be understood that the ICS is flexible. If the incident calls for three complete divisions, great. If one individual can fulfill many responsibilities effectively, that is also acceptable. In jurisdictions that must operate with limited personnel, one individual may have to wear many hats.

It is vitally important that the inner workings of the ICS be fully understood by those who must use it. The medical personnel compose the EMS division or group and are responsible for patient triage, treatment, and transportation. Fire service personnel that compose the fire safety group provide appropriate fire suppression, institute basic on-scene safety measures, and are responsible for management of hazards present. Those who work directly with the vehicle rescue equipment become the rescue or extrication group.

The complete model ICS also designates these command staff officers and duties whenever the IC cannot effectively handle any of these functions:

Information Officer (IO): Deals with the media and keeps them apprised of the particulars of the incident.

Liaison Officer: Acts as contact with such agencies as the Red Cross, Public Works Department, and any other cooperating agency.

Safety Officer: Monitors and assesses hazardous and unsafe situations and develops measures for ensuring personnel safety.

The five ICS functional areas include command, operations, plans, logistics, and finance. The responsibilities of the plans, logistics, and finance section officers include the following:

Planning Officer: Assists the commander by preparing alternative strategies and keeping track of the situation as it unfolds. Any technical specialists brought to the scene report to the planning officer. Personnel of this division track the status of all resources, display the current incident size and predicted escalation, and advise the IC about technical advice received from the advisors.

Logistics Officer: Provides necessary support such as facilities, services, and equipment to the working units. The logistics division establishes proper communications to and from the scene as well as among operating forces on the scene through the communications sector. This division develops adequate equipment and supplies to support the needs of the incident and commands the staging of resources assigned to the incident.

Finance Officer: Bears responsibility for all financial aspects of an incident, for example, when a special outside private contractor agency would be required in the rescue.

The accident scenario cited in Chapter 2 illustrates the ease with which the Model ICS can be implemented at vehicle rescue emergencies. Two vehicles had collided, leaving a station wagon on its edge. The ICS is established as the first emergency service person, a police officer, radios his arrival, positions the police vehicle properly, and begins to survey the accident scene while assuming temporary command (Fig. 4-2).

Medic 30, an advanced life support ambulance with two EMT-Ps aboard, arrives next. The police officer makes direct contact with the medics, reports the situation as it is known at this point, and turns command over to the senior member of that crew (Fig. 4-3). The

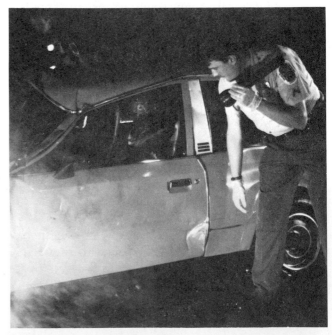

FIG. 4-2 Police officers work as a team as they cautiously move closer to an accident vehicle during initial scene size up. Their approach position demonstrates basic street survival skills necessary for law enforcement and EMS work.

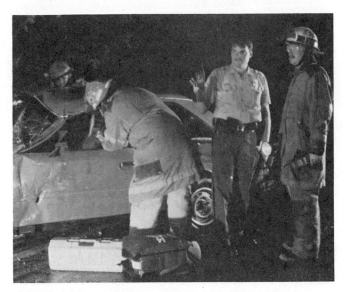

FIG. 4-3 Police officer confers with medical supervisor relaying known information.

medics represent the EMS group; the senior medic now serves as both temporary IC and EMS officer. Both medical crew members work to fulfill their responsibilities at the accident scene. The police officer, representing law enforcement, assumes responsibility for security, traffic control, and crowd control measures. The fire department engine company arrives, bringing a supervising fire officer to the emergency scene. At this point the senior EMT-P makes face-to-face contact with the fire officer, reports on the situation, and passes overall command to the officer. The medic can now fully concentrate on patient care activities. As IC the engine company officer establishes effective command and control, conducts a full scene survey, and ensures that efforts to accomplish the overall goals necessary to provide care for the patients are initiated. A senior firefighter with the engine company now acts as fire suppression crew leader for the firefighting safety crew while their officer commands the overall incident.

During a large-scale rescue incident, it is possible to have all members of the initial arriving crews delegated as officers. This is commonly done when, for example, EMS personnel are confronted by a multi-casualty incident. In these special situations the medical crew members may be assigned by the EMS branch officer or the IC to act as triage or treatment group officers rather than individual providers of care. It is important to realize that the situation itself and not a standard operating procedure is the final determining factor in how each crew and each indi-

vidual is used. The greater the knowledge of the members of each emergency service agency about the functions of the ICS, the better the level of service provided.

The action continues in this scenario as the rescue company arrives. The rescue officer contacts the IC and either is assigned as the rescue and extrication group officer or accepts command. Either rescue crew members work under the direction of their officer or the team's senior person acts as the extrication crew officer.

A chief officer may arrive on the scene and, make direct contact with the IC. Command may switch to the higher ranking officer, or the present IC may continue to command with the superior ranking officer simply monitoring the situation as it occurs. In minor incidents, allowing the junior officer to remain in command permits that individual to gain valuable experience in a command function. The higher ranking officer steps in only if conditions deteriorate or the situation warrants an assumption of formal command.

A transportation group may be established if many casualties are involved and multiple transportation is needed. If aircraft are to be used in patient transport, a Medevac or air transportation group may be established to handle arrangements to safely accommodate the aircraft. If a private contractor must be called to render assistance at the scene, an individual can be assigned to coordinate this, acting as a one-person logistics officer. As the news media appear on the emergency scene, the public information officer becomes the contact person for the needs of the press. Any emergency service personnel and vehicles not immediately needed at the scene are controlled by the staging officer in a clearly accessible area, at least one city block or its equivalent away from the emergency scene. Any person assisting the IC by recording information and documenting incident events becomes a one-person planning section (Fig. 4-1, *E*).

As a command and control management tool, the ICS provides for the greatest degree of safety and efficiency for all operating personnel at emergency scenes. The chain of command is well defined and known to all present. The IC is the boss, the supervisor responsible for all functions being completed. As the IC's span of control grows, certain functional responsibilities are delegated to others who manage and supervise smaller working teams or areas and report to and coordinate with the IC. This minimizes confusion and maximizes efficiency and safety. It cannot be emphasized enough that lack of a command system or willing violation of the installed command system will cause conflicts, misunderstandings, and confusion that may well result in an ineffective, unsafe operation. All assisting agencies summoned to the incident scene as additional resources, *must* be required to function within the scope of the existing ICS when operating at the scene.

Uncoordinated "freelance" rescue and medical operations are a prime example of the failure of a command system. The adoption and implementation of essential portions of the ICS at vehicle rescue incidents provides the most effective solution to proper management of today's rescue situations.

RESPONSIBILITIES OF COMMAND AT VEHICLE ACCIDENTS

The IC at a vehicle accident is responsible for completing an incident assessment. The IC or an individual assigned by the IC to do this must complete a 360°, walk-around scene survey with a flashlight and portable radio readily available. The officer *must* have full personal protective clothing on with all components properly donned. The size-up information, coupled with the wisdom of the officer's experience and training, allows the IC to make preliminary predictions of rescue problems and needs. This assessment establishes an incident "profile" that reflects the specific personality that each accident assumes.

Each vehicle rescue incident can be classified as a minor incident, a working rescue, or a major incident (Fig. 4-4). In a minor incident, available resources will be entirely capable of controlling the accident without additional assistance or complex operations. Some responding crews may even be directed by the IC to return to quarters before their arrival or report to a staging area.

If the commander sees and feels that many needs — both immediate and long-term — will have to be addressed, the accident becomes a working rescue incident. As with a working fire emergency, all assigned resources are committed to action at the scene, and additional resources will be staged for possible use. Whenever the incident exceeds the capabilities of the initial assignment of personnel and equipment, additional resources must be alerted and advanced to a staging area.

When the commander's assessment classifies the incident as major, arriving resources may be completely overwhelmed, either by the large geographic area that the accident encompasses or by the multiple number of vehicles, patients, or problems, as with a multi-casualty plane crash or passenger train derailment.

All information gathered during size up and assessment, regardless of the incident's profile, can be fitted neatly into one of three basic information categories: fire/safety, medical, or rescue. This gives a clearer picture of what is going on and allows standardized solutions to be generated.

High-priority hazards in the fire/safety category include fire, a fuel spill or leak, the hazards of electricity from a vehicle or downed power transmission wires, the presence of hazardous materials, and the instability of vehicles or structures at the scene. Other potential fire/safety hazards include spilled fluids, sharp metal and glass, inadequate lighting, poor work surface traction, and the inherent dangers of traffic and crowd conditions. Fire/safety hazards generally pose the most serious threat to the safety and survival of emergency service personnel working on the scene. Any safety hazard may completely halt all other actions until it can be corrected. All of these problems can generally be handled by fire department engine company personnel.

Medical size-up information includes determining the number of existing or potential patients that will require attention, their location, the nature and degree of injury, and the particulars of their entrapment at the scene. Medical problems and activities are handled by EMS personnel on the scene.

Rescue information gained from the initial size up includes anticipated problems of providing access to the patients and an estimation of the disentanglement and extrication work needed for proper removal of the injured. Entrapment problems resulting from the collision are dealt with by the rescue-trained personnel. Individuals may have to be "borrowed" from one crew to supplement in other areas. For example, a firefighter may be assigned to assist with patient packaging or longboard work.

During size-up survey work the IC has a close opportunity to observe hazards that exist in, on, and around the scene. The IC completes a full circle around all involved vehicles, maintaining an approximate 10-foot distance from the closest vehicle. This distance identifies the *action circle* and takes on an important significance as the action unfolds. Crowd control measures, such as rope or banner tape, must be placed around the accident scene perimeter as

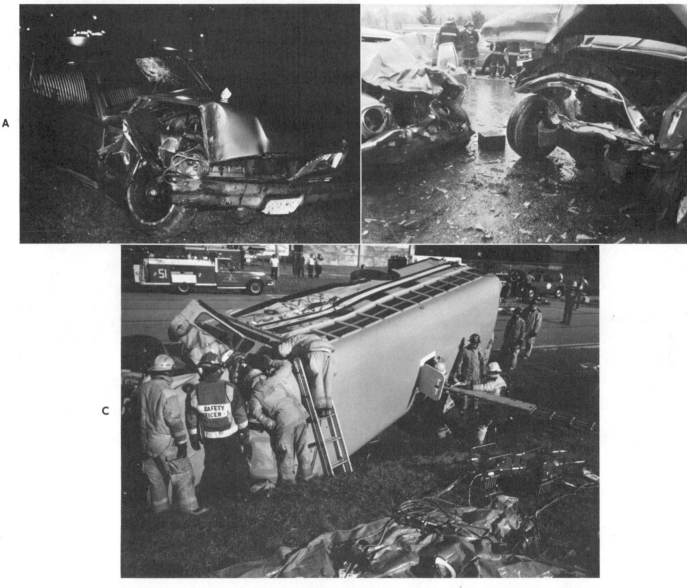

FIG. 4-4 A, A minor incident with the vehicle sustaining head-on collision damage, producing injuries to occupant. **B,** A working vehicle rescue incident typified by this multivehicle, multipatient collison with trapped occupants. **C,** At major vehicle rescue incidents, first-arriving equipment and personnel may be inadequate to handle the situation due to a large geographic area involved or multiple numbers of vehicles, patients, or rescue problems.

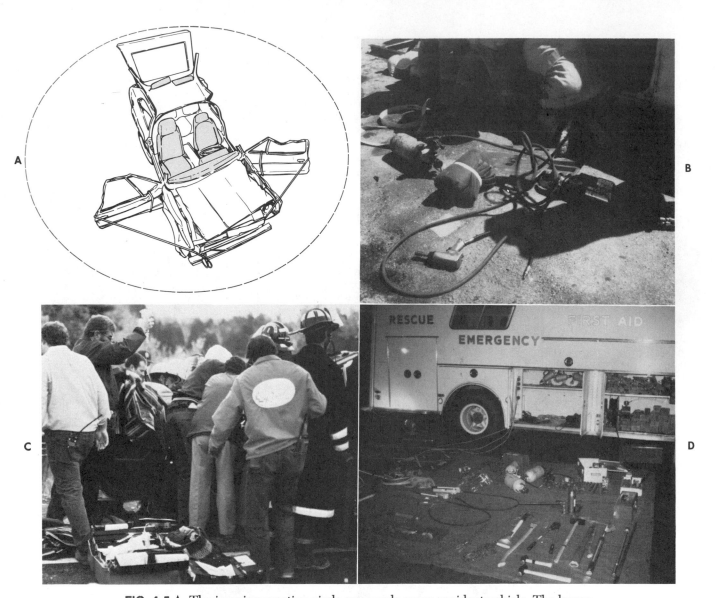

FIG. 4-5 A, The imaginary action circle surrounds every accident vehicle. The larger this clear area is, the more efficient rescue operations will be and the greater the degree of safety for emergency service crews. **B,** Tools and equipment should be returned to the tool staging area outside the action circle. **C,** EMS equipment litters the action circle, as emergency personnel mix with bystanders to congest this scene. **D,** An efficient, well-illuminated, and readily accessible tool-staging layout.

soon as possible, thereby establishing an *outer circle.* Only those personnel assigned to work within the action circle enter the control point. All standby crew members and equipment must be maintained beyond this circle of safety (Fig. 4-5).

The IC moves around the perimeter of the action (or inner) circle, glancing back and forth from the accident vehicles to the areas surrounding the scene. In scanning this area the IC may detect previously unseen accident victims or important safety hazards.

As it becomes safe to do so, the IC looks at all eight sides of each involved vehicle — inside and outside, top and bottom, left and right sides, front and rear — while being prepared to react instantly to any unexpected problem during this survey. The IC communicates with other team members on the scene as all report their findings. When several crew members survey portions of the scene simultaneously and share their findings, the size-up process can be very quick and thorough (Fig. 4-6). They must, however, be

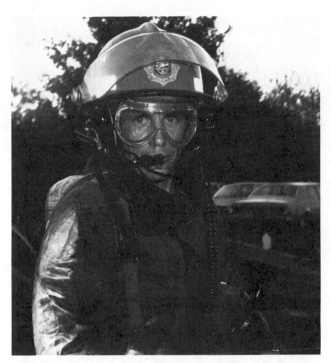

FIG. 4-6 Metro-Dade County Fire Rescue Division members use portable radios, microphones, and headsets to communicate directly with rescue crew members at the emergency scene.

cautious when communicating accident information while in close proximity to injured patients or bystanders. Size-up information is confidential and should be kept strictly between emergency personnel. It is not for the eyes or ears of bystanders or patients.

The IC sees to it that communication is established with the patients as soon as appropriate and that it remains constant throughout the entire rescue, extrication, and transportation process. At least one crew member must remain dedicated to the patients to ensure both their physical and mental safety. This individual also provides the patients' medical care.

Upon concluding the initial scene size up, the command officer moves *away* from the damaged vehicles to make a final assessment of the overall accident scene. The failure of an IC to physically back away from the action is a common and very serious shortcoming. Human nature draws the IC close to the vehicles. The presence of people who need attention lures them into staying where the action is. Action-oriented officers feel most comfortable when they are doing something. A position close to the action, however, will have a serious detrimental influence on

the IC's ability to continue commanding the incident at this early stage and hamper further size up. Step back and get the big picture!

The initial survey, from first arrival to the point where a complete 360-degree circle has been made around the scene, should generally take 60 seconds or less. During this vital minute the foundation is laid for every action that will evolve. The unknown becomes the known, and both real and potential scene hazards are identified, as are existing or anticipated rescue and medical problems (Fig. 4-7). During this 60-second period, the patient or patients are located and contacted if possible. After completing the initial walk-around survey, the IC compares the fire, safety, medical, and rescue problems discovered or anticipated with the resources at hand or responding to the emergency scene. Available resources must be sufficient to gain control of the situation. Adequate resources of trained emergency service personnel must be responding, along with apparatus and equipment sufficient to control the immediate and future needs of the emergency. If the needs exceed the resources, the IC must establish priorities, and use available resources to their best advantage.

As scene operations evolve and crews work to perform various initial tasks, the IC continues gathering information by conducting *sustained size-up* surveys. These reconnaissance missions allow the IC to upgrade or downgrade the situation to reflect progress or lack of progress on the scene. The situation should move toward a more stable and controlled emergency. Remember, it is the accident victim who is having the emergency, not the responding personnel. Sustained size up conducted by the IC continually monitors the actions and reactions of emergency personnel, patients, and all scene developments. Regular radio status reports should be broadcast from the scene to the communications center, updating the status of personnel and equipment and reporting progress or lack of progress with the rescue.

The IC must continually think ahead to anticipate what may be needed to remain in control of the incident. Ongoing size-up activities enable the IC to stay on top of the accident's challenges.

VEHICLE RESCUE STRATEGY AND TACTICS

With the initial scene size-up work completed and the IC identified and functioning, it is time to develop a basic plan of action and specific procedures to be followed. The plan becomes the vehicle rescue *strat-*

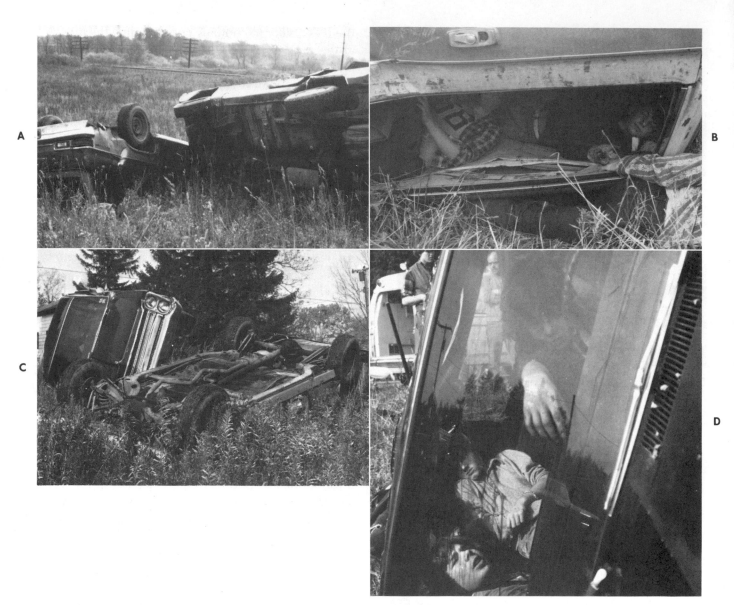

FIG. 4-7 Initial scene circle survey. **A,** Observations from only one point of view do not reveal the true nature of the incident. **B,** Only by circling accident vehicles are special injury and entrapment situations apparent to command personnel. **C,** Size up also reveals the driver's side of the rollover vehicle in contact with front of the vehicle on edge. Commander should anticipate more complex efforts to extricate patients in front seat area of upside down vehicle. **D,** Close observation of vehicle on edge quickly reveals at least three occupants inside, with driver suspended on high side near wheel and column.

egy, and the specific procedures used to carry out the plan compose the rescue *tactics.* The most common strategic goals or plans of action at an accident call for the following:

- Preventing further death or injury.
- Safely stabilizing the incident.
- Making the patient readily accessible.
- Treating the patient.
- Making the patient readily removable.

- Extricating the patient in the safest and most efficient manner.
- Delivering the patient to the appropriate trauma surgical team within the golden hour.

Although the many variables at a vehicle accident scene make each accident slightly different from the next, the single most important goal of all rescue incidents is to prevent further death and injury. Maximum safety is achieved by first ensuring the safety and well-being of all emergency service personnel. Responders must accept full responsibility for their actions and act safely and professionally at all times when working an incident. Concern for the safety and well-being of uninvolved citizens is another priority. These people are not trained to be aware of real or potential accident scene hazards. It is the responsibility of emergency service personnel to maintain safety for citizens at an accident scene. The greater the distance between these people and the accident scene, the greater their level of safety. A third area of concern for preventing further death and injury is ensuring the safety of a vehicle's occupants, whether uninjured or trapped and injured. If the accident victims receive the entire focus of attention from the rescuers, a hazard can go undetected that may cause additional injuries or deaths at the accident scene. The primary responsibility of the IC is the safety of all persons at a motor vehicle accident.

When personal safety is ensured, the second strategic priority becomes incident stabilization, which includes effective command and control of the accident scene and completion of all phases of the vehicle rescue life cycle. As other basic incident strategies are met, the incident becomes effectively managed.

The IC must develop an overall strategy for the specific accident. Balancing the needs of victims, medics, and rescue personnel with resources available now and those available in 5 minutes and in 30 minutes sets the stage for an overall mode of operation. The basic modes of vehicle rescue operation are *offensive*, *defensive*, or combinations of the two.

Medical and rescue personnel normally operate in an offensive mode. Most experienced rescue personnel find it difficult to relate to anything but what would be classified as an all-out, aggressive rescue process. After all, they argue, it is just a car accident! Yet the reality of vehicle rescue today tells us that not all accident situations can be aggressively attacked. A conservative strategy, our defensive rescue mode, is justified in situations that either overwhelm available resources or threaten the life safety of emergency service personnel.

The process for determining which rescue mode operation will be initiated involves sizing up the situation and balancing the resources needed against those available. If resources are adequate and safe operations can be ensured, an offensive rescue operation is required. If the immediate needs exceed the available resources or if safety to operating personnel cannot be immediately ensured, a defensive or combination

rescue operation is adopted. The adequacy or inadequacy of resources is based on the initial incident size up and the experience and perceptions of the situation by the IC.

An offensive rescue strategy mode, where the initial assignment of personnel, equipment, and apparatus can control the entire situation, yields an aggressive attack on the situation. On-scene forces perform all required tasks properly and efficiently and quickly gain control of the incident. All needs of the patient are met.

The offensive/defensive rescue strategy mode calls for the command personnel to be somewhat conservative. The IC commits available personnel and equipment to action yet summons standby crews or directs additional resources to stage in anticipation of future needs. Calling for additional resources "just in case" typifies the offensive/defensive rescue strategy. If you require help, call for it. Do not take it as a sign of personal failure. All actions must be directed toward gaining the upper hand of the situation while additional resources are responding. Whether or not these reserve forces will ever be used at the scene is not important. What is important is maintaining a margin of safety. This same concept is used on the fireground when the IC calls for additional alarms. In offensive or offensive/defensive operations the resources available are maintained to exceed the resources needed.

The defensive/offensive rescue mode is called for when rescue crews are overwhelmed by the situation or when there is an immediate threat to life safety of the operating crews, as in a collision where an involved vehicle is burning. Action taken to minimize the safety threat posed by the fire takes priority over all other events and possibly delays patient care and rescue operations momentarily. Once the hazard is controlled, personnel commit themselves to a conventional offensive approach to handling the incident.

In a defensive/offensive rescue operation the IC commits all initial resources, summons additional resources, and attempts to "hold" the problem until it diminishes or additional resources of personnel and equipment arrive.

The final mode of vehicle rescue strategy is the defensive rescue mode. A highway accident may be called in, with the caller reporting simply "a person trapped." The call may sound routine enough, an example of an expected offensive rescue operation. That basic strategy may prevail in the minds of responding personnel until they actually arrive at the scene and find an accident involving a tractor-trailer truck placarded as transporting hazardous materials with a fire involving a large portion of the vehicle. In this situation, work to rescue anyone trapped within the wreckage becomes virtually hopeless. The defensive rescue mode describes such incidents as "losers" in terms of committing resources in hopes of the successful rescue of a viable patient.

It is the responsibility of the IC to issue a "go or no-go" decision to pursue an offensive, defensive, or combination strategy mode of operation based on preliminary, initial, and sustained size-up information. The overall strategy defines the broad goals of the operation and in what order they are to be accomplished. Setting the incident strategy is one of the most essential components of an effective, coordinated ICS.

Once the problems have been identified and the strategic objectives and modes of operation selected, it is time for the IC to assign rescue tactics or tactical objectives to group or division leaders and crews. Tactical objectives are carried out by companies or crews and are narrower in scope than strategic objectives. The basic objectives, which must be coordinated with the tactical objectives assigned to other crews, include scene stabilization, safety, support, access, emergency care, disentanglement, extrication, and termination.

Once the IC has selected a strategy, assigned tactical objectives, and worked to ensure a safe operating environment, the supervisors of groups, divisions, and crews must work together to determine exactly what will be done to meet their objectives (Fig. 4-8). Radio procedures should diminish to where the IC manages by exception. Team personnel work under the safety supervision of their leaders, who coordinate directly with the IC. If everything is going well, the IC and operating forces stay off the radio to eliminate unnecessary radio chatter. Only EMS personnel communicating with the medical facilities and the IC in contact with the control center should make more radio transmissions after their arrival than before. Subordinate officers report to the commander with information only if they have met their objective and are available for other assignments, they cannot meet their assigned objective, or a safety problem or need for more resources arises (Fig. 4-9).

Command or Combat

The first-arriving officer or crew chief at a vehicle accident needs to make many quick decisions, decisions that will have both short-term and long-range effects on the outcome of the entire incident. One such

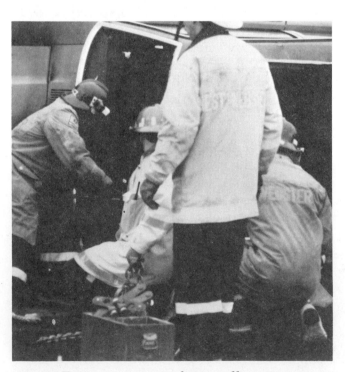

FIG. 4-8 Extrication group or division officer oversees extrication activities and communicates with IC or Operations Chief.

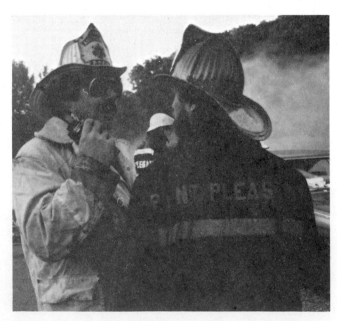

FIG. 4-9 Safety Officer confers directly with the IC and can order tactical changes when safety is compromised.

decision is whether to "command" or "combat." The individual who decides to command, to become a commander of the incident, no longer participates as a team leader or a working member of a team. The decision to combat, by contrast, means that the individual continues as a working member of a team. In some cases, command and combat modes are combined.

The decision of this key individual significantly influences the safety of personnel on the scene. Many rescue disasters, in terms of both the level of safety and the performance of emergency service personnel, have been attributed to the lack of initial command and control. When each team or crew leader arrives on the scene and simply goes into the combat mode, necessary supervision and coordination is neglected.

When an individual leader or a senior person becomes overwhelmed by the accident scene, there are three possible courses of action. One reaction might be to do nothing, taking no effective action to mitigate the incident. These officers tread water until something or someone changes the situation. Second, the individual may revert to do what comes naturally regardless of whether it is appropriate. For example, a fire officer becomes the firefighter on the nozzle, or a supervising rescue officer operates the rescue equipment. An overwhelmed senior medic might render individual care to the first patient they contact, disregarding other problems or patients at the scene. These actions jeopardize the safety and well-being of everyone at the scene.

When an officer does decide to go into combat with the team, this "quick attack" mode should not last more than a few moments and will end with one of the following:

- The situation is stabilized.
- A more qualified or higher ranking officer arrives and assumes command.
- The situation is *not* stabilized, and the officer removes himself/herself from the hands-on action and assumes command.

Typically, the most appropriate course of action when confronted by an overwhelming rescue situation is for the first-arriving officer or crew chief to pull away from the action and take responsibility for supervising the incident initially. A portable radio can be used to facilitate contact with the operating team while the officer meets command responsibilities. The following questions illustrate the steps involved in the command or combat decision-making process:

1. Will immediate operations totally control or minimize the problem?

If the answer is "yes," the incident is minor, and the initial officer or crew chief will be able to adequately command and control the incident using assigned resources and standard rescue and medical procedures.

In this scenario, the officer will do the following:

- Assume the role of initial IC.
- Establish the ICS.
- Develop offensive rescue management strategies following the vehicle rescue life cycle.

If the answer is "no," the incident is moderate (a working rescue) but controllable by available resources once they arrive and carry out their assignments. The senior crew member or officer initially commands and controls the incident using available resources and standard procedures. Additional resources may be either staged or committed to control the incident. Higher ranking or more qualified officers are expected on-scene momentarily.

In this scenario, the officer will do the following:

- Assume the role of IC.
- Establish the ICS.
- Develop defensive/offensive rescue management strategies following the vehicle rescue life cycle.

The officer assigns group, division, or crew leaders, requests additional assistance or resources as needed, and deploys all immediate resources in a holding or defensive action until resources become adequate. At that point, effective offensive activities can be initiated and the situation brought under control. As a higher ranking officer takes command, the initial officer assumes a subordinate role such as Operations officer or a group leader.

The second IC will do the following:

- Assign the initial commander where most appropriately needed.
- Further develop initial defensive/offensive and subsequent offensive rescue scene management strategies as resources become adequate.
- Expand the structure of the ICS, to command and control the incident as necessary.
- Request additional assistance or resources, to control the situation as necessary.

2. If the problem is of such magnitude that control is not possible, are on-scene forces initially overwhelmed? Is immediate assistance urgently needed? Is the problem so massive that it will require intricate coordination of numerous crews from various agencies?

If the answer is "yes," the incident is of major proportions and is probably a multi-casualty or disaster incident.

In this scenario, the first officer will do the following:
- Assume the IC role.
- Establish the ICS.
- Request additional resources.
- Develop initial defensive rescue management strategies following the vehicle rescue life cycle.

Whenever additional assistance is called for, the officer in charge must plan how and where these responding resources will be used. When these units arrive, someone must direct them to the staging area or give them specific individual assignments. Without direction, they are likely to choose their own course of action, which can result in *their* objectives being met and those of the IC being abandoned. This means duplication of effort, loss of accountability of work, greater overall losses, and possible injury or death. Staging and specific tactical assignments are imperative.

When confronted with the urge to get involved in the hands-on action, the first-arriving officer must first remember the advantages of assuming command. Only later, and only if able to do so without compromising command responsibilities can this individual fulfill a subordinate role. Everyone's safety, including the officer's, depends on this immediate decision to establish a strong and effective command posture.

INCIDENT COMMAND POST

An effective command structure at an accident scene must have both a designated IC and an incident command post. By definition, a vehicle rescue incident command post is the overall command center in the field. Information that comes to and goes from this point is instrumental in successful control of the accident situation. The magnitude and the nature of the emergency influences the degree of sophistication of the command post itself. As with the ICS, the size, location, and number of personnel are commensurate with the incident's needs or anticipated needs.

The command post must meet a number of basic requirements, most important of which is to keep the officer in charge adequately informed of the situation as it evolves. In vehicle rescue incidents the location of the command post should afford a good view of the action area, since being within eyesight of unfolding events assists the IC's decision-making processes. Everyone at the command post must be protected from extremes of heat, cold, precipitation, and wind to lessen distractions by physical discomforts. Typical command post locations include the passenger area of

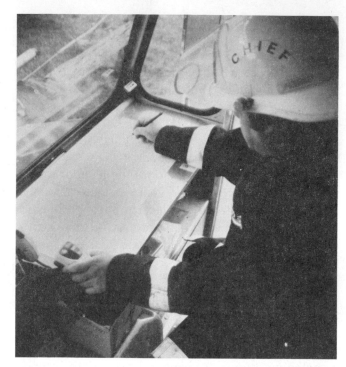

FIG. 4-10 Command post rescue vehicles allows tracking of activities and communication.

a pumper or rescue truck or the officer's personal vehicle.

The inside rear areas of heavy-duty rescue trucks are now being designed and equipped to function as command posts (Fig. 4-10). This can present a problem, however, when the coming and going of personnel to get or return equipment in the compartments *inside* the vehicle distracts command post personnel. Specialty van or buslike vehicles designed as field command and operations centers also serve well as command posts, although a typical vehicle accident rarely warrants the response of a specialty vehicle of this type.

The command post must be readily identifiable. Having a command post is one thing; knowing its location can be an entirely different matter. If the first-arriving ambulance or fire vehicle is the designated command post location, the IC would generally be located in or near that vehicle. Portable identification markings can help to identify either the command vehicle or area designated as the command post. An orange traffic cone on the hood or roof of a vehicle, a bright-colored flag on the antennae, or a flashing green light are examples. Some heavy-duty rescue vehicles are equipped with an elevating light of a unique color not found on any other vehicle on the

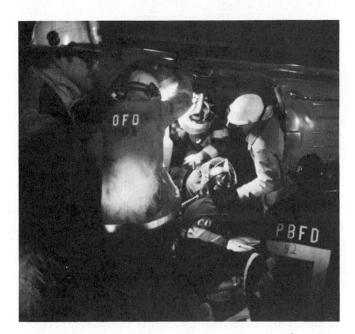

FIG. 4-11 Communication among and between the group officer as immediate supervisor, safety officer, and IC (not shown) is essential.

accident scene. This flashing lamp allows for rapid visual identification of the command vehicle. The location of the information officer should also be advertised to draw the news media away from the command post operation and toward a readily identifiable location and proper contact for incident information.

The IC must be well identified. Protective clothing that includes a distinctive color helmet or coat commonly identifies officer personnel in the fire service. The use of the high-visibility ICS vests can denote command, staff, group, and division officers.

Because the magnitude of a vehicle accident is usually less than that of a working fire emergency or a hazardous material problem, the IC who is equipped with a portable radio for communications, protected from the weather, and readily identifiable to all personnel working at the scene can function effectively, moving about the accident scene as rescue work progresses. The IC's effectiveness as a supervisor, evaluator, and strategy developer at the accident scene can often be enhanced by having accessibility to all areas of the accident scene (Fig. 4-11).

Although moving around the accident scene allows the IC to see action or conditions from a personal perspective, a drawback to this "two-legged" command post is that the IC may tend to wander excessively. Constant movement reduces the ability of other personnel to readily locate and communicate with the supervisor. At an accident scene, it is discouraging to ask a firefighter, "Where is the Chief?" only to have them reply, "I don't know exactly. The last I saw of him he was going clockwise!" Roving the scene also tends to get the IC involved in the action. This is not acceptable. Hands-on commanders limit their view of the incident and can lose perspective of accident events. Command and control can quickly be lost.

The IC needs several essential pieces of equipment to command effectively. A vehicle radio is vital for transmitting and receiving radio messages. For vehicle rescue incidents, a good multichannel portable radio is also recommended. Pencils, pens, paper, and a clipboard can easily be carried as standard items on any emergency vehicle. A key document for the IC to have is the local *incident control chart* on which to record specific information about the emergency. The chart, which may be handwritten or preprinted, allows for documentation and tracking of vehicles, equipment, and personnel. Magnets, chalkless marker boards, or even china marker pens can be used with the control chart to provide accountability of resources used at a scene. This list of available local resources can be a valuable memory jogger for the IC who may need additional rescue or medical equipment and cannot remember exactly what particular equipment a certain rescue company has.

The incident control chart can also list actions that need to be addressed or anticipated. Printing the schematic for the vehicle rescue life cycle on the back of the chart is one way to arrange this information.

Miscellaneous information that needs to be documented can be written on additional pieces of paper. At a major fire or disaster incident, a planning division is established to record such data. At an involved vehicle rescue incident the IC running a one-person command post can talk into a small portable cassette tape recorder, noting times, places, and events for transcription at a later date. This information can also be logged onto a master tape recorder at the central communications center if a radio transmission or phone call is made on a monitored line.

The IC should also have a pair of good quality binoculars available for situations such as sizing up a transportation incident involving suspected or known hazardous materials or looking down a steep mountain incline. Good quality highway maps of the area, with detailed information on all roads, bridges, railroads, and waterways, are also important to have at hand, as is the DOT *Emergency Response Guidebook*. For documentation of wind direction and velocity conditions, a portable weather flag or wind sock is necessary.

The usual command post at a vehicle accident consists simply of a senior officer in a white coat and helmet who is standing at a specific spot on a roadway with portable radio in hand, directing and supervising the operation. From this basic beginning, the command post can become larger and more sophisticated in design. Regardless of appearance, however, its function remains the same: a central location for those in command of the incident to contact each other and give and receive information.

CHALLENGES TO THE VEHICLE RESCUE INCIDENT COMMANDER

The IC's first and foremost role is that of being an effective leader. Certain personal qualities are thus essential. Effective commanders get respect by both their actions and their example. Their leadership inspires confidence in others and enables them to get maximum performance from their personnel. The chaos of an accident scene must be sorted through and organized into a safe and efficient operation. Amidst the typical crowd of spectators, traffic pile-ups, and unpleasant sights and sounds of an accident, the IC must remain in control both personally and professionally.

The ability to remain a professional requires a resourceful and flexible leader. The IC must know what to do and how to get it done. Decisions must be made with absolute determination, leaving nothing to chance. Experienced commanders never assume *anything*.

The IC can easily be overcome by the emotion of the situation and not realize it. The need for logical thinking and reasoning may become impaired. Judgment can become inaccurate as the leader becomes a psychological victim of the incident. All command personnel must strive to remain in control of their own mental and emotional state and stay calm, cool, and collected as they act and react to the situation. The IC in particular must be able to see beyond the emotion of the moment to make the correct, rational decisions that yield the best and most effective methods of operation. More than any other person on the scene, the commander, must have the ability to see beyond the immediate problems and envision solutions to present and anticipated problems.

At an accident, everyone may have a different idea of how things should be done. The final authority, however, is the IC who must calmly consider all points of information, analyze what will and will not work, assign priorities, and arrive at a well-balanced plan that provides necessary personnel safety and still accomplishes the task. Although decisions about which piece of rescue equipment to use for which task are left to those working directly with a specific problem, the IC must approve of the overall techniques being employed.

Because experience is one vitally important component of a successful rescue operation, an IC who is new at leading rescue operations should seek the advice and counsel of the experienced working crew members, who represent a valuable depth of experience and have a keen insight into what is necessary to meet the particular problems that may present themselves.

All supervisory personnel are challenged to look for simple solutions first when tackling a complex or difficult evolution. Maintaining a balanced, common-sense approach to problem-solving, while not easy, produces more efficient and safer overall accident activities. Commanders should see to it that emergency teams try the obvious first. This general rule applies to most rescue operations. If a simple solution to a problem does not work, more complex actions can be taken. For example, when a rescue team reports that a given vehicle door is jammed, the IC, playing "devil's advocate" or "doubting Thomas," can ask, "Have you tried the inside handle? Is the door unlocked? *Why* is the door jammed?" These questions must be properly answered before further actions are taken.

Command personnel must also remember that the workers involved in hands-on contact with a vehicle have a limited view of the overall problem. Their close position makes them susceptible to tunnel vision, a close-minded perspective on a given problem. The commander, not directly involved in any of the specific evolutions, has an excellent view of the scene from a physically more distant and overall perspective. The ability to step back to look at the whole problem — "to get the big picture" — is an important attribute of a good commander.

Issuing an order is only half of the challenge of properly directing a person or crew. The term *command feedback loop* describes the process of issuing an order and being kept informed of the status of the work being done to accomplish that order. As the IC or other individual leaders assign tasks, they must either observe these tasks being carried out themselves or have other persons report the progress or lack of progress back to them. This information must be continually cycled back to the supervising officer. A good leader always has a back-up procedure in mind for cases when the report advises that something has not worked or cannot be accomplished. Command personnel must remember the motto of the Boy Scouts of America and always "Be prepared."

The IC is also challenged with the responsibility of establishing and maintaining communications with a communications center and establishing communication and cooperation among agencies and personnel on the actual scene. Communications under emergency conditions must be clear, concise, and deliberated. Know what you want to say and then communicate to those working for you exactly what you want. There is no reason to be pompous or demanding. A firm but tactful approach is best, especially when dealing with other agencies. Effective leaders often will ask a subordinate officer for an opinion about a given problem before issuing a command order. This provides good information to the commander, allows the subordinate to become involved in the decision-making process, and assists that individual to gain command experience as they progress within the organization.

When communicating with others either face-to-face or by radio, effective leaders are best understood when they speak calmly, even when others around them are shouting and overly excited. The mental discipline it takes to look and sound calm when deep inside you are shaking in your proverbial boots is a skill that can be learned. This approach will cause those around the leader to calm down as they too reflect the leader's coolness and professionalism.

When dealing with excited crew members on the radio, "screamers" must be told to calm down and asked to repeat the original garbled message. When told they are not properly communicating, they may suddenly realize that they are overexcited and repeat their message in a calm and more easily understood tone of voice.

Command personnel must also require identification of personnel responsible for various command functions within the individual groups. This is particu-

larly important with the medical group and its personnel. Clearly labeled, high-visibility vests or arm bands effectively identify individuals fulfilling the various command functions at an emergency scene. The vests can be modified to serve as subtle memory-joggers for those wearing them. Attaching a laminated card in a holder to the vest, much like a hunting license on a hunter's jacket, reminds the wearer of the responsibilities necessary for that individual to fulfill the assigned function. The unused vests that the IC still holds represent positions or functions that are either not needed at the incident or are not fulfilled at that point in time.

Another important responsibility for the IC is determining when the services of a particular emergency unit or crew are no longer needed. Certain services may not be required at a minor incident. The heavy-duty rescue company, for example, may be returned to quarters before arrival if on-scene resources can adequately handle the situation. As activities wind down at the scene, an alert leader assesses the further need for particular personnel, equipment, and emergency vehicles. If the IC determines that a vehicle and its crew are no longer needed, it is wise to promptly return them to in-service status. Remaining at the scene for a prolonged time is a waste of that crew and may also expose the crew unnecessarily to inclement weather or stressful situations. If there is any doubt about whether the services of a particular crew are needed, the unit remains. Otherwise, a prompt return of that company is indicated.

SUMMARY

The personnel that supervise and manage the accident scene must always be *analytical* in their work, *bold* in their strategy and tactics, and *caring* in their responsibilities. Adopting and implementing the vehicle rescue ICS, sized to match the profile of the incident, allows the officers to fulfill vitally important functions. This system of managing each accident scene improves interagency coordination and provides for a safe, controlled working environment. When emergency service personnel within a community believe in the ICS and are led by an individual with the courage and ability to put the ICS in place in an emergency situation, the system *works*.

5

Collision Trauma

OBJECTIVES

At the end of this chapter, you will be able to:

- Explain the practices and procedures necessary for providing safe and efficient care to a vehicle accident trauma patient.
- Correctly define and describe kinematics.
- Correctly describe the basic types of vehicle collisions and their related mechanisms of injury.
- Correctly describe entrapment problems anticipated with each basic type of motor vehicle accident involving occupants in various locations within the vehicle at the time of the collision.
- Correctly define the golden hour, and explain how the concept of the golden hour can influence vehicle rescue activities for a given trauma patient.
- Accurately describe the correct procedures for rapid trauma patient assessment.
- Describe the necessary practices and procedures for the rapid extrication of a selected trauma patient.

Chapter 5 will help you to understand safe and efficient emergency medical procedures and techniques for motor vehicle accident victims. Its medically oriented focus is on various types of vehicle accidents from the point of view of the vehicle occupant. The events that take place in fractions of a second during the collision are detailed to describe the mechanisms of occupant injury, why occupants become trapped within the wreckage, and the special needs of the accident trauma patient.

The relatively new philosophies presented by the nationally recognized continuing education course "PreHospital Trauma Life Support" provide an important understanding of the injury-producing events that take place during an accident. This training program and its companion text, *Prehospital Trauma Life Support* (PHTLS), are primarily oriented toward the advanced-level emergency medical technician. Basic trauma life support or critical trauma care training programs have recently been developed to meet the needs of the basic-level EMT provider. The referenced text is a product of the efforts of the PreHospital Trauma Life Support Committee of the National Association of Emergency Medical Technicians in cooperation with the Committee on Trauma of the American College of Surgeons. Their fascinating study of the science of trauma gives the EMS provider an excellent understanding of the unique needs of the serious trauma patient.

Along with the golden hour concept of trauma patient survival, the PHTLS text emphasizes the need for rapid assessment of the critical trauma patient and the importance of basic treatment for shock and hypoxemia. The challenge for EMS and vehicle rescue personnel lies in the need for rapid removal and transportation to an appropriate medical facility in selected cases of multisystem trauma. Vehicle rescue personnel must complete all their tasks in concert with the EMS crews at the accident scene quickly and efficiently (Fig. 5-1). Efforts must be concentrated on life-threatening patient conditions. Nonthreatening conditions must not distract or delay the delivery of the trauma patient to the medical facility within the golden hour of life.

The preface of the PHTLS text contains a critical statement on patient-handling procedures that is worth repeating here: "A current maxim seems to be that the higher the level of the EMT's certification, the longer the patient is kept in the field. This is a fatal error with trauma patients." Many EMS and vehicle rescue authorities agree with this statement and endorse the excellent PHTLS Course text. The people who worked long and hard for several years to produce this material are to be commended for their courage, dedication, and vision. All medical care providers responsible for patient care in prehospital situations should consider taking this training for the positive impact it will have on their work.

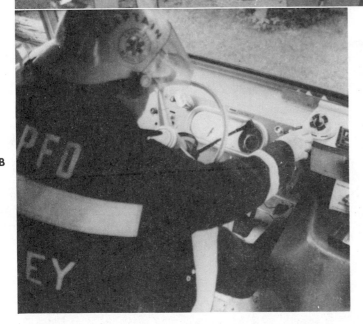

FIG. 5-1 A, EMS crews work with vehicle rescue personnel and law enforcement agencies. **B,** Vehicle operator turns egg timer to 60-minute setting when starting the response to the incident to monitor the trauma patient's golden hour.

KINEMATICS

Think of a motor vehicle accident as a giant real-life puzzle. What you find on arrival is the end result of the collision. Knowledge of the events that preceded the arrival of the emergency crews can tell you how to proceed to solve existing problems. All the pieces of information that fire, medical, and rescue personnel need to accomplish their assigned tasks can generally be found at the accident scene if they are aware of what to look for, how to look, and where to look. Improving your ability to read a wreck and understand the dynamics of a vehicle collision from the occupant's point of view will help you provide better service at the next motor vehicle accident call.

A moving vehicle possesses *kinetic energy* — its energy of motion. When two objects interact, as during a collision, exactly equal and opposite forces result (Fig. 5-2). When the vehicle contacts something that suddenly and violently stops its forward progress, its kinetic energy is transformed into damage to the vehicle. The occupants of the vehicle suffer their traumatic injuries as these energy forces are further transmitted through the vehicle to them. It is the trauma injury that plays the most significant role in this nation's annual automobile injury and death statistics.

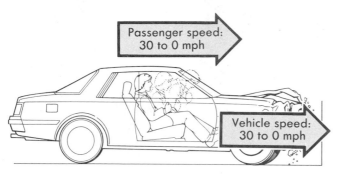

FIG. 5-2 Occupants are traveling at the same speed as the vehicle until the moment of collision.

Collisions within a Collision

A vehicle can be involved in a collision in four basic ways: the deadly head-on or frontal crash, the hazardous rear-end collision, the T-bone or side impact collision, and the rollover (Fig. 5-3). Any vehicle in an accident can undergo several types of collision in the same accident or be involved in two or more collisions in a single accident. A vehicle might be hit broadside, for example, and then roll onto its roof, producing injuries and entrapment problems related to both the side impact collision and the rollover crash. Each accident type presents distinct disentanglement and extrication challenges for vehicle rescue personnel.

For every vehicle collision, there are a series of distinct collision impacts. A typical accident begins when one vehicle contacts another or some stationary object such as a tree or bridge pillar. This impact, the *vehicle* collision, will be either a head-on, rear-end, side impact, or rollover collision. The initial collision

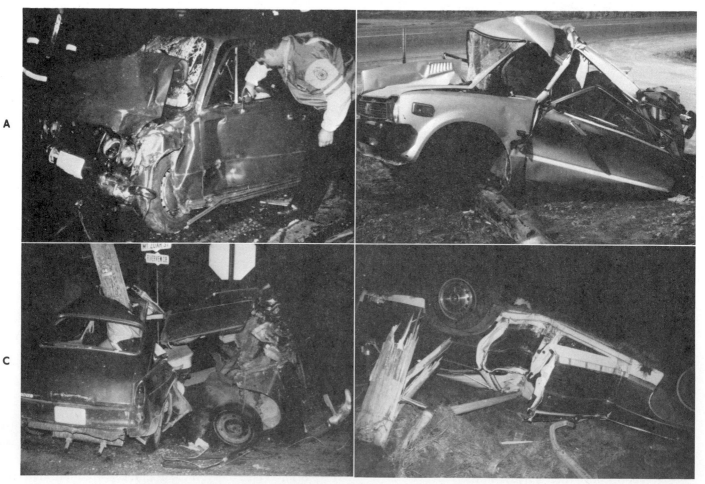

FIG. 5-3 Types of vehicle crashes. **A,** Head-on collision. **B,** Rear-end collision. **C,** T-bone collison. **D,** Rollover collision.

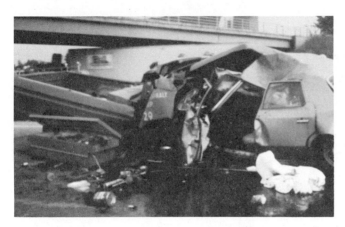

FIG. 5-4 The vehicle collision transforms the energy of motion into a crushing and crumbling of metal. This accident resulted from the automobile driver's decision to commit suicide by driving against expressway traffic at high speed until colliding with a truck. Occupants of both vehicles died in the crash.

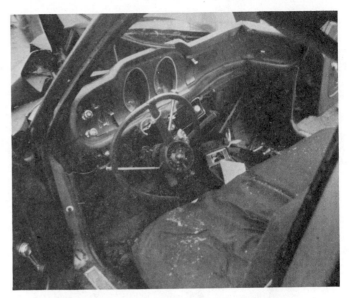

FIG. 5-5 The occupant collision directly injures those inside the vehicle. Note the extreme deformity of the steering wheel ring and supporting spokes by the driver's body as he was thrown forward. The unrestrained front seat passenger was trapped in and under the dash.

transforms the energy of the moving vehicle into damage as it is absorbed first by the exterior body material and then by the vehicle's structural components (Fig. 5-4). Damage to the shape and structure of the vehicle causes potential occupant entrapment within the wreckage as doors jam, roofs crush, and floorboards buckle.

Up to the moment of impact, the occupants of the vehicle are traveling at the same rate of speed and in the same direction as the vehicle itself. A fraction of a second after the initial collision, a second impact occurs — the *occupant* collision, in which the occupants move toward the impacting force until they crash against interior components of the vehicle, smash into another occupant, or collide with loose objects flying about the passenger compartment (Fig. 5-5). Restrained occupants initially impact their seat belt restraint system. Unrestrained occupants move dramatically toward the impact source and then away from it as they collide violently with other passengers or objects in the vehicle's interior (Fig. 5-6). The occupant collision is the principal reason occupants receive traumatic injuries in an accident and explains why they may be trapped by such interior components as the pedals, dashboard, steering wheel, or steering column.

The accident is not over yet. A third distinct impact follows, the *internal organ* collision, which involves the occupant's internal organs hitting the open cavity areas inside the body. The internal organ collison causes many of the serious internal trauma injuries that

the occupants receive. As the human body absorbs portions of the collision energy, it experiences its own compression, bending, tearing, and fracturing forces, both externally and internally. The ensuing effect on the patient depends upon such factors as the individual's age, position within the vehicle, total amount of energy expended during the collison, and use of passenger restraint systems. Table 5-1 shows the number and type of injuries sustained by 139 people involved in frontal collisions compared to the restraint system used.

Thus, in each type of accident, the individual inside the vehicle experiences *at least three separate and distinct collisions.* Each one presents potential injury and entrapment problems that must be dealt with by emergency service personnel on the accident scene. Realizing what has happened to the patient during the brief seconds of the accident event plays a significant role in providing proper care for the collision trauma patient.

MECHANISM OF INJURY

Severe vehicle collisions present great probabilities for fatal injuries. In a typical frontal collision scenario, for example, the vehicle stops or radically slows its forward movement as the occupants, whether restrained or not, continue to move forward within the

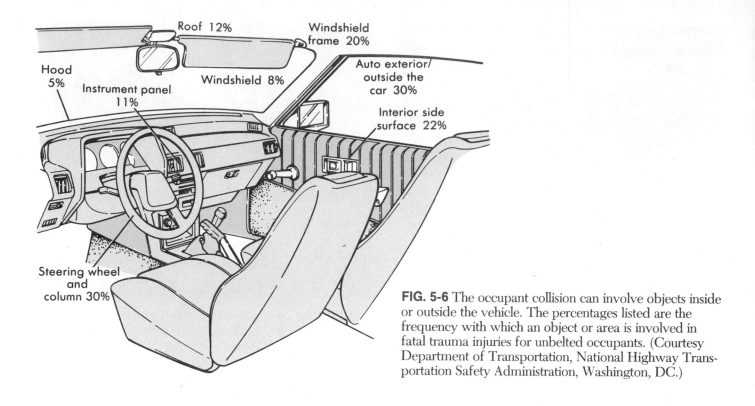

FIG. 5-6 The occupant collision can involve objects inside or outside the vehicle. The percentages listed are the frequency with which an object or area is involved in fatal trauma injuries for unbelted occupants. (Courtesy Department of Transportation, National Highway Transportation Safety Administration, Washington, DC.)

TABLE 5-1 Comparison of Injuries of 139 Unrestrained, Lap-belted, and Lap/Shoulder-Belted Occupants

	Uninjured	Minor Injuries	Moderate Injuries	Severe Injuries	Total
Unrestrained Occupants	4	20	17	16	57
Lap-Belted Occupants	1	16	5	28	50
Lap/Shoulder-Belted Occupants	2	12	10	8	32
TOTAL	7	48	32	52	139

Modified from National Transportation Safety Board: Safety study: performance of lap belts in 26 frontal crashes, Pub No 917006, Washington, DC, 1986.

passenger compartment. Those riding in the front seat have a high probability of receiving serious head injuries. The American College of Surgeons Committee on Trauma reported in 1983 that brain damage occurs in more than 50% of all vehicular accident fatalities, noting that what may seem simple or trivial head trauma can produce lethal intracranial hemorrhages. Head injuries therefore require continued observation and evaluation throughout the medic's contact period with the patient.

The driver may sustain head injuries from contact with the steering wheel, steering column, front windshield, side windows, dashboard, even the interior portions of the roof or roof posts. Other front seat occupants, whether belted or unbelted, may also contact the interior roof headliner area, roof posts, or dashboard components nearest them (Fig. 5-7). Occupants in the rear of the vehicle are also thrown forward in a head-on collision. The major difference between these occupants and those in the front seat is that they are less likely to contact the vehicle's injury-producing dashboard area components. Rear seat occupants, if restrained by lap belts or rear seat lap and shoulder belt combination systems (Fig. 5-8), can still receive head injuries from contact with the back of the front seat as it may be displaced rearward by

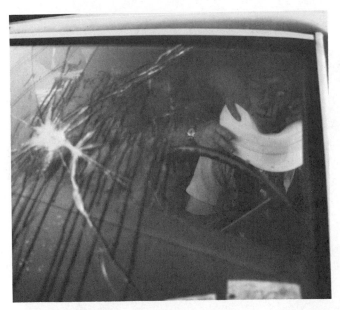

FIG. 5-7 Head injuries occur during occupant collision.

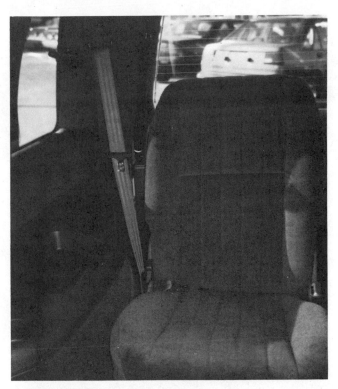

FIG. 5-8 All but the driver and front passenger seats in GM's newest plastic vans are readily removable bucket seats, each with its own lap and shoulder harness restraint.

the collision forces. These passengers are also susceptible to injury from objects placed on the rear window shelf or the cargo areas as these items rocket about the interior passenger compartment area.

Unrestrained rear seat occupants may be thrown forward or rearward, bounced up or down, or even ejected from the vehicle during the collision dynamics. If thrown into the front passenger area, they too become susceptible to injury from vehicle glass, steering wheel and column, dashboard, and roof structure. Injuries resulting from contact with the front windshield safety glass may cause massive external damage to the head, face, and scalp. These contusions and lacerations can make for a very ugly accident scene. The presence of an extra plastic lamination layer on newer windshields significantly reduces these terrible windshield-induced injuries. Internal head trauma injuries, less readily visible, may include hematoma, cerebral edema, decreased oxygen perfusion of the brain, concussion, increased intracranial pressure, and fractures.

Any head injury indicates the need for head, neck, and spine immobilization measures to be undertaken. EMS personnel need to be proficient in immobilization procedures for all sizes, ages, and shapes of occupants who could become trapped within a wreckage (Fig. 5-9). Immobilization procedures for accident victims who have been ejected or are otherwise outside the vehicle must also be practiced (Fig. 5-10). Accident victims found standing outside the

vehicle when first contacted by EMS workers may require implementation of the "standing take down" longboard immobilization technique to receive appropriate care.

Airway management problems can develop with a traumatic head injury if the upper airway becomes obstructed by the individual's tongue, edema, or a foreign body such as food or teeth. The blunt chest trauma injuries sustained by vehicle occupants in head-on collisions are caused by the impact between the thoracic area and the portions of the vehicle. The driver is apt to be thrust into the steering wheel and steering column, resulting in injuries like multiple rib fractures, fractures to the sternum, and flail chest. Cardiac compression occurs when the heart is crushed between the sternum and the vertebral column. A fractured rib may puncture the lung, resulting in a pneumothorax condition. Compression forces working against the internal organs may also yield tremendous tearing or shearing stresses inside the body, damaging the aorta and causing the patient to bleed to death internally if surgical intervention is not provided in time (Fig. 5-11).

Collision victims, particularly the driver, can also

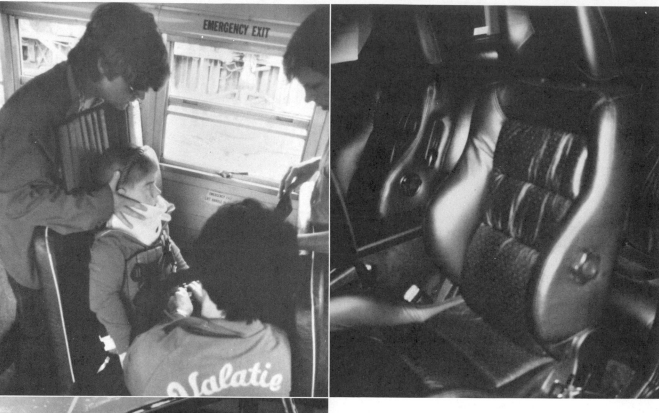

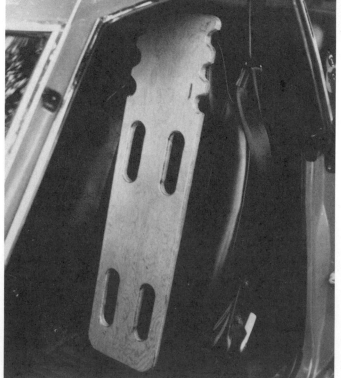

FIG. 5-9 A, A lifelike rescue mannequin allows EMS personnel to safely practice patient packaging and handling. **B,** Curvature and high sides of bucket seats popular with sports car manufacturers require EMS personnel to provide flexible immobilization device. **C,** Homemade "skinny board" used to properly immobilize seated patient.

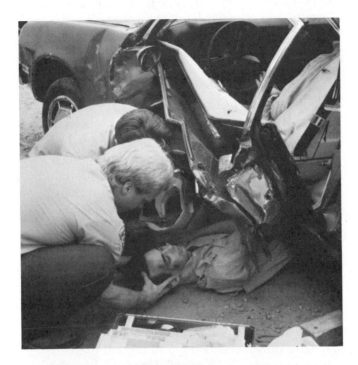

FIG. 5-10 EMS personnel must be proficient in immobilization and proper handling techniques for patients ejected or otherwise outside of vehicles.

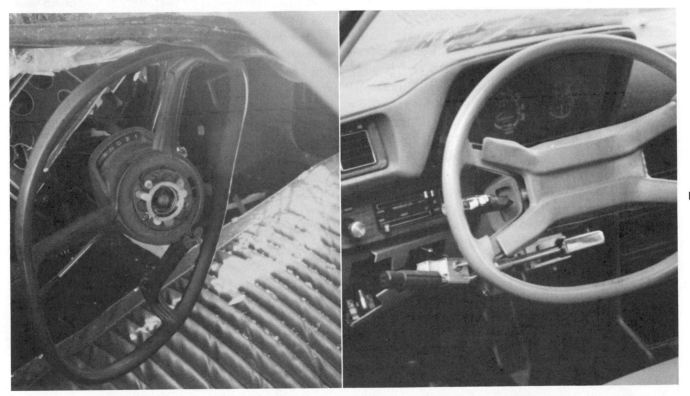

A   B

FIG. 5-11 A, Contact with interior vehicle components can produce internal trauma injuries. **B,** A vehicle designed for a disabled person may give clues to the patient's handicap. The presence of driver control equipment, however, does not always indicate that the driver is handicapped.

receive blunt or penetrating trauma injuries to their abdomen during occupant collisions. Many of the body's major organs are extremely vulnerable to damage in the head-on crash scenario. Blunt trauma may result from abdominal compression against the occupant's seat belt and lap belt assembly, contact with the steering wheel ring, the steering column, the dashboard, or other objects inside and outside the vehicle. Crushing of the internal organs may even cause the spleen and liver to fracture and hemorrhage.

The EMS and rescue community now knows that the lap-belt-only style of passenger restraint systems still in use can cause injury or death, particularly in frontal collisions. Deceleration stresses induced by these systems may damage internal organs such as the spleen, kidneys, bowels, and stomach, any of which may rupture and hemorrhage. The occupant's pelvis may also be severely fractured resulting in internal hemorrhaging. The National Transportation Safety Board performed a safety study in 1986 and addressed this issue. The Safety Board believes that many emergency medical personnel (including those operating ambulance services), police, fire/rescue personnel, emergency room nurses and physicians, and others called on to treat motor vehicle crash victims remain unaware of the possibility and gravity of seat belt-induced injuries. Although the Board found many articles in leading medical journals concerning this problem, it appears that there is still a widespread lack of understanding in this area. In 6 cases reviewed by the Board, out of the 26 in which a lap-belted person was involved (nearly 25%), there was serious question about the adequacy of the medical handling of the lap-belted victim. In some cases there was little doubt that poor diagnosis and inadequate treatment contributed to the death of a person who might well have survived with prompt, appropriate treatment. As more people begin to use their belt systems, it becomes important for the medical community to educate itself about the type of injuries they may be called on to diagnose and treat and take action to ensure that this knowledge is rapidly and effectively disseminated to those who will need it.

Trauma patients who have received such internal injuries may appear stable upon visual examination, only to suddenly deteriorate. There may be no early signs of shock because internal blood loss, contained within the body cavity, slows the onslaught of shock. The conscious, "walking wounded" patient, even with potential cervical spine injuries, may attempt to persuade medical care providers at the accident scene that medical attention is not necessary. Only by reading the vehicle closely and accurately and making an effort to check for all potential mechanisms of injury can EMS personnel anticipate these internal injury problems. As these trauma patients deteriorate physically, they become walking time bombs. Possible trauma in the abdominal area alone can be serious enough to cause death.

Internal trauma injuries induced by lap belts can be difficult to diagnose by medical personnel in the field. Any vehicle accident victim who was wearing a seat belt of any type should be evaluated for internal injuries, especially to the vulnerable abdominal region. Any person involved in a serious auto accident who was wearing a lap-belt-only restraint should be transported to a medical facility regardless of a lack of complaints or apparent injury symptoms. Internal injuries may not be apparent until several hours after the accident. Rapid assessment at the scene and prompt transport to a medical facility are crucial to the survival of patients with serious injuries. They truly may have only a golden hour of life left to live.

In one case studied by the Safety Board an 82-year-old woman was involved in a side-impact collision with a bus; the woman was restrained by a lap belt only. About 28 hours after the crash, medical personnel observed a drop in blood pressure that was accompanied by the onset of a rapid pulse. Internal x rays were taken almost 3 hours later, followed by an exploratory laparotomy. The woman died on the operating table. She was found to have sustained multiple tears in the mesentery, perforation of the bowel, and a major contusion of the abdomen. The probable source of these injuries was the lap belt.

When field-level EMS providers deliver the trauma patient to a medical facility, a brief report must accompany the patient history information advising the attending physician what type of passenger restraint system was in use at the time of the collision and how it was worn (high or low, loose or snug) on the occupant. As a result of mandatory seat belt legislation, some vehicle occupants reluctantly wear their shoulder harness seat belt assembly but use it improperly. It is becoming more common to find occupants, especially shorter-height individuals, with the shoulder harness belt placed under their arm in an attempt to be more comfortable. This procedure, besides being unauthorized, can lead to serious internal injuries. The occupant's ribs can be fractured by the blunt trauma of a collision, driving the free ends of the ribs into the lung or heart.

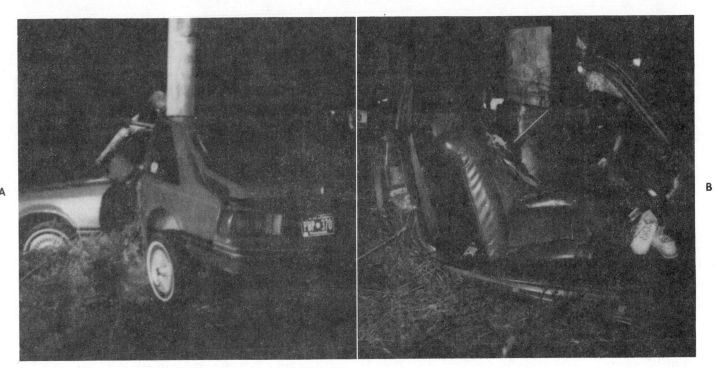

FIG. 5-12 Photographs accompanying patients to the trauma or medical facility showing **A**, the exterior view and **B**, the interior view.

Understanding where and how the patient was injured is important not only for those in the field but also for those at the trauma center or medical facility. To assist doctors and surgeons in understanding the mechanism of injury to a particular patient, some EMS or rescue units carry an instant print camera in their equipment inventory. The rescuers take at least two photos, one of the damaged exterior of the vehicle and a second of the damaged vehicle interior (Fig. 5-12). These photos are transported with the patient either by ambulance or air transport to the medical facility and delivered as part of the patient's medical report.

People who realize that a collision is imminent will spontaneously tense all their body muscles, instantly inhale, and hold their breath through the brief crash scenario. All these reactions stem from our basic animal instinct for survival and occur almost automatically. Think about an unsuspecting person's reaction when you sneak up from behind and startle the person. The tensing and inhaling reflexes are very similar. When you hold your breath, your lungs are inflated. The energy from a collision impact may then cause these hollow organs to rupture violently. This is referred to as the "paper bag effect" by EMS authorities.

The instantaneous tensing of the body's muscles can result in fracture and dislocation injuries because of a rigid body. Collision victims, stiff-legged and bracing for the crash, have actually had their legs and feet driven right through the floorboards. Professional emergency vehicle driving instructor Richard Turner, who once worked as a movie stunt driver, was asked how he routinely survived such planned collisions. His reply bears remembering. Using unusual mental discipline, Dick Turner trained himself to go completely limp at the exact moment of the collision. With a secure lap and shoulder belt restraining him, his limp body was able to roll with the punches time and time again.

While operating under the influence of alcohol, drunk drivers survive some relatively serious crashes with surprisingly few injuries because of their dulled reflexes. Their comprehension of the events unfolding before them is slowed to the point that they do not tense in anticipation of the crash. They simply ride out the collision dynamics. This is no endorsement to drive while intoxicated. On the contrary, it must be remembered that it is the intoxicated condition that got the individual into the crash situation in the first place.

Penetrating trauma injuries may result from contact with sharp, piercing, or cylindrical-shaped vehicle

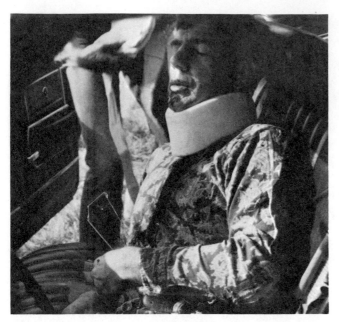

FIG. 5-13 EMS personnel must be trained in proper procedures for handling impaled objects such as glass shards or metal objects.

components. For example, impalement may occur if the gear selector lever, mounted either at the steering column or on the floorboard area, impales the patient. Occupants may also be impaled by turn signal levers, dashboard protrusions, emergency brake controls, broken glass, brake or clutch pedals, and even solid, one-piece radio antennas (Fig. 5-13). Parts flying off other vehicles or outside items such as highway fence posts, railings, trees, or buildings may protrude into the vehicle during the collision. A vehicle rescue instructor from Texas tells of an accident in which the lone driver of a pickup truck had three screwdrivers impaled in his body. The screwdrivers were from an open tool box that was in the passenger compartment of the truck before the rollover collision.

It is extremely important for the injured patient that medical personnel recognize the possibility of head, brain, and spinal injury during the initial assessment work. The serious potential of this type of trauma injury must be a central focus of all emergency scene activities evolving around the patient. EMS personnel that underestimate the potential for spinal injury are negligent in their duty to both the patient and the medical profession. Each motor vehicle accident patient must be treated as if that person has received spinal injuries. Failure to do so can cause problems for both patient and medical personnel. The central nervous system does not regenerate. We cannot afford mistakes in patient care with these types of injuries.

Multimillion-dollar lawsuits have been successfully argued in jury trials against good-intentioned EMS providers when their action or lack of action was found to have caused spinal system damage resulting in crippling or fatal injuries. When personnel are in doubt about the need for spinal immobilization, the most prudent medical philosophy is to initiate spinal immobilization procedures, regardless of the patient's lack of motor or sensory deficits. Physicians can attest to the fact that a spine injury cannot be ruled out just because a patient is walking, standing, or moving normally. The patient may have no apparent motor, sensory, or circulatory deficit and report no obvious spinal system pain, point tenderness, or deformity. A spinal injury can only be ruled out by x-ray and other neurological examination work at a medical facility.

The more vehicle damage created during the collision, the greater or more severe the probable injuries to the occupants. Remember, some of the energy possessed by the vehicle in motion manifests itself as a powerfully destructive force that acts directly against the patient. A 150-lb person in a relatively low-speed collision can have in excess of 4500 lb of force exerted on the body. The weight of the average human head alone can apply over 750 lb of force to damage the cervical spine.

The impact of these forces on the occupant's spine can yield a variety of injuries depending on the type of vehicle accident, the exact forces generated by the collision, the person's age and physical condition, and the position in the vehicle at the time of the initial and subsequent impacts. Those closest to the impact zone, the area nearest the source of the impact, are most prone to severe injury. The potential for spinal injury is always there, regardless of the type of collision or the crash dynamics. It is not just a rear or front collision that causes head, neck, and spine trauma.

The head, neck, and spine of front seat occupants involved in a collision are susceptible to injury from many different sources. For the driver, direct contact with the steering wheel and column, resulting in facial and abdominal injuries, may also result in spinal column injury. The violent force of the body striking the components of a vehicle can transect the spinal cord either partially or completely. The crushing of the structure of the vehicle into and onto the occupants inside may compress their spinal column, resulting in a pinching injury to the spinal cord. This same compression impact can also produce compression fractures of the vertebrae at any point along the spine.

As the occupants move and strike interior portions

of the auto, the stresses may dislodge small fragments of bone from a fracture of the vertebrae or twist and turn the body with enough force to displace the vertebrae. Whiplash injury is an example of such spinal displacement. It can also indicate violent cervical extension/flexion injuries to the spine, that may actually stretch the spinal cord. Occupants also receive bruises as they collide with various objects inside the vehicle, causing swelling that can quickly cause a reduction in blood supply to portions of the body.

Rear seat occupants can also receive serious spinal injuries. In a head-on collision, these persons can receive head, face, and upper body injuries when the back of the front seat, roof, door posts, roof posts, and other components of the vehicle are forced rearward and inward. Rear seat occupants restrained by lap style seat belts may strike the back of the front seat, forcing the head backward and severely stressing the spinal column.

Experience has demonstrated that, with all other factors being equal, occupants not restrained within the vehicle are more likely to receive injuries. Spinal immobilization procedures should be undertaken when the mechanism of injury is apparent, the patient has received an injury above the clavicle, or a head injury has produced a change in mental status. Rescuers should ensure that every effort is made to meet the patient's needs for the ABCs of basic life support while at the same time not compromising any further injury to the spinal system.

In most vehicle accidents, whether the patient is trapped within the wreckage or not, protection and immobilization of the head, neck, and spine can and should be accomplished in the location where the patient is found by medical personnel. If this location is inside the vehicle, EMS personnel must work in conjunction with rescue personnel to maintain the integrity of the patient's spinal column. If, however, patients are in a location that presents an immediate threat to their continued survival, they may be rapidly extricated from the vehicle.

In a classic example of just such a situation, a woman driving a two-door vehicle pulled into a gas station along a busy highway. While approaching the gas pumps, an 18-wheel tractor-trailer careened off the expressway, jackknifed across the parking lot of the gas station, and smashed into her car, crushing it against the fuel pumps and igniting a quick, hot fire burning under her vehicle.

In dramatic photographs of the incident taken by a passing amateur photographer, the woman is seen trapped inside the wreckage screaming for help while flames begin to surround her. The windshield glass had blown out of its opening upon impact with the truck. This allowed the gas station attendant and another citizen to use a garden hose to spray a meager stream of water inside the car and onto the woman.

Under these circumstances, it would have been proper for the citizen rescuers to try to remove the woman from her burning vehicle before she received any medical treatment. Her life was in great jeopardy at this point, as were the lives of the helpers. But the people on the scene were unable to get the woman, who was obese, out of the vehicle. Instead, they wet her down enough with the garden hose to keep the fire from harming her. The fire department arrived, extinguished the fire, stabilized the scene, and treated the woman in the vehicle. Standard disentanglement procedures were then used to remove her from the wreckage.

Emergency service providers may also move a patient before complete immobilization when life-threatening injuries are present. A widely distributed photograph used in campaigns to rid our highways of drunk drivers shows an accident victim being rushed into a hospital emergency room. A close look at the medical attention the patient is receiving reveals that there is no cervical collar, backboard, or longboard in place. Although this is a serious omission in most situations, this patient has had both legs traumatically amputated above the knees. The rush is a justifiable one to save this person's life.

Rapid extrication before completing spinal immobilization procedures is also justified for patients in cardiac arrest, respiratory arrest, or other unstable conditions. It is generally accepted that CPR is difficult or ineffective when the patient is in a sitting position. The decision to move a patient before standard immobilizing and packaging is a judgment call that must be made quickly by medically trained personnel (Fig. 5-14). A patient should not, however, be moved before immobilization work simply for the convenience of medical or rescue personnel. Such negligence signifies a lack of training and education on the part of the emergency service providers.

Medical personnel working on a trauma patient must possess the skills necessary to rapidly administer basic life support measures, provide proper treatment for shock, and initiate effective and proper C-spine immobilization. They must also be sufficiently aware of vehicle rescue procedures to operate safely within the tangled wreckage and to know which procedures

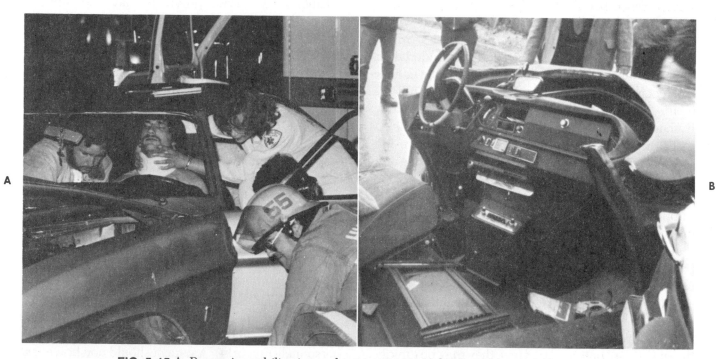

FIG. 5-14 A, Rapid patient extrication is warranted when the condition of the patient is deteriorating rapidly and surgical intervention is required to save a life. **B,** Total roof removal permits rapid patient extrication.

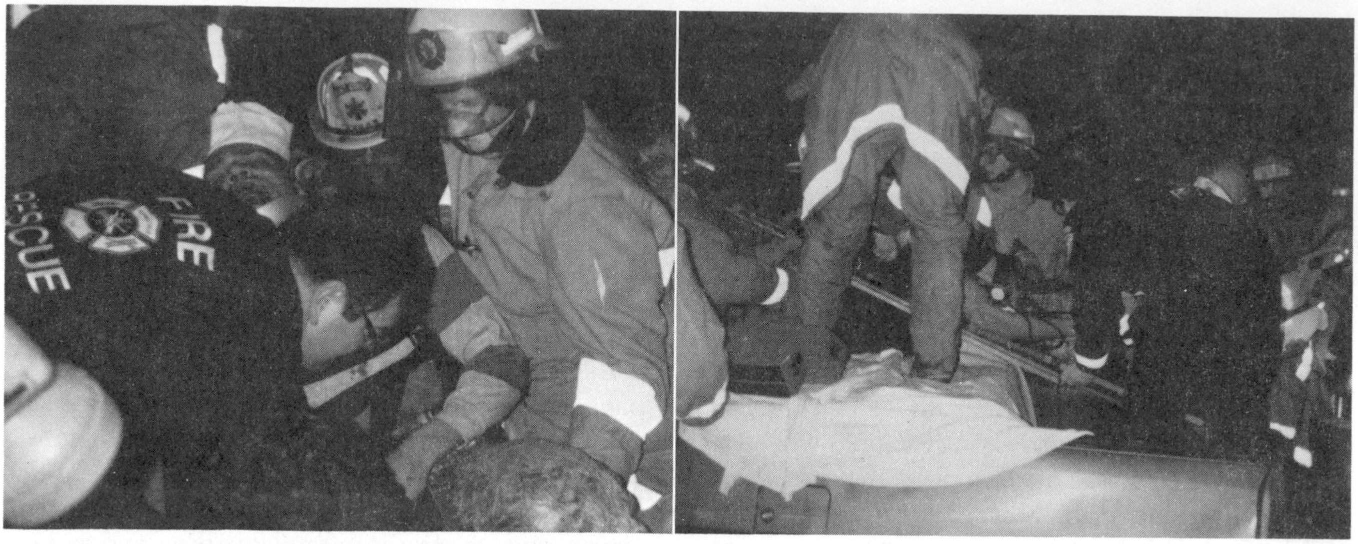

FIG. 5-15 A, Proper immobilization and extrication procedures are hampered by delays in roof removal. **B,** Remove the vehicle from the victim before removing the victim from the vehicle.

will aid them in their patient care and extrication. Successful spinal immobilization of a trapped person is difficult or impossible to achieve deep inside a damaged vehicle. This is particularly true when a vehicle's roof is buckled downward or crushed inward. Rescue personnel, working in a coordinated effort with the medical personnel, can remove the offending portions of the vehicle in a brief period of time. The time invested by rescue personnel in removing all of the roof, for example, allows for the most effective and time-efficient spinal immobilization procedures to be accomplished, with noticeable benefits to overall patient care (Fig. 5-15).

Accident victims often receive traumatic injuries to

their extremities that appear very grotesque, such as open wounds, contusions or hematomas, sprains, strains, dislocations, fractures, and burns. These extremity injuries are likely to receive much attention because they are easily recognized, readily accessible, and familiar to medical care providers.

Critical, life-threatening conditions must always, however, take precedence over less serious injuries. EMS and vehicle rescue personnel must not let extremity injuries distract them from potentially critical trauma injuries. Only two extremity injuries are considered by medical authorities as having the potential to be life-threatening. Serious external bleeding is one, requiring priority action by medical personnel, and the presence of internal bleeding in the upper leg associated with a fractured femur is the other.

Assessment of the accident patient by EMS crews indicates whether the patient has received an isolated local extremity injury or is instead a multisystems trauma injury patient. Multisystems patients must be rapidly immobilized on a longboard as their life-threatening conditions are addressed. Medics must not lose time treating a low-priority injury in the field. Their focus must be on what is critical for the patient's survival.

Motor vehicle accidents can result in burn injuries to vehicle occupants, bystanders, and emergency service personnel. Thermal burn injuries stem from contact with hot engines, engine fluids such as oil or antifreeze solutions, hot exhaust systems, and catalytic converters. Death or serious electrical burn injuries can result from contact with downed electric wires or the vehicle's electrical system. Chemical burn injuries can also occur when, for example, contact is made with the liquid acid solution leaking from a damaged vehicle battery. In addition, an automobile's trunk may contain pesticides, chemicals for pool chlorination, or other compounds that can cause respiratory or skin chemical burn injuries on contact.

Acceptable, state-of-the-art prehospital care for burn injuries must be thoroughly understood by vehicle rescue personnel. Their training must give them the conditioned ability to act quickly and correctly to assess the accident situation without exposing themselves or others to injury. Effective action must be taken to stop the burning by moving the patient from contact with the heat source and cooling the burn injury. Effective life support measures must be maintained through continuing contact with the patient. As with all multisystems trauma injury patients, there should be rapid evaluation, adequate medical intervention and life support, and transportation without delay to an appropriate medical facility.

SPECIAL TRAUMA CONSIDERATIONS
Rear-End Collisions

Each motor vehicle collision has its own inherent style, almost an identifiable "personality" of destruction to the vehicle and injury and death to its occupants. Injury-producing events that occur during certain collisions need to be looked at with respect to their special considerations of injury trauma.

For those inside a vehicle, a rear-end collision is actually two collisions in one. Consider the movements that we make when riding in a vehicle that brakes hard to come to a complete stop. As it slows, we move forward. When the motion of the vehicle stops completely, we feel ourselves suddenly moving in the opposite direction. The vehicle itself may even rock back and forth.

A rear-end collision causes this same back-and-forth movement. The initial rear-end impact throws the occupants toward the rear of the vehicle, but at the second the momentum stops, they are rocked away from the source of the impact. The energy of the rear-end collision may propel the impacted vehicle forward, causing it to hit something in front of it and subjecting it to both a rear-end collision and a frontal impact (Fig. 5-16). This typically happens in a chain

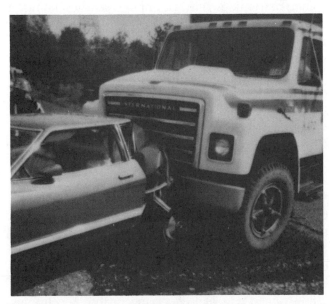

FIG. 5-16 Occupants of vehicles involved in rear-end collisions undergo severe forward and rearward flexing of their heads, necks, and spines.

FIG. 5-17 A, Rear-end collisions involve potential entrapment concerns when the body of the vehicle is shortened or compressed. **B,** The mechanisms of injury include head, neck, and spinal trauma; contact with the vehicle glass or structure; and crushing trauma.

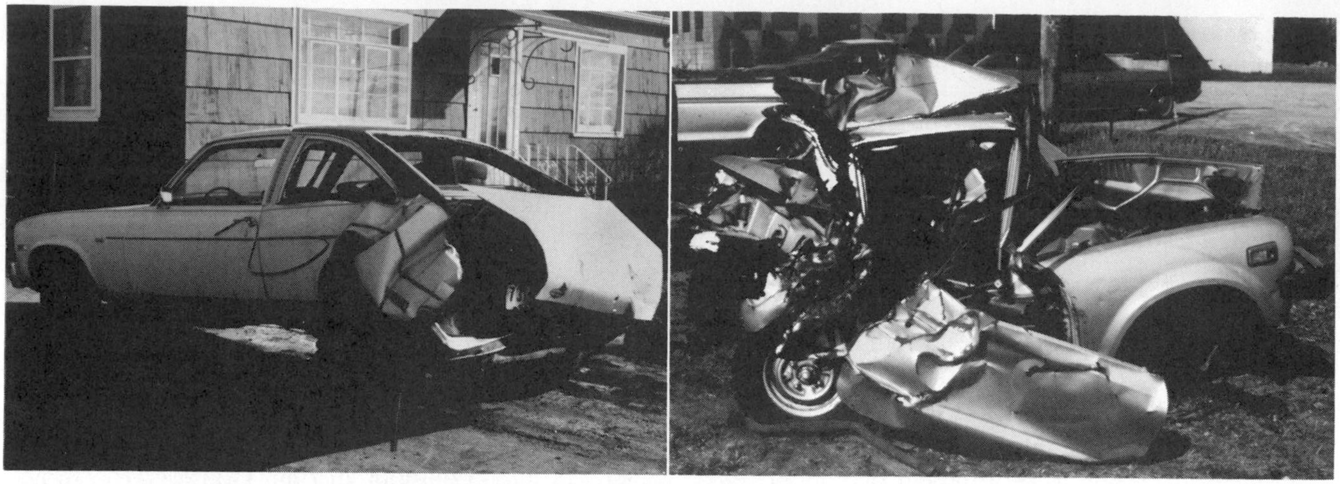

reaction collision involving a series of vehicles in a single line.

In a basic rear-end collision, injuries occur as the vehicle being struck moves instantly and sometimes violently forward. The occupants inside are suddenly pressed backward into their seat by the rearward acceleration forces as their legs and lower body move with the vehicle. At the same time, their arms and upper body are stretched upward and rearward as they are thrust toward the point of impact at the rear of the vehicle. This action places extreme stresses on the person's body, particularly the head, neck, and spine. Extremities may be injured as they come in contact with components of the vehicle. Internal injuries occur as the forces generated during the collision impact against the patient's body.

In the next instant, the momentum abruptly changes direction, throwing the occupants forward and causing injuries typical of head-on collisions. These injuries affect the head and face, spine, chest, and abdomen (Fig. 5-17). The occupant's spine can receive extension and flexion cervical injuries. Unrestrained occupants are violently moved inside the vehicle until the collision runs out of energy. They are entangled by components of the vehicle being damaged, or like unguided missiles, they are ejected from the vehicle. Experience has shown that those persons who are ejected during collisions are more likely to be fatally injured than those who remain inside the vehicle. Unrestrained rear seat occupants or those occupying the rear areas of such vehicles as station wagons or mini vans can, upon impact, be instantly ejected

through rear or side window openings. Unrestrained front seat occupants may be thrown out side windows or door openings or tossed into the rear passenger areas of the vehicle.

Side Impact Collisions

The T-bone or side impact collision occurs when a vehicle is struck along one of its sides, generally at a point somewhere between the front door hinge and the rear door latch area. When impacted, this vulnerable area can greatly distort the entire structure of the vehicle. The T-bone collision can damage a vehicle so that its make and model are barely recognizable.

According to the National Highway Traffic Safety Administration, nearly 8000 people die in side impact crashes each year in the United States. Of the total, 47% die as a result of head injuries, which often occur because they are ejected from the vehicle. This is approximately 30% of all U.S. automobile occupant deaths. Another 23,500 persons are severely injured. Two thirds of side impact fatalities occur in vehicle-to-vehicle collisions. Crashes into poles, trees, and other fixed objects like bridge abutments claim the rest. EMS personnel know that high-speed side impact collisions can cause tremendous death and destruction.

For the occupants of the vehicle struck broadside, the collision is a combination of impacts. Regardless of whether the vehicle moved toward a fixed object or was impacted by a moving vehicle, the occupants initially move toward the source of the impact. This is true of all types of collisions. In the T-bone collision

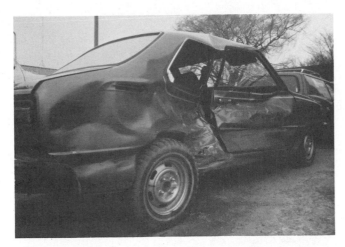

FIG. 5-18 In a T-bone collision the reaction forces occupants toward the initial thrust then moves them away from the initial impact area.

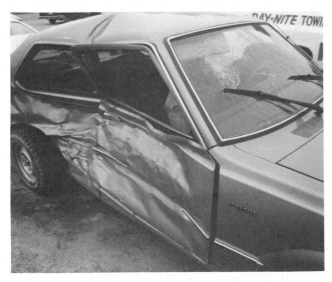

FIG. 5-19 Potential mechanisms of injury in T-bone collisions include vehicle door impingements, glass breakage, and facial contact with laminated windshield glass.

the reaction forces to this initial thrust then move the occupants away from the initial impact area (Fig. 5-18). In essence, the occupants undergo a "one-two" punch as they are hit first from one side, then from the other.

Injuries that evolve from this "action-reaction" scenario include trauma to the patient's head and face from impact with interior vehicle components, broken window glass, other occupants, loose items inside the vehicle, or contact with outside objects (Fig. 5-19). Spinal injuries may occur as the person is torqued back and forth inside the vehicle. Occupants

of side impact collisions require immediate attention to the head, neck, and spine. Chest, abdominal, and other internal injuries occur as those seated nearest the initial collision side are hit and pressed against the inside of the side door and roof post. If the vehicle is hit on the driver's side, an unrestrained front seat passenger may be thrust across the front seat toward the impact. During this movement, they can hit the steering wheel and column, the gear selector lever, or other vehicle components inside or outside the vehicle. Restrained or unrestrained occupants can receive injuries to extremities, again from the stresses and contact of the side-to-side impact action.

When severe impact forces are generated during the collision, occupants may be impaled by interior door knobs, cranks, or armrests. The vehicle's own side door collision beam may impale the occupants. Vehicle rescue and EMS personnel must constantly be on the alert for the presence of impaled objects, especially with side-impact collision patients.

Rollover Collisions

The rollover collision is truly a combination of accident types. Unlike trained circus animals, vehicles cannot roll over by themselves from a stationary point. They must be acted upon by outside forces that create the momentum necessary for the vehicle to complete the rollover maneuver. A vehicle can rotate or roll in three different ways. Most commonly, vehicles roll in line with their long axis, such as when a vehicle rolls onto its side or its roof. The forces may be strong enough for the vehicle to actually complete a 360-degree rotation one or more times.

A vehicle involved in a rollover collision may also rotate about its center axis, such as when hit broadside at a point near the front or rear of the vehicle. In the more unusual rollover accident, the vehicle rolls end over end about its short axis, as when a moving vehicle leaves a roadway and plunges down an embankment toward a lower level. The vehicle hits the ground first in a frontal collision, and the rear of the vehicle then rotates upward and forward, turning the vehicle upside down (Fig. 5-20). The rear of the vehicle then hits the ground as the end-over-end rotation continues. As the momentum ceases or an object such as a tree stops the travel of the vehicle, this violently destructive accident comes to an end. This collision scenario is fortunately not a frequent occurrence.

The extent of occupant injuries and entrapment in a rollover collision is influenced primarily by the

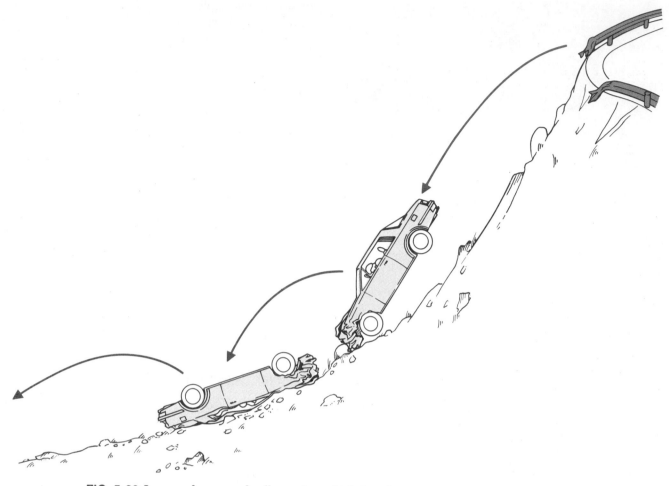

FIG. 5-20 In an end-over-end rollover the vehicle hits the ground first in a frontal collision, rotates upward and forward, turning the vehicle upside down. The vehicle hits the ground again as the rotation continues.

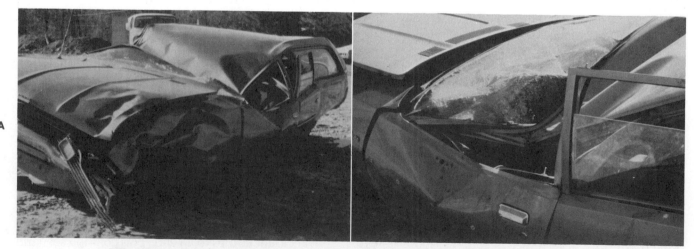

FIG. 5-21 A, Rollover collisions can produce complex vehicle extrication problems. **B,** Sufficient energy can be generated to crush the entire roof structure into the passenger compartment.

amount of force released during the rollover. A gentle 90-degree roll onto one edge is quite different from a series of complete high-speed, end-over-end rolls down an embankment. The destruction of both the vehicle and its occupants is directly related to the energy involved in the rollover crash (Fig. 5-21).

As a rollover occurs, the occupants either move first toward the initial impacting force or are thrust toward the lower side of the vehicle. If an accident takes place at an intersection, for example, the first impact might be a side impact collision along one side of the vehicle. The impacted vehicle immediately begins to rotate like a spinning top while its wheels remain on the roadway. As the spin continues, the occupants are thrown to the outside areas of the passenger compartment. Given sufficient momentum, one side of the vehicle may raise off the ground causing not only a spinning rotation but a rolling action. Any unrestrained persons and loose objects inside the vehicle are tossed around like clothes tumbling in a clothes dryer. The injury potential increases with each and every roll sequence. In a high-speed rollover the centrifugal force is so great inside the vehicle that passengers and loose objects literally stick to the vehicle until the rolls slow down. The next-to-the-last or final roll may be slow enough for the tumbling action to occur.

Restrained occupants inside a rollover accident vehicle generally remain inside during the crash sequence. Unrestrained passengers, however, are likely to be ejected if there is significant speed associated with the rollover. During the rolling of the vehicle, these passengers are thrust outward by centrifugal force. A nearby window or door opening may be sufficient to eject them from the vehicle. The restrained passenger who rides it out can survive this accident in most cases.

The rollover collision can be very destructive to the vehicle. Side structural areas, along with doors and roof areas, buckle inward, trapping the occupants inside a *shrink wrap* package. Vehicle rescue and EMS personnel have their work cut out for them in successfully providing patient care, effective disentanglement, and safe patient extrication (Fig. 5-22).

If the final resting position of the vehicle is upside down, rescue and medical personnel are confronted with another challenge. Rescue personnel must perform their tasks on a vehicle that is not only damaged but upside down. This positioning causes orientation problems in that components are upside down and backwards from their conventional positions.

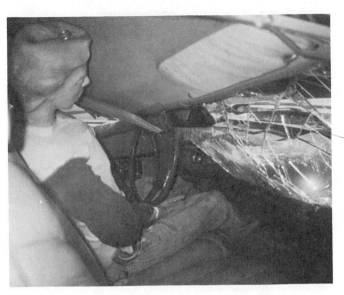

FIG. 5-22 Mechanisms of injury in rollover collisions (as depicted in this simulation) include crushing of the vehicle's structure, entrapment by interior components, and contact with broken or shattered glass.

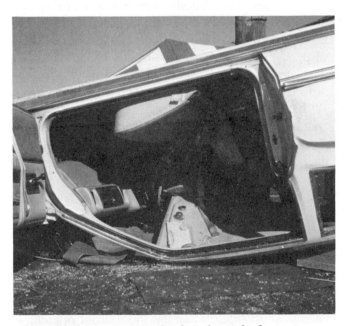

FIG. 5-23 Occupants may be found upside down, restrained by their lap belt or shoulder harness assembly. Note the removal of the back of the front seat to extricate the patients.

Given the current trend of increased use of vehicle seat belts, occupants may be more frequently found suspended in the upside-down position, restrained by their belt inside their overturned vehicle (Fig. 5-23). Medics must practice providing proper care for injured patients located in this unusual position. Because

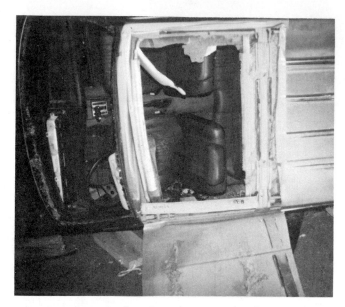

FIG. 5-24 A sunroof evolution may not be the most effective method of opening the roof for patient extrication.

medical immobilization procedures from simple C-collar placement through shortboard and longboard work are more difficult when the patient is suspended, emergency care providers should practice this special type of extrication in training sessions before having to accomplish it at real-world incidents. With the United States and some Canadian provinces enacting mandatory seat belt legislation and many states adopting mandatory child restraint legislation, the possibility of finding a suspended patient becomes increasingly real.

If the vehicle that has rolled over is found on its side or edge, patients can be extricated through the area formerly occupied by the roof. *Total roof removal* allows for maximum access to the passenger compartment and the greatest degree of efficiency and safety during the extrication process. There are still rescue teams who work to remove occupants from a vehicle on its side by making the sunroof opening in the sheetmetal of the roof skin (Fig. 5-24). This is a noisy and time-consuming task. For injured persons and medics inside it may well be the single noisiest rescue job that could possibly be performed on the vehicle. These well-intentioned rescue teams must change their practices and procedures from the old sunroof method to the state-of-the-art technique of total roof removal. There is no excuse for anything less.

Rollover collisions of any variety are complex problems for responding emergency service providers.

Injury scenarios include all possible combinations, and the degree of destruction to the vehicle can turn even the most basic disentanglement and extrication procedure into an involved operation that will challenge trained crews to their fullest.

EMS RESPONSIBILITY AT MOTOR VEHICLE ACCIDENTS

Once an injured or trapped person is contacted, the medic/patient relationship is officially established. The injured person is now technically our patient and, legally and morally, becomes the direct responsibility of the emergency medical care providers. With this understanding comes the realization that EMS personnel must accept certain responsibilities at an accident scene and fulfill certain assignments. Correct fulfillment of these tasks results in the most appropriate care being rendered to the patient with the greatest regard for safety of all concerned.

If first to arrive at the emergency scene, EMS personnel must establish command, issue a brief report on the situation, and complete an incident size up (Fig. 5-25). At some time during all this early activity as hazards are controlled and the scene is stabilized, contact with the injured patient must be established. The medic/patient contact continues

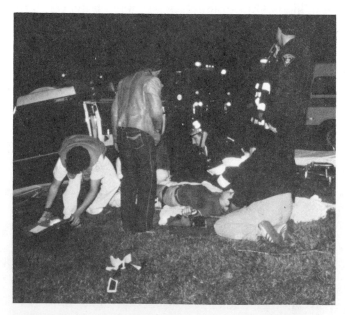

FIG. 5-25 Size-up activities for EMS personnel include determining the number and locations of patients, assessing degrees of injury and entrapment, and establishing priorities for patient care.

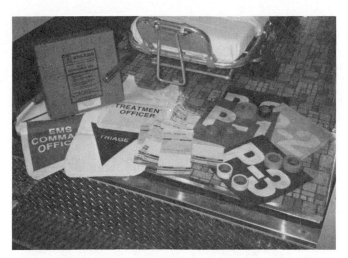

FIG. 5-26 Basic field unit MCI response and triage kit.

from that point throughout the entire process of rescue and extrication until delivery to a medical facility. Generally, the senior ranking or most experienced medically trained person is placed in command of care, treatment, and handling.

EMS personnel must also evaluate the overall condition of multiple accident victims and quickly develop a priority sequence for caring for the injured through the process of assessment and triage (Fig. 5-26). Depending on their level of training and certification, EMS workers are responsible for initiating primary medical care in accordance with the priority assigned to these patients. In carrying out this assignment, the medics accept responsibility for maintaining and supporting the patient's needs, both physical and psychological. All injuries to accident victims include a psychological injury as well as a physical injury. Treating only physical injuries without consideration for the human being underneath is a cold and shallow attitude for any emergency care provider to adopt.

A woman injured in a head-on collision may suffer serious physical injuries to her face. She may remain quite cooperative, not truly realizing the seriousness of her injuries. Suddenly, she may explode with rage or become uncontrollably violent because during the care phase she happened to glance at her reflection in the rearview mirror. Rearview mirrors should be moved or removed by inside medical personnel under these circumstances. As another example, child passengers in their parent's automobile may suffer emotionally for the rest of their life from the trauma of seeing their dead parent's mutilated body in the wreckage. The failure of EMS and vehicle rescue

personnel to consider the patient's psychological needs is a too-frequent error. We cannot let the routine of accident after accident lull us into feelings of complacency. We must always put ourselves in the place of the patient when considering the psychological well-being of the injured.

Medics who are good at what they do take their responsibility seriously and are constantly aware of what their patient sees, hears, and feels while being tended. They make sure that someone is always there to comfort the patient even when the patient seems to be unconscious. Remember, the last sense people lose as they lose consciousness is their sense of hearing. The calming voice, the medic's hand that comforts the patient, or just the feeling that there is someone out there who cares can be the most important assistance that any EMS provider ever renders to another human being. The goal is to do everything possible to prevent further injuries and keep from aggravating existing injuries.

Emergency medical care at the scene of an automobile accident evolves in several stages. Initial patient assessment work is accomplished first. The patient's life-threatening injuries and conditions are recognized, corrected, or stabilized. Work on airway management, respiration, blood circulation, initial spinal immobilization, and prevention of shock are done at this early rescue stage. Airway management may be *the* most important intervention needed to save a life or buy additional survival time for a trauma patient who is being extricated. All medical training stresses the importance of the ABCs. What we must remember is that the most advanced medical care team will not have a chance to save the patient if the open airway is not maintained. All emergency service personnel, regardless of their agency affiliation, must be familiar with basic airway management maneuvers (Fig. 5-27). The procedures are simple. Learn them.

As further access to a trapped patient becomes available, secondary assessments and additional spinal immobilization procedures are carried out by personnel. At this point the patient may be ready for removal. EMS personnel, in cooperation with the vehicle rescue crew, determine the need for any disentanglement activities necessary to free the patient.

The responsibility for patient packaging — the packaging of injuries and immobilization of limb fractures as well as spinal immobilization of the overall patient — generally lies with EMS personnel. As medics stabilize and immobilize the accident victim,

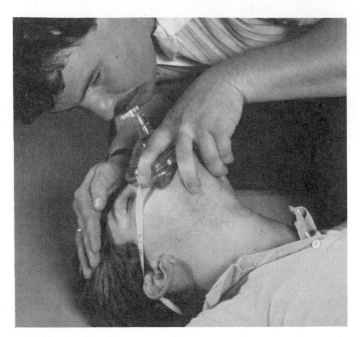

FIG. 5-27 Emergency service personnel must understand basic airway management protocols.

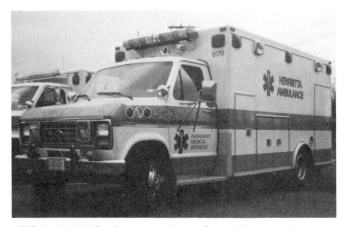

FIG. 5-28 Medical care continues from the time the patients are removed from accident vehicles until they arrive at a medical facility.

they are then involved in the disentanglement and extrication of that patient from the vehicle. At this point the medics are assisted by additional persons. Fire department personnel, for example, generally perform the necessary vehicle rescue work and assist

with other physically demanding tasks. The attending medic should stay at the patient's head or upper torso area and coordinate any efforts to protect and move the patient. It is particularly important that the medic take charge of the emergency service personnel assisting with the longboard extrication work.

Medical personnel attending to the patient are responsible for safe transport of that person to an appropriate medical facility. The best means of patient transport could include air transportation when available and appropriate. Whether transported by land or air, the patient receives continuing emergency medical care from first contact through removal from the wreckage to arrival at the medical facility (Fig. 5-28).

Once started, emergency medical care in the field must not stop until the patient is transferred physically and legally to the medical facility or pronounced dead by a responsible authority.

SUMMARY

The collision trauma patient with significant multiple trauma injuries must be perceived by medical and rescue personnel as being different from a patient who has received localized injuries. Even the basic philosophy of multisystem trauma patient care is different. This unique individual requires rapid assessment, aggressive intervention, and immediate transportation to an appropriate medical facility that can provide suitable treatment.

When accidents are less serious and patient injuries are less than life-threatening, all activities can appropriately be paced as rescue and medical work proceeds. But the most important guideline for EMS personnel is that the treatment time frame for a seriously injured collision trauma patient is very short, sometimes only approximately 10 minutes. Within this incredibly short interval, all accident activities receive new priorities. The ultimate goal is to deliver a salvageable patient to the appropriate medical facility in the safest and most efficient manner and within the patient's golden hour of life. When all emergency service personnel from all agencies work closely together and are united in their desire to meet this goal, lives are saved.

Rescue Tools and Equipment

6

OBJECTIVES

At the end of this chapter, you will be able to:

- Correctly list and describe the eight basic families of vehicle rescue-related tools and equipment.
- Correctly categorize a given rescue tool or appliance by its proper rescue tool family.
- Accurately define the relationships between tools within a given family and among tools from different families.
- Describe the function of a given vehicle rescue tool or appliance and how it applies to the field of vehicle rescue work.
- Identify and describe the functions of the various component parts of a given rescue tool or appliance.
- Correctly explain the safety considerations that must be met for the well-being of operating personnel and injured patients when employing a given rescue tool or appliance in a particular vehicle rescue evolution.
- Correctly explain all necessary or recommended preventive maintenance procedures applicable to a given rescue tool or appliance.
- Correctly and efficiently diagnose the possible operational problems that a given rescue tool or appliance can develop under actual field situations at vehicle rescue incidents.

Hundreds of tools and appliances are used by emergency service personnel to free persons trapped within damaged automobiles. This rescue equipment is grouped into several categories or *families,* based on whether they operate by pressurizing a hydraulic fluid, compressing air, providing electric power to a motor, using power directly from an internal combustion engine, burning compressed gases, or by using simple mechanical means.

There are two families of hydraulic-powered rescue equipment: power rescue tools and hydraulic jack tools. The other six families include pneumatic (air) tools, electric tools, compressed gas tools, gasoline-powered tools, vehicle-mounted tools, and hand tools. This chapter discusses the tools composing each family and their important safety considerations, recommendations for proper operation of the equipment, and suggested areas of preventive maintenance. It also provides a troubleshooting guide for diagnosing problems that may occur.

A tool such as the H.K. Porter Arsenal or the Rescue Gator tool uses compressed air yet operates by receiving pressurized hydraulic fluid. This type of tool is classified as a hydraulic-powered tool rather than an air-powered rescue tool. Hydraulic-powered rescue spreaders may use a gasoline motor to run a hydraulic pump, but because the tool operates by controlling the flow of pressurized fluid within, it is listed in the power rescue tool family and not in the gasoline-powered family. For our purposes, what makes a tool move determines its family.

Those directly involved in using rescue equipment must be trained in its safe and proper application and be able to understand and operate a multitude of different types and styles of equipment. They must have the depth of knowledge to initiate "primary" and "backup" alternative techniques as necessary.

Agencies providing vehicle rescue services must develop equipment inventories to address each rescue problem. The necessary tools and equipment should be arranged on emergency vehicles in a logical manner and should be easily accessible. Rescue personnel must be able to work with a primary tool in a primary technique and, when constrained by vehicle damage, patient conditions, or tool failure, must know how to employ backup tools or backup techniques to complete the task. This skill can only be acquired by fully understanding how the rescue equipment functions, how its operation relates to other rescue equipment, and how, when, and where to use it.

HYDRAULIC-POWERED RESCUE EQUIPMENT

The two distinct families of hydraulic rescue equipment used by rescue teams are the *power rescue tool* family, and the *hydraulic jack tool* family (Fig. 6-1). Both are operated by the flow of a hydraulic fluid under pressure. The determination of which family a specific rescue tool fits into is based on the date the equipment became available to the rescue market in North America.

The hydraulic jack tool family includes the standard hydraulic jack and the remote-controlled hydraulic jack, commonly referred to by the trade name Porto-Power. (Although the name Porto-Power is a registered trademark of the Blackhawk Corporation, in this text it refers to all of the many units of various manufacturer origin.) Hydraulic jack tools are those introduced to the North American rescue service *before 1970*. The hydraulic rescue equipment classified in the power rescue tool family were introduced to the North American rescue service *after 1970*.

Power Rescue Tool Family

The name for this general classification of equipment reflects the feature that makes them so valuable for today's rescue applications: their power. The term *power rescue tool* is used throughout this text in lieu of slang names or trademarks. This is the only place in this text that the reader will see the word *JAWS*. This reference arose with the introduction of the first power rescue tool introduced into the United States by the Hurst Performance Company of Pennsylvania. Truly a stroke of pure marketing genius by the Hurst company, the name JAWS is now so well known that even the general public uses it to describe the equipment. The Office of the Fire Marshall in Ontario, Canada, referred to power rescue tool equipment as "heavy hydraulics" when establishing their vehicle rescue program in the early 1980s. Regardless of training terminology or product trademarks, this chapter's power rescue tools include but are not limited to the following alphabetical listing of equipment and manufacturers:

- Amkus Rescue System — Amkus, Inc., Downers Grove, Illinois
- Arsenal Rescue System — H.K. Porter, Inc., Somerville, Massachusetts
- Bahco Rescue Tools — Bahco Kraftverktyg, Enkoping, Sweden
- The Boss — Special Services and Supply, Inc., Chenoa, Illinois
- Holmatro Rescue Tools — Holmatro, Inc., Millersville, Maryland
- Hurst Rescue System — Hale Fire Pump Co., Conshohocken, Pennsylvania
- Hydra-Spred'r Rescue Tool — Allied Tool Corporation, Sharpes, Florida (This manufacturer has ceased operation.)
- Kinman Rescue Tool — Kinman of Indianapolis, Indianapolis, Indiana
- Lancier Rescue Tool — Lancier, Inc., Pittsburgh, Pennsylvania

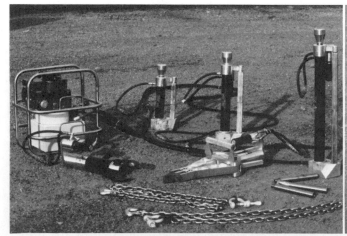 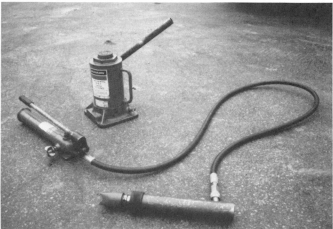

A   B

FIG. 6-1 A, Typical components of a power rescue tool system include power plant, cutter, spreader, ram, hydraulic hoses, and chain accessories. **B,** Standard 12-ton capacity hydraulic jack with handle inserted and the remote-controlled hydraulic jack 4-ton capacity porto-power unit compose the hydraulic jack tool family.

- Lukas Rescue System — Lukas of America, Inc., Stamford, Connecticut
- OWI — Orion World Industries, Melbourne, Florida
- Phoenix Rescue Tool — F.M. Brick Industries, Inc., Horsham, Pennsylvania
- Rescue Gator — Lincoln Safety Products, St. Louis, Missouri
- "Rescue 10" Rescue Tool — Sweed Machinery, Inc., Gold Hill, Oregon
- Viking Rescue Tool — Viking Rescue System, Inc., Villa Park, Illinois

There are distinct differences as well as many similarities in operating features, characteristics, performance, and quality among today's power rescue tool systems. Their common components are discussed because these are found on most typical rescue systems.

POWER PLANT

The power plant (Fig. 6-2) is the means by which the system pressurizes the fluid that operates the accessory tools. The power plant's function is to do the following:

- Operate the hydraulic pump to provide pressure to the hydraulic fluid.
- Direct the fluid under pressure through hydraulic hoses as necessary.
- Store needed quantities of hydraulic fluid.
- Provide the means to relieve fluid pressure in the hydraulic lines.
- Provide the means to shut off power to the system.

A power plant for a power rescue tool generally consists of six major components:

- Hydraulic fluid reservoir
- Quantity of hydraulic fluid
- Hydraulic pump
- Means of power for hydraulic pump (gasoline, diesel, electric, or water turbine engine)
- Directional and relief controls
- Hydraulic hoses

Power can be provided to the hydraulic pump of the power plant in many ways. In the more sophisticated systems, power is provided by 2-cycle or 4-cycle gasoline engines or by the use of electricity for 12-volt, 110-volt, or 220-volt motors. Most complete

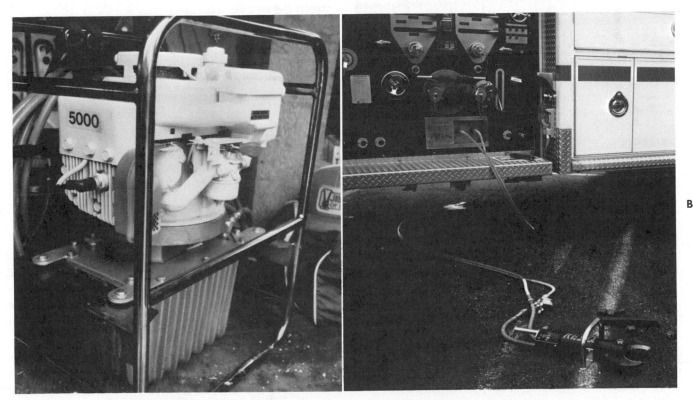

FIG. 6-2 A, This power plant consists of 4-cycle, gasoline engine-driven hydraulic pump operating at 5000 psi maximum fluid pressure. **B,** Water-driven hydraulic fluid pump delivers power to components of the power rescue tool system.

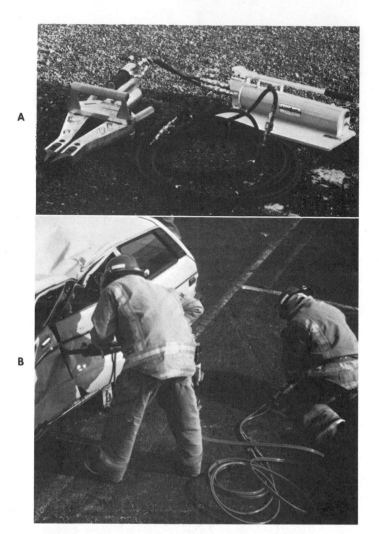

FIG. 6-3 A, Manual pumps are designed as backup or auxiliary power units or are used as a separate pump for simultaneous rescue tool operations. **B,** Power spreader unit is receiving pressurized hydraulic fluid from manual pump being operated by crew member.

power rescue tool systems also provide manual hydraulic pumps, either single-stage or two-stage models, to sufficiently pressurize the fluid to operate the rescue equipment. They are labor intensive and considerably slower than gasoline or electric power plants (Fig. 6-3).

Personnel operating power plants must have a basic understanding of several important operating features to be certain that safety prevails at all times. If the power plant uses a gasoline engine, rescue personnel must be able to locate and operate the engine "run" and "choke" controls and know the exact location and operation of the shut off or stop control. This control must be found without hesitation in the event of emergency and should therefore be distinctly marked

or painted a bright fluorescent color for quick and easy identification.

The engines of gasoline-powered units must be started with caution. All hydraulic pressure relief or control levers should be in the "neutral" or "relief" position, and the throttle and choke lever should be properly set for starting. To prevent the starting rope from being pulled completely out of the recoil housing assembly of the power plant, the rescuer should pull the rope in one hand while firmly gripping the cage of the power plant with the other hand. This positioning keeps the rescuer within arm's reach of the power plant and reduces the chance of the starter rope being overextended. The rescuer must remember to use good posture to avoid a possible back injury during engine starting.

Once the power plant is in operation and if rescue personnel are adequate in number, a crew member should be assigned to remain with the power plant. This individual stops and starts the unit as necessary, operates the fluid directional lever or relief lever, and ensures that the power plant operates safely at the scene. This crew member also monitors the position of a gasoline- or diesel-powered unit to ensure that engine noises and exhaust fumes are directed away from the rescue work area.

The rescuer at the power plant also ensures that the vibrating power plant does not vibrate around or "walk away" as it sits on the ground. This traveling can be minimized by mounting rubber cleats, foot pads, or even a piece of old tread from a snowmobile to the bottom cage rail of the power plant.

Concern must also be given to power plant operating time. Gas power plants equipped with relatively small fuel tanks may provide only 20 minutes of operating time. Units with larger capacity fuel tanks can run for well over 60 minutes. Rescue personnel should operate their power plant conservatively because of the limited running time of some units. Starting the unit long before it is to be used or allowing it to run when the crew members have stopped working with the rescue tools wastes resources, causes unnecessary noise at the scene, and increases the chance of running out of fuel if the unit is needed again during the rescue.

All rescue team members, especially the member assigned at the power plant, must be able to readily recognize the sound that their particular power plant makes just before it completely runs out of fuel. The widely used Chrysler 2-cycle industrial engine, the original power unit for the Hurst Rescue systems, has a very distinct fast throttle "racing" of the engine just as the last quantity of fuel is consumed. This sound signals that the fuel supply has been exhausted and that refueling is necessary.

Refueling of a hot gasoline or diesel power plant should be avoided if at all possible because a cool unit is safer to refuel. "Hot refueling" should only be done when absolutely necessary and never as a routine. The individual performing the refueling operation should shut off the power unit, don proper protective clothing including eye protection, and pour the fuel from an approved fuel safety can. Hardware store gasoline cans are unsafe for storing flammable liquids such as gasoline. The refueling should be done in a safe location, downwind and downhill from the accident work area to minimize vapors traveling toward the work area. The fuel mixture should flow from the safety can into an adequately sized funnel and then into the fuel tank. Pouring from a gas can directly into the small opening of the fuel tank can cause a fuel spill. The funnel minimizes spillage of fuel onto portions of the hot engine and exhaust system. During hot refueling, a firefighter in full protective clothing should be standing by with either a charged hoseline or an appropriate fire extinguisher ready for immediate use.

The maintenance associated with rescue system power plants depends on whether the unit is electric or gas powered and on who manufactured it. Electric power plants require that all electrical connections and switches be maintained properly and that the hydraulic fluid in the reservoir of the power plant be at the proper level. Spare quantities of hydraulic fluid should always be available at the emergency scene. If an electric power plant fails to function when turned on, personnel should quickly check to see that the unit is indeed receiving electricity. The generator, as well as all electrical connections, circuit breakers, and electric cables, should be inspected to ascertain the problem.

Gasoline or diesel power plants also require that fluid levels be maintained. If it is a 4-cycle engine, the proper engine oil levels must be maintained. If it is a 2-cycle engine, the proper mixture of gasoline and oil needed to lubricate the pistons of the engine is necessary. All gasoline engines also require proper maintenance of the choke and throttle control, correct carburetor settings, and a properly functioning spark plug. Several spare spark plugs and a spark plug wrench must be available at all times.

Gasoline engines for rescue systems are usually started by pulling a rope. The recoiler unit securing the rope is prone to failure. The small rope can break because of fraying, or the recoil device can malfunction and jam. A complete spare rope and recoiler unit can be provided with the power plant at very little expense. In a field situation, when a failure of the rope or recoiler occurs, the existing recoiler housing unit can be removed and the spare installed. It is possible to plan for this potential breakdown and actually modify the recoiler attachment screws by replacing the existing sheet metal screws with inverted machine screws and wing nuts, simplifying the rope recoiler replacement process and permitting rapid replacement in the field.

If a gasoline power plant fails to start, the problem is usually a fouled spark plug, an empty fuel tank, or a flooding of the carburetor. If the spark plug has fouled, rescue personnel should immediately install a new one. If the tank is empty, replacement fuel should be added. If the carburetor has flooded, the air inlet cover may be removed, the choke left in the "open" position, and the unit allowed to sit while the vapors dissipate.

If it is not possible to start the engine after all obvious field techniques have been tried and a separate manual pump unit is not available, a last resort effort allows for manual operation of the power plant. All rescue tool systems that have electric or gasoline power plants use a positive-displacement, direct-drive hydraulic pump submerged within the hydraulic fluid reservoir of the power unit. Every time the pump moves, fluid is pumped. Knowing this, rescue personnel can remove the spark plug from the gasoline engine to eliminate internal engine compression and pulling resistance. Without a plug, rescuers must then repeatedly pull the rope, causing the engine crankshaft and the direct-drive hydraulic pump to move. This will actually pressurize the fluid. If the pressure controls are set and the trigger of the attached tool operated, each pull on the rope results in slight tool action. This technique is obviously a last resort procedure, designed only to be used to allow personnel to remove equipment if the power plant fails during operation. The spark plug cylinder will require maintenance after this emergency operation, plus the cause of the original power plant failure must be determined.

All power rescue tool systems use a fluid under pressure to activate the rescue accessories. Table 6-1 shows that this fluid can be a phosphate ester, ethylene glycol, automatic transmission fluid oil, or a mineral-based standard hydraulic jack oil fluid. Under

TABLE 6-1 Power Rescue Tool System

Manufacturer	Hydraulic Fluid Used
Amkus	Mineral-base hydraulic oil
Amkus-Hurst compatible	Phosphate ester or glycol
Arsenal	Mineral-based hydraulic oil
Bahco	Mineral-based hydraulic oil
Boss	Mineral-based hydraulic oil
Holmatro	Mineral-based hydraulic oil
Holmatro-Hurst compatible	Phosphate ester or glycol
Hurst	Phosphate ester or glycol
Kinman	Automatic transmission fluid oil
Lukas	Mineral-based hydraulic oil
Phoenix	Phosphate ester or glycol
Power-Pry	Mineral-based hydraulic oil
Rescue Gator	Mineral-based hydraulic oil
Rescue 10	Mineral-based hydraulic oil
Titan	Mineral-based hydraulic oil
Viking	Mineral-based hydraulic oil
Webber	Mineral-based hydraulic oil

pressure, the fluid circulates from its source through hoses to and from rescue equipment, allowing the equipment to function when the tool controls are activated. Rescue personnel must be fully aware of the significant differences in fluids used by different manufacturers.

It is possible to be injured by exposure to power rescue tool hydraulic fluid in several ways. Personnel can inhale, ingest, pressure inject, or externally contact the fluid. The severity of the particular injury depends on the nature of the hydraulic fluid and the degree of exposure. Inhalation can occur when a fluid leak develops while the hydraulic system is pressurized, causing the fluid to be sprayed and a rescuer to breathe the vapors or mist into the respiratory system. Ingestion can occur when fluid touches a person's face near the mouth. Fluid spilled on work gloves, turnout coats, or work rags may be ingested into the body if the contaminated item is inadvertently used to wipe the face or mouth. External contamination can occur when a person working with a power rescue tool has fluid spilled or leaked onto exposed skin. This contamination injury is most common and generally results in irritation, infection of cuts, and minor rash symptoms.

Pressure-penetration injuries occur when a leak or component rupture occurs within any pressurized part of the system. The leak or failure at a coupling on a hydraulic hose, for example, could spray fluid under enough pressure to "inject" into soft tissue portions of the body. Areas of exposed flesh, even eyeballs, are vulnerable to fluid penetration injuries. The injured patient trapped in the wreckage, the medical worker attending the patient, and the rescue personnel operating hydraulic equipment must all be properly protected from this possibility.

The original fluid used in the Hurst rescue systems is sold as Hurst RT-23/Aerosafe 2300, a phosphate ester-based hydraulic fluid. This synthetic fluid is known for its applications in the airline industry as an aircraft hydraulic system fluid. The information in the box below was provided by the rescue system manufacturer.

Several of the rescue tool systems offer a choice of hydraulic system fluid. The Kinman Rescue system is unique in that Type A automatic transmission oil is used to power the system. Most rescue systems use a mineral-base oil as the hydraulic fluid. The common oil, a hydrocarbon derivative, is considered non-toxic and presents minimal hazards to operating personnel. One manufacturer of a mineral-based hydraulic oil is the Shell Oil Corporation of Houston, Texas. Their hydraulic oil is sold under the tradename Shell Tellus T Oil 23. Information regarding this product is

---

HURST RT-23/AEROSAFE 2300

CHARACTERISTICS
Stable under normal atmospheric conditions
Indefinite shelf life under sealed conditions
Specific gravity at room temperature (77° F): 1.008 (specific gravity of water: 1.000)
Fire flash point: 330° F
Auto-ignition temperature: 1020° F
Functional range: –60° F to 220° F
Electric conductivity: low

HEALTH AND SAFETY INFORMATION
Ingestion causes nausea, vomiting, cramps, diarrhea, and irritation of mouth, throat, and gastrointestinal tract.
Contact with either liquid or vapor causes immediate burning sensation.
Skin contact causes irritation; prolonged contact causes inflammation.
Inhalation of mist or spray causes upper respiratory tract irritation with coughs, sneezing, and swelling of nasal passages.

TELLUS T OIL 23

HEALTH INFORMATION

Ingestion

Based on component information, product is no more than slightly toxic if swallowed.

Skin Contact

Based upon component information, product is presumed to be practically nonirritating to the skin. Prolonged and repeated contact may result in skin disorders such as dermatitis. Accidental release under high-pressure applications may result in injection of oil into skin causing local necrosis. Condition may be evidenced by delayed onset of pain and tissue damage a few hours following high-pressure injection.

Inhalation

The inhalation of vapors (generated at high temperatures only) or oil mist may cause a mild irritation of the mucous membranes of the upper respiratory tract.

Eye Contact

Based on component information, product is presumed to be practically nonirritating to the eyes of users.

Aggravated Medical Condition

Pre-existing skin and respiratory disorders may be aggravated by exposure to this product.

OIL EXPOSURE: EMERGENCY MEDICAL CARE PROCEDURES

Ingestion

Do not induce vomiting. In general, no treatment is necessary unless large quantities of product are ingested. Get medical attention.

Skin Contact

Remove contaminated clothing. Wipe excess from skin. Flush skin with water. Follow by washing with soap and water. If irritation occurs, get medical attention. If material is injected under the skin, get medical attention. To prevent serious damage, do not wait for symptoms to develop.

Inhalation

Remove affected person to fresh air and provide oxygen if breathing is difficult. Get medical attention.

Eye Contact

Flush eyes with water. If irritation occurs, get medical attention.

obtained from Shell's Material Safety Data Sheet and shown in the box above.

F.M. Brick Industries, manufacturer of the Phoenix tool, can assemble its rescue system to operate with either phosphate ester fluid or a glycol fluid. The glycol, essentially an antifreeze solution, again presents minimal health or safety concerns when compared with the active ingredients in a phosphate ester hydraulic fluid.

Protection for personnel working with any hydraulic equipment includes donning proper protective clothing, including approved safety glasses with side shields or safety goggles. The standard 4-inch flip-down eye shield mounted on structural firefighting helmets does not adequately protect the wearer from eye injury at motor vehicle accidents. These shields offer protection *only* when used in conjunction with safety glasses or goggles.

Transmitting Fluid under Pressure

During operation the hydraulic fluid moves from one component of the rescue system to another by circulating through hydraulic hoses. It is the function of these hoses to safely and reliably deliver fluid under pressure throughout the system and return the fluid to the power plant reservoir.

Power rescue system hoses are generally manufactured from either thermo-plastic or rubber materials. Most of the hydraulic hoses are nonperforated and electrically nonconductive. Typical system hoses generally have a ¼-inch inside diameter and consist of several layers of hose and reinforcement material meshed together to form the finished product. A critical point of information regarding these hoses is their pressure ratings. All hydraulic hoses have a listed burst test pressure, the pressure at which the hose fails. The operating or working pressure is the pressure at which the hoses are normally designed to operate. When rescue personnel compare their system's hose burst pressure with its operating pressure, an indication of the safety factor designed into their system can be calculated. The higher the ratio of the two pressures, the greater the margin of safety for personnel working with or near the power equipment.

TABLE 6-2 Sample Power Rescue Tool Hose Ratings				
System	Maximum Hose Operating (psig)	Operating (psig)	Hose Burst (psig)	Safety Factor
Amkus	5000	10800	20000	2:1
Arsenal	–	10000	35000	3.5:1
Hurst (original white hose)	–	4200	1000	2.5:1
Hurst (orange hose)	–	5000	20000	4:1

Dash (–) signifies information not available.

Personnel operating with power rescue tools or those considering purchasing these systems are advised to be fully aware of all safety features that may or may not be designed into each system by the manufacturer (Table 6-2).

Hydraulic hoses and couplings connect the tools of the rescue system to the power plant. It is the function of the hydraulic coupling to provide a connection that will not fail under the operating pressure of the system. The coupling must withstand the many conditions present at a rescue scene and remain functional at all times.

Each hydraulic connection contains two different units joined together to make the complete assembly. Each coupler is either a male or female type, with the male half of the coupling designed to insert into the female coupling. Once the couplers are properly seated together, hydraulic fluid flows through the connection. There is no standardized male or female coupling and therefore no compatibility between systems among the many power rescue systems.

The female coupler is provided with a swivel ring that rotates and also moves back and forth in a direction parallel to the coupling. Pulling back on the collar (thereby moving it away from the end of the hose) allows the coupler to receive the companion male coupler. Once coupled, the female collar moves forward, making a leak-proof connection. This movable locking ring on the female coupler maintains the integrity of the connection between the two coupler halves. On better quality hydraulic hose couplings, an important safety feature minimizes the chance of accidental hose disconnection. The better female couplings use a swivel collar with a slot and have a pin located in the coupler itself. The collar can only be moved back and forth to hold or release the male coupler when the slot and the pin are properly aligned. Once coupled, the collar should be rotated so that the slot does not align with the pin, thereby "locking" the two coupling halves together.

Couplings that have locking collars may present difficulties in connecting or disconnecting if the slot and pin are not properly aligned. Instead of actually looking at the female coupling to attempt to see if the slot and pins have lined up, you can pull back slightly on the swivel collar while slowly rotating it. When the slot and pin line up properly, the collar will automatically move rearward and unlock, allowing for insertion or release of the male half of the connection. Personnel should have their protective clothing and eye protection properly in place and connect or disconnect the couplings only while holding them away from and below their face.

Rescue personnel sometimes find it difficult to connect the hydraulic hoses even with the locking collar properly set. If the hoses cannot be coupled, it is possible that the male coupler has become pressurized. The hose can become pressurized if the operator continues to operate the trigger control even after the power tool has completely closed or retracted. The tool "loads" pressure into the hoses and the couplings, making them difficult to connect or disconnect. The male coupler can also be pressurized if fluid is directed into a hydraulic line that has not been completely connected to another tool or hose. Also, a coil of hydraulic hose may pressurize itself if subjected to a rise in temperature such as when placed on a hot asphalt or concrete roadway or exposed to direct sunshine for several hours. The fluid heats up inside the hose coil and expands, creating its own internal hose pressure.

In these situations, pressure must be relieved before the couplers will properly function. This can be accomplished quickly by operating any fluid pressure relief valve, control valves, or changeover valves designed into the rescue system. Unscrewing threaded hydraulic connections at the hose coupling or at the connection to the power plant can also relieve unwanted pressure, although this action will cause a loss of fluid and will expose personnel to possible fluid contamination. A final emergency pressure-releasing procedure that is not endorsed by all system manufacturers or vehicle rescue instructors involves covering the male hose coupler with a cloth and pushing the nipple end against a stationary object. This action is intended to unseat the nipple, thereby reducing fluid pressure in the line. Potential problems with this emergency technique are that it causes the pressurized fluid to squirt out under high pressure, again placing personnel at risk of fluid exposure, and may damage the nipple of the male coupler. This technique should therefore be considered a last resort and avoided if possible.

The hydraulic couplings may also be damaged by exposure to contaminants. For example, disconnecting a coupling and then dropping the end to the ground permits dirt to enter the coupling. Granules of dirt inside the coupling end can damage the coupler's soft internal components, contaminate the fluid, and prevent the couplings from properly joining together, resulting in a possible fluid leak. Gasoline, diesel fuel, engine oil, water, and antifreeze are all typically found at an accident scene and can quickly contaminate exposed couplings. Rescue personnel should always maintain control of the open-end couplings while connecting or disconnecting to avoid any contact with contaminants. In addition, the couplings should be connected together as much as possible, or plastic or metal end caps should be installed if provided.

If contamination of a coupling occurs, crew members should not blow the dirt out of the coupling by mouth. This risks personal injury because of fluid contact in the mouth, eyes, or skin. The coupling should be cleaned by flushing in a can or pan of clean hydraulic fluid, brushed with a soft bristle brush, and wiped dry with a clean cloth. The contaminated hydraulic fluid should then be discarded.

Other system components that can move fluid through the rescue system include manifold blocks, hose reels, and various fluid valves and control levers. If available for a particular rescue system, manifold blocks form a means of circulating fluid to and from multiple tools connected in series to the same power plant. Personnel operating with manifold blocks must be sure that a complete hydraulic "circuit" is made because the fluid must travel from the power plant through the manifold, into and out of all hose lines and rescue equipment, and then to the power plant reservoir. Improper connecting of the hoses short circuits the flow of fluid, which will cause a tool to function improperly or not at all.

The hydraulic hose reels available for rescue sys-

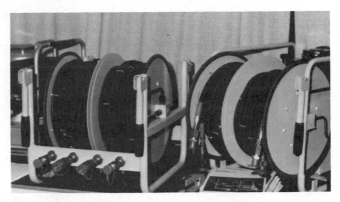

FIG. 6-4 Hydraulic hose reels allow a quieter, less cluttered work area.

tems allow for up to 100 feet of hose to be stored and used directly from the reel (Fig. 6-4). The long hose lines require that greater quantities of fluid be available at the power plant to meet the needs of the expanded system. The advantages of the long hose and reel are that it can reduce hose clutter at an accident scene, it can be quickly returned to service, and it allows operating personnel to work at greater distance from the noise of gasoline power plants or rescue vehicles. Its disadvantages include the long hose being more readily exposed to physical damage and the inherent loss of fluid pressure (friction loss) in the long length of hose running from the power source to the operating equipment. The resistance of the fluid moving through the hose can cause noticeable changes in the responsiveness of the power tools and reduce their operating capacities.

A significant safety improvement in power rescue tool systems came with the introduction of manual relief valves. This feature, located either at the power plant or on the hydraulic lines supplying fluid to the tools, allows operating personnel to quickly and safely relieve hydraulic fluid pressure in hose lines or tools by simply moving a lever. Many power rescue systems have additional fluid transfer valves, (called changeover valves) to control the flow of fluid from one pair of hydraulic hoses to another. The valve should be in the "open" or "neutral" position when starting or stopping the power plant to minimize the load on the power plant.

Much like an air bubble within the bloodstream of a human being, air may become trapped within the hydraulic system causing tools to function erratically or fail to hold their position when triggers are released. Removing the trapped air is accomplished by connecting all hose lines to all tools and operating each tool through its complete operation cycle several times.

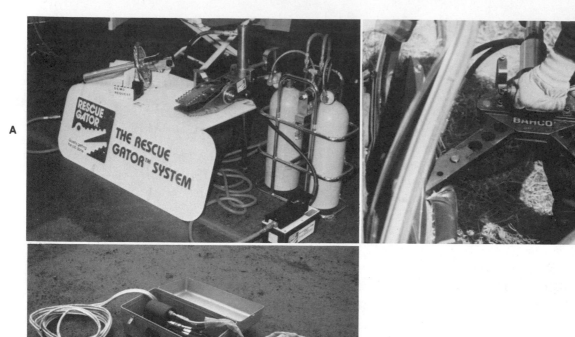

FIG. 6-5 A, Single-acting power rescue spreader. **B**, Double-acting spreader. **C**, Multipurpose or combination tool.

SPREADER

The component of the power rescue system known as the spreader is a hydraulic-powered rescue tool consisting of a piston connected to metal arms that open and close as the piston moves. The spreader applies a force outward as the arms open and, in more sophisticated systems, exerts forces inward as the arms close. Large spreaders have a "wet" weight of approximately 70 lb with hoses and couplings attached and fluid filling the tool and a total overall tool spread of 30 inches or more with the arms closed. Small spreaders commonly weigh between 45 and 55 lb and typically open 24 inches. Either size spreader can incorporate a single- or double-acting piston and be a single purpose or multipurpose tool.

Single-acting spreaders apply force in the outward direction only and use springs to return the arms to the closed position (Fig. 6-5, *A*). The Arsenal spreader, Boss spreader, and Hydra-Spred'r are examples of single-acting spreaders. Double-acting spreaders, the most common type, use hydraulic power to both open and close the arms (Fig. 6-5, *B*). Single-purpose spreaders have standard style arms with metal tips at the ends, and push or pull as power is applied, depending on their design. The spreader arms with cutter blades integrated into the design are used with multipurpose or combination power rescue tools (Fig. 6-5, *C*). These units both push and pull and perform a cutting function as the arms close.

The basic components of a hydraulic spreader are the following:

- Hose, couplings, and valving controls
- Tool body with hydraulic piston inside
- Spreader arms
- Spreader arm tips and accessories

Spreader Controls

The hydraulic controls for the power rescue spreaders direct fluid through the tool and throughout the remaining components of the system. All manufacturers use controls designed with a neutral or "deadman" position along with the open and close positions. Most rescue systems use an actual hydraulic control valve, which allows the tool operator to control the speed of operation directly. The further the valve is moved to one side of the neutral position, the faster or more powerfully the unit moves. With a few rescue systems, such as the Arsenal, Gator, or Boss, compressed air is actually controlled by the tool operator. The flow of compressed air directs the hydraulic fluid throughout the system to open or close the attached tool.

With the electric-powered Kinman tool, the tool operator uses a very different type of spreader control system. The operator uses an electrical contact switch to start or stop an electric-powered hydraulic pump, moving oil from the pump to operate the attached tool. With this electric control, "feathering" the movement of the tool by slight movement of the control trigger is next to impossible. The electric switch is either open, breaking the electrical circuit, or closed, completing the electric circuit and powering the single-speed hydraulic pump.

Spreader Accessories

Tips of power rescue tools may be permanently machined components of each arm or interchangeable accessory components that use pins to secure them to the end of the arm. In systems that have interchangeable tips, various designs of tips and accessories can be added. The automotive tip, which is used for most spreader operations, is a wedge-shaped metal tip with serrations in its working surfaces. Several manufacturers encourage users of their tools to reverse the automotive tips on the arms, putting the long side of each tip facing outward to increase the maximum opening distance of the arms. Some interchangeable tips are designed for specific rescue applications. The most common alternate tip design provides a narrow tip and a companion wide-shaped tip to be used together to rip or tear sheet metal. Users of the Hurst rescue system refer to these tips as aircraft aviation tips.

The most common accessories to attach to the spreader are those designed for pulling functions. The various systems use either shackles, grab hooks, and rescue chain or shackles, synthetic nylon or polyester strapping, and ratchet devices (Fig. 6-6). The pulling attachments allow the spreader to exert a pulling force as its arms are closed. There are a number of shackle designs. Amkus and Viking systems use a shackle with

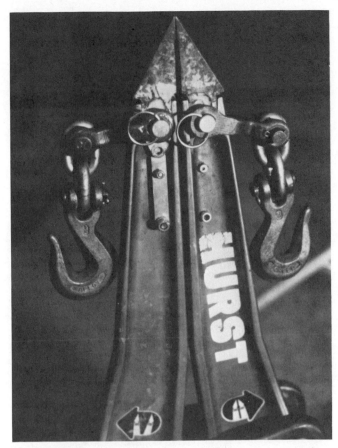

FIG. 6-6 Rated chain, shackle assembly, pins, and grab hooks are the most common attachments for accomplishment pulling evolutions with power spreaders.

the pins permanently attached. Lukas employs a European grab hook, called the shortening claw, that is attached to a square pin. The square pin and shackle are inserted inside the open box-shaped ends of the Lukas spreader's steel arms for pulling (Fig. 6-7). Other systems use pulling accessory kits with open shackles, several links of chain, and a rated grab hook. The shackle attaches to the arm with locking pins that are usually completely detachable from the shackle unit. Additional attachment pins should be available as spares in case the primary set is misplaced.

Three critical procedures must be followed when using a power spreader equipped with these detachable locking pins, chain, and hooks. First, the grab hooks attached to the shackles must be positioned so that both hooks have the open sides facing out or away from the arms of the spreader tool. Second, the pins that secure the shackles to the arms of the tool must be inserted from the bottom side of the arm of the tool so that any load applied to the pins from underneath forces the pins to seat themselves in the

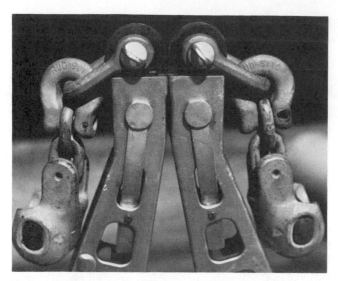

FIG. 6-7 European style of grab hook, called *shortening claw*, used with Lukas spreaders in pulling evolutions.

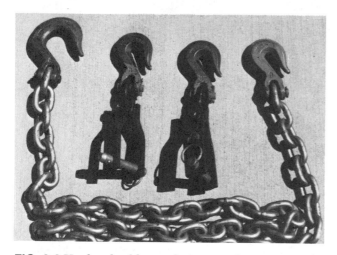

FIG. 6-8 Hooks, shackles, and pins must be set properly to ensure that evolution is done safely.

arms. If the pins entered the shackles and arms from the top side, pressure from below could pop the pins up through the lower portion of the shackle (Fig. 6-8). A final safety feature requires that as the rated rescue chain is attached to the grab hooks, it must be positioned to pass through the grab hook with the free end of the chain remaining accessible on top of the arm. Positioning both chains in this manner results in a balanced pull on the arms of the spreader. If one chain were to be inserted from the bottom and the companion chain placed down from the top, a serious imbalance could occur, placing excessive stress on the arms of the tool during pulling. Imbalanced chain

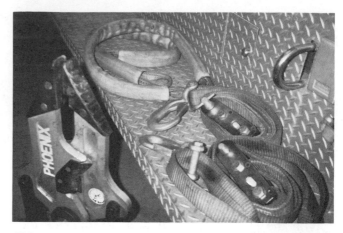

FIG. 6-9 Phoenix power rescue system strapping, slings, and ratchet shackles.

hookups have caused spreader arms to completely fracture in a sudden and violent action.

Pulling with the Phoenix or Holmatro rescue tool involves the use of synthetic strapping (Fig. 6-9). Unlike chain, these straps are susceptible to damage from sharp glass, metal, or contaminants such as gasoline, oils, or acids. Personnel using strapping must continually protect the integrity of the strap by removing contamination hazards, padding vulnerable areas, and placing blocks near sharp-edged hazards.

When pulling with power rescue system spreaders, rescue teams working with chain must use chain and hook assemblies that are equal to or greater in quality and load rating than those supplied by the manufacturer for the product. Hurst rescue equipment, for example, requires chain with a link diameter of ½ inch. The chain is alloy quality and has a working load rating of 12,000 lb. Other systems typically use ⅜-inch chain with less pulling capacity.

All power rescue system spreaders should be stored with the arms slightly open to allow for quick and efficient tip changes when necessary. This position also does not create excessive fluid pressures during storage of the tool.

Power Output

Power rescue equipment has three different force capacities that can be measured. As measured theoretically by design engineers, the *calculated* power rating of a tool may not accurately represent the performance of the equipment, although this rating is commonly advertised by rescue system salespeople. All power rescue tool manufacturers desire to show their product in its best light. To many, this means

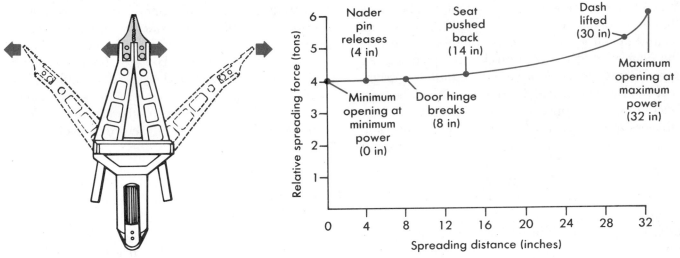

FIG. 6-10 The power output of all spreader units varies throughout operation of the tool.

promoting the power of the spreader. A figure such as 12,000 lb or 18,000 lb is used to attempt to indicate the work that the particular spreader can deliver. For rescue personnel desiring an accurate description of the power rating of their spreader, these numbers are misleading.

The output of a rescue tool as measured while the tool is actually moving is its *dynamic* power rating. Establishing this rating requires sophisticated measuring equipment to monitor the output of the tool. As a power rescue tool is used, the dynamic power rating forces fluctuate dramatically. This change in power output for a spreader unit is because of the change in the relative position between the moving piston and the tips of the tool. All spreaders increase their power output as the arms open and also exert greater force at points further down the arms than at the tip.

The third tool rating is its *static* power rating. This figure represents the power of a tool while motionless and is generally greater than the dynamic rating. All tools are more powerful when held stationary than when they are moving due to losses incurred during the physical movement of the component parts.

Rescue personnel need an accurate description of the tool's performance as measured at various arm positions and at several points along each arm. This information is best depicted in graphic form and is referred to as the rescue tool's "power profile". On a graph depicting the performance of a power rescue spreader, the vertical axis indicates tool power output and the horizontal axis reflects the opening distance of the spreader arms (Fig. 6-10). The graph's fluctuating

power profile line demonstrates the increase in power output as the arms are opened and decrease as the arms reach the closed position. Accurate depiction of the force of a particular spreader in the various operating positions requires two separate power profiles. One reflects measurements taken at the very tip of each arm, and the other displays power available at a point on each arm 4 inches below the tip where readings are higher.

Power rescue spreaders are less powerful when pulling than when spreading or pushing. One model of rescue spreader from Amkus, Inc., for example, has a rating of, 16,500 lb maximum opening force and a closing force of 14,600 lb at full open position. One spreader from Holmatro, Inc. has an opening force rating of 10,340 lb with the arms fully opened and a closing power rating of 7700 lb with the arms in the same position. In some cases, power output ratings for pulling are only 50% of the spreading power. It is important that rescue personnel be fully aware of the actual power output of their particular system, from the completely open to the fully closed position, during both pulling and spreading operations, and during both dynamic and static operation. Vehicle rescue personnel should stop accepting theoretical power-rating information as gospel truth. Tool manufacturers should be required to list only those tool power ratings that they have proved.

Safe Operation

Spreaders approaching 70 lb or more in wet weight can be operated by one or two rescue crew members.

When two rescuers work the one tool, one becomes the *control operator,* the other, the *assist operator.* The control operator, the only crew member to operate the control trigger, is responsible for planning the specific strategy necessary to accomplish the assignment and actually places the tool in position. The assist operator simply supports the weight of the tool. Many smaller size and lighter weight spreader units available today can be used safely by a single rescue crew member.

Rescue team members operating rescue spreaders must place their hands only on the tool's handles or control levers, never on or between the arms of the tool, which can result in serious injury. Balance and good body placement are important when operating power rescue spreaders. For example, during efforts to force open a jammed automobile door, a spreader tool may slip while under a load. It generally kicks backward, and any crew member whose upper thigh or groin area is tightly pressed against the back of the body of the spreader tool can receive painful injuries.

It is also unsafe to get between the spreader tool and the structure of the vehicle being worked on by personnel. The tool may shift or twist into a position that can easily trap and injure anyone located there. Because this problem can develop so quickly, almost before the worker realizes it, all personnel should make it a rule never to place themselves in this dangerous area. There should also be an alert crew officer and an assigned scene safety officer on hand to monitor these activities.

Personal protection for members operating power rescue equipment should include safety glasses with side panels or safety goggles. Plastic 4- or 6-inch flip-down eye shields mounted on firefighting helmets or the two-piece Bourke style of eye shields on fire helmets are inadequate to protect against hazards present around power rescue equipment. In addition, hoods made of fire-resistive materials that are commonly worn for structural firefighting operations increase upper body protection because they cover exposed body areas not protected by structural firefighting coats or helmets.

Preventive Maintenance and Inspection

Visual inspection of the spreader unit, component parts, and accessories should be performed routinely and after each use of the equipment. This inspection should check for proper fluid levels and for any cracks or dents that may have developed in the body of the tool or on the arms. Cracks or stress marks, particu-larly in units that use aluminum or aluminum alloy arms or tool bodies, are a critically important sign of possible tool failure. The alignment of the arms should also be visually checked. The tips should close and meet each other evenly. If there is a detectable difference in the alignment of either arm, there is reason to suspect that the unit has been subjected to overload conditions and is in need of factory inspection and service.

POWER CUTTERS

It is extremely important for rescue personnel at a motor vehicle accident to be able to cut or sever various materials. Changes in the quality and thickness of metal in vehicles and increasing use of plastic materials are making it more difficult to force our way into a vehicle by pushing or spreading. Cutting away strategic portions of the vehicle will become the main ingredient of our vehicle rescue evolutions during the 1990s and beyond.

The first cutting accessory for power rescue systems was developed by the Hurst Performance Co. for use with their model 32 spreader. Called the Power Shears, the accessory resembled a giant pair of scissors constructed of metal and attached to the ends of the arms of the spreader with lightweight metal clips. The power shears functioned as the spreader was opened or closed.

Rescue personnel have since encountered many potential safety problems when using the original power shears. They could be opened too far and become jammed in the open position, or the metal wire clips designed to hold the shears on the arms could fly off during use. As the shears aged in the field, continued use increased the probability of shear blade failure during cutting operations. A modified design introduced several years later incorporated a limiting collar to control opening of the blades, screw-in knurled knobs to better secure the shears to the spreader arms, and shorter, sturdier blades (Fig. 6-11). Another design cutting shear assembly also became available for use inside the arms of certain Hurst spreader tools.

The final chapter in the power shears story was written when Hurst introduced spreader units designed with more power than the original shears could withstand, prompting their recall. Unfortunately, some rescue teams still use the original shears for their cutting operations.

Although all rescue tool manufacturers have since developed their own cutting tools, no other manufacturer has ever marketed shears designed to be added onto the arms of the spreader. All power rescue system cutters available today are either separate units designed to perform basic cutting functions or combination spreader-cutter tools.

Power cutter units consist of the following basic components:

- Hose, couplings, and valve controls
- Tool body with hydraulic piston inside
- Cutter blades

Operation and Function

Cutters can be classified as either single-acting or double-acting hydraulic units, depending on whether the cutter blades return to the open position by hydraulic power or by means of a mechanical spring. With the more common double-acting cutter units, the hydraulic piston in the body of the tool is extended or retracted to move the cutter blades to the open or closed position (Fig. 6-12).

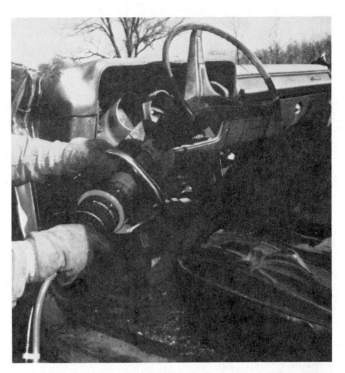

FIG. 6-12 A more powerful, efficient, and reliable cutter unit is a double-acting type that cuts (closes) and opens under hydraulic power.

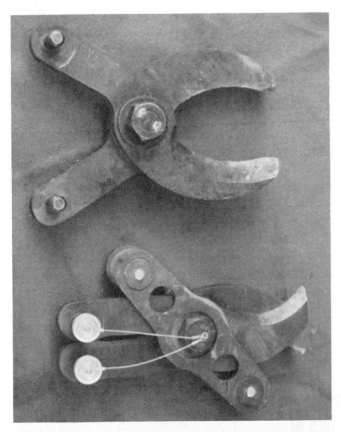

FIG. 6-11 Problems developed with the original cutting accessory for the Hurst Model 32 tool *(top)*, resulting in a second generation cutter accessory with improvements *(bottom)*. Because of additional improvements, both cutters are now obsolete and must not be used.

The cutter unit manufactured by H.K. Porter for the Arsenal rescue system is an example of a single-acting cutter tool. The drop-forged tool steel blades of the cutter are operated from the open to the closed position by the action of a hydraulic piston. The blades, however, do not return to the open position by the same hydraulic piston. Instead, as with most single-acting cutter units, large springs pull the cutter blades open. This can be a serious shortcoming because the cutter blades are likely to jam in the closed or "cut" position. Personnel working with single-acting cutters must always prepare their work by removing lightweight metal trim material, cloth headliner material, or seatbelt strapping before any cutting is started. These items can become lodged between the blades, causing them to jam (Fig. 6-13).

Not all power rescue system cutters cut metal the same way. The cutter manufactured by the Amkus Co. is typical of units that have machined cutting blades with a tapered design. The unit functions with such close operating tolerances that the blades cut by a metal shearing action, just as a conventional pair of scissors cuts paper. It is important for rescue personnel to realize that this shearing principle imparts energy into the object being cut. At the moment the cutter finishes the severing action, the pieces separate with a

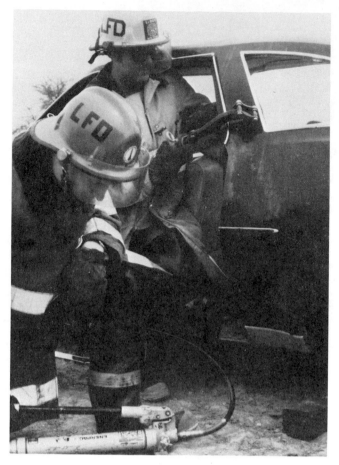

FIG. 6-13 A single-acting power cutter unit operated by a manual hydraulic pump.

release of energy that can be explosive. The more the material being cut resists the efforts of the cutter, the greater the potential for a sudden release of energy as the cut is completed.

A cutter unit from F.M. Brick Industries, Inc. is now available with one stationary and one movable cutter blade. The material is cut as one blade closes against the other.

Most cutters are designed to use curved and tapered blades. The blades cut as they draw the material into the "throat" area of the tool. There may also be a recess designed into the throat of the blades at the point where the most cutting power is developed. For example, Holmatro claims that its multipurpose spreader can cut cold-rolled steel bars up to ⅝-inch in diameter using this recessed opening area. Another cutting principle used by manufacturers such as Hurst, Holmatro, and Lukas uses straight cutting blades. The cutting is accomplished with specially developed notches machined into the blades (Fig. 6-14).

Safety and Efficiency

Rescue crew members who operate power cutter units must take several basic measures to ensure their safety and to make sure that the tool is used efficiently. Full protective clothing including safety goggles or safety glasses must be in use. The cutter units, typically lighter than the spreader tools, can be safely operated by one fully protected rescue crew member. Injured patients and attending medical personnel near the cutter work area must be effectively insulated from any threat posed by the cutting evolution.

For maximum efficiency, personnel should position the blades of the tool completely around the object being cut and maintain the blades in a position as perpendicular as possible to the material being cut. The rescue tool operator must be alert for the possible movement of the tool into a slanted position as the cutting progresses and be ready to react accordingly. If this shifting is appreciable, the tool operator should reposition the unit to a location several inches from the first attempted cut and again operate the tool. If an operator were to continue to cut with the blades in an off-angle position, several things could happen. In an off-angle cutting action, the blades spread outward from each other, transmitting cutting stresses from the entire blade to its outer edges. This can reduce cutter efficiency and cause blade destruction. Additionally, as the off-angle pressure causes the blades to spread apart, the material being cut is twisted and forced between the blades. This action twists the cutter and may damage the blade. The tool can then suddenly move or jerk if the cut is completed, snapping the tool away from the operator.

Operators working with cutting tools should make every effort to avoid cutting unsupported or "free" ends of objects. Cutting once through an automobile roof post, for example, separates one portion of the metal from another. But, making a second cut a short distance away from the first cut introduces the potential for the object to move. The energy imparted into the object being cut may launch its unsupported free end. Holmatro, Inc. cautions personnel using their cutter units about the hazards of free ends by stating "…the parts will come apart with such a force that they can cause great physical damage." Portions of metal roof posts weighing 4 to 5 lb have traveled more than 20 feet from the vehicle in actual case histories. Personnel should plan their work to avoid having to make second cuts on free ends.

If long, continuous cuts need to be made, such as when severing the wide roof posts of an automobile,

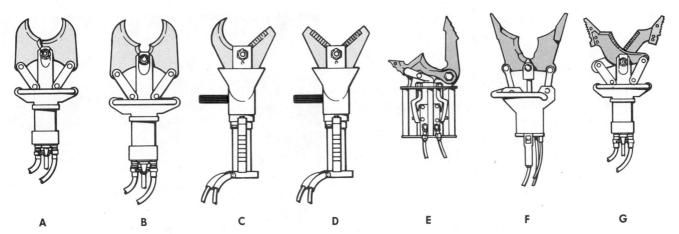

FIG. 6-14 A, Standard curved-blade model (Hurst Model 0-90). **B,** Curved-blade cutter with recessed throat (Hurst Model 0-150). **C,** Curved-blade and serrated-blade cutter (Lukas LS-600). **D,** Straight serrated-blade cutter (Lukas LS-700). **E,** Curved-blade and straight-blade cutter with one stationary blade (Phoenix 30/12). **F,** Curved-blade cutter with recessed throat integrated with spreading tool (Kinman). **G,** Serrated straight-blade cutter integrated with spreading tool (Hurst Paladin).

one of two methods can be used. In the first, an initial cut is made deep into the sheet metal, using the full depth of the cutter blades. The tool operator then makes a second cut from a slightly different angle that takes out a "piece of pie." With this pie-shaped metal portion removed, the cutter is then moved deeper into the "V" of the starter cut. Additional cuts are made in this fashion as the unit progresses across the area that needs to be cut.

The second method begins with a full-depth initial cut. The cutter is then withdrawn, and only the lower blade is inserted into the cut. The body of the tool is then held at an approximate 45-degree angle to the surface of the metal being cut. As the blades are closed, the top blade is maneuvered ahead of the original cut, making a new cut. The process, called *walking a cutter,* is continued until the desired distance has been covered. This technique is required for use with the newest generation of power cutters, called "continuous" cutters. Their one curved blade and its companion straight blade work to make long-length cuts, such as when working a cut from one side of an automobile roof to the other.

When the power cutter unit is not being used or is prepared for storage on the rescue vehicle, the cutter blades should be closed just enough so that the outer edges of the blades touch each other. The blades of a standard power rescue cutter form a closed circle when properly stowed. This closed blade position protects the working surfaces of the blades and

reduces the unwanted hydraulic pressure that can build up when the blades are closed too tightly.

Capabilities

Most power cutter problems are attributable to abuse of the tool by rescue personnel. The blades are specifically designed to cut certain metals, such as the sheet metal found on vehicle door and roof posts. When the cutter is used to sever solid metal objects such as concrete reinforcing bars, unwanted tool stress and blade damage can result. Potential problem areas on a typical automobile include the following:

- Cold-rolled steel, ¾-inch thick steering column
- Torsion bars
- Solid cast brake pedal or clutch pedal shaft
- Cast white metal door hinge
- Seat belt mounting bolts and reinforcing plates
- Hardened steel Nader lock bolts and reinforcing plates

Small nicks or indentations may be found in the cutting edges of the blades as a result of cutting these solid metal materials. When the cutting edge is damaged, the forces generated during cutting are no longer transmitted along the entire length of the blades. They are instead concentrated at these imperfections, which can cause premature fatigue of the blades and lead to blade failure during routine sheet metal cutting operations at a later time.

Although heavy duty metal components on a vehicle can readily be cut, moved, or removed with other tools or techniques, rescue personnel that intend to use their power cutter for severing heavy solid metal objects should obtain the relevant information from the manufacturer of that particular unit. Some tools can cut it, others cannot. The tool manufacturer's advice should be taken into consideration, as should the effect of the composition of the material being cut on the system's warranty or replacement terms. For example, one exception to the warranty on Amkus rescue system tools is "damage from failure to follow instructions contained in your owner's manual." The Amkus owner's manual for their model 25 power cutter specifically states, "The cutter is capable of cutting door posts, door struts, seatbacks, steering columns, and brake pedals. We do not recommend cutting steering columns under most conditions, but the capability is there." The manual goes on to state, "Although the Amkus cutter is extremely powerful, it is recommended that hardened steel not be cut. Small indentations may develop on the blade surface and possible blade breakage may occur. Items such as the steering wheel and the brake pedal are case hardened or surface hardened and can be cut." Holmatro, Inc states in a technical bulletin that their cutters "... should not be used as a demolition tool." Rescue personnel must understand the possibility of physical damage to their cutter and be aware of the liability risks associated with exceeding the manufacturer's criteria when operating this equipment.

Maintenance and Troubleshooting

Preventive maintenance for power cutter units includes checking proper fluid levels within the rescue system, cleaning and visually inspecting the component parts of the cutter unit, and checking to see that all nuts, bolts, retainer rings, screws, and pins are in place and securely fastened. Scheduled 6-month preventive maintenance for these units should include visually checking the blades for damage and wear. Owners of power cutters are advised by some manufacturers to check the blades of their units annually by submitting them to magnaflux or penetrant dye testing. Blades that show unusual wear or fatigue should be replaced as necessary.

POWER RAMS

In the early 1980s, North American crews operating with power rescue tool systems were introduced to a new rescue accessory with a simple design and important new capabilities, the power rescue system ram

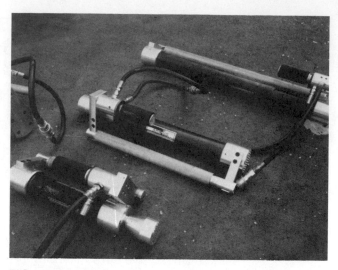

FIG. 6-15 Power rams can harness up to 20 tons of pushing, spreading, or lifting force.

(Fig. 6-15). Since then, power rams have become available for almost all of the major power rescue systems. These rams are sophisticated adaptations of the standard hydraulic jack unit. When they are available at an accident scene, rescue crews can rapidly push or pull with greater amounts of power and over longer distances than ever. As the saying goes, "If you can't spread it, ram it!"

A power ram consists of these basic components:
- Hose, couplings, and valve controls
- Tool body with hydraulic piston and plunger inside
- Ram base, plunger head, and interchangeable ram accessories

Design and Function

Most power rams are single plunger units with a stationary base at one end and a movable plunger end opposite. The plunger is the movable piston that travels in or out of the hydraulic cylinder that makes up the body of the tool. Holmatro and Viking rams are examples of twin plunger units, which have two independent plungers incorporated into one tool. Both extend and retract independently from each end and are controlled by a single control hydraulic valve located at the center of the ram. The latest generation power rams, presented first by the F.M. Brick Industries, Inc., now use a two-piece telescoping plunger unit (Fig. 6-16).

Power rams can be classified as single-acting or double-acting hydraulic units. A single-acting ram

Capacities

Power rams are manufactured in various sizes and capacities. Short-length rams have retracted lengths of between 12 and 24 inches. Medium-size rams are between 24- and 35-inches long when retracted. The largest rams have retracted lengths in excess of 35 inches. Extended overall lengths range from the shortest (Hurst Mini Ram) at 22 inches to the longest (largest Holmatro ram) at 65 inches.

Power capacities of rams vary with the physical size of the ram and the operating pressure of the hydraulic fluid in each particular system. Regardless of manufacturer, all power rams are more powerful while extending or pushing than when retracting. This power variation is inherent in the design and construction of the basic hydraulic piston assembly. Rams have a flat disk situated at the bottom of the plunger rod, inside the body of the ram. One side of this piston disk is completely exposed; the other side has the plunger rod attached to its center. The square-inch area of the open side of the disk is generally twice the useable area of the plunger side.

To extend the ram, the tool operator diverts hydraulic fluid under pressure against the full side of the disk. The available hydraulic fluid pressure is multiplied by the available surface area of this piston disk to create a given force rating for the ram. To retract the ram, the operator diverts the fluid against the other side of this disk, the side with the rod attached to it. Even though the fluid pressure remains the same, there may be up to 50% less surface area, which is why rams cannot retract or pull with the same force as when they extend or push. On average, rams develop only one half of their maximum power during their closing mode.

Many power ram manufacturers offer accessory attachments to increase the versatility of the tool. Accessories include plunger heads, bases, chain hook and shackle attachments, and extension tubing. Interchangeable plunger heads include conical point heads, flat bases, "vee" heads, wedge heads, and serrated heads. The chain and shackle attachments allow rams to be used to perform pulling evolutions. The extension tubing was developed as a means of extending the useable reach of the individual ram and may be either solid 10-inch lengths or assorted-length hollow tubing.

If operating personnel encounter difficulty while threading or unthreading any of the ram attachments, the problem may be due to the plunger itself turning

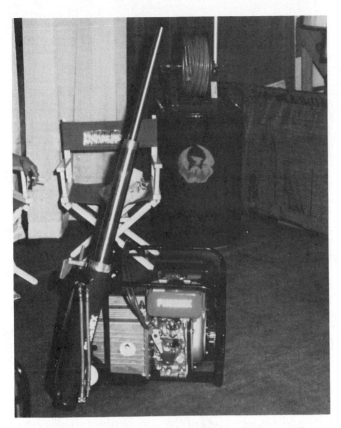

FIG. 6-16 The F.M. Brick Industries, Inc.'s Phoenix Super Ram, which extends from 25 to 60 inches in length, has a telescoping feature.

extends its plunger by hydraulic fluid pressure. The return of the plunger is generally accomplished by means of mechanical springs. Double-acting rams, the most prevalent and reliable type, use hydraulic fluid to both extend and retract their plunger.

Another important difference between power rams is whether they are direct control or remote control types. Direct control rams, which are the most common, have their hydraulic control valves mounted directly on the ram itself. In addition, grip handles are located directly on the tool body. The Phoenix ram, a remote-controlled power ram, has its control valve on a short hydraulic hose attached to the tool. One advantage of this style of remote control ram is that its lower tool profile allows it to be positioned in more restricted spaces than conventional direct control rams. Operating personnel can also situate themselves in a somewhat safer location when operating the remote control ram under actual rescue situations. One disadvantage is that it may require two hands to hold the ram in position initially and a third hand to operate the ram's remote control.

while the threading is being attempted. To correct this problem, personnel can fully extend or retract the plunger, increasing pressure against it. Under this pressure, the plunger will stop turning so that the attachments may be put on or taken off properly.

Safety Considerations

Rams are used to lift, spread, push, pull, or assist with stabilization efforts. As with all rescue equipment, operating personnel should be fully protected. Because rams are relatively light in weight by comparison to the larger power spreaders, one fully protected rescue crew member can safely operate the ram. All necessary safety precautions should be undertaken to insulate the trapped patient and attending medical personnel from any danger posed by operation of the ram.

The ram should only be held or maneuvered by using the grip handles or by the body of the tool itself. Hands should never be placed on the moving plunger because this action can contaminate the surface of the plunger with dirt and subject personnel to possible pinching injuries.

In vehicle rescue operations, there are very few situations where it is appropriate to say "never." One of these situations, however, involves operations with rams, which should never be used as the sole means of stabilizing an object or lifting a load. Under real-world applications, additional safety equipment must be committed to render the operation safe. At a minimum, wood blocking should be deployed at strategic locations to secure the object in its new position. Rescue and medical personnel should never place themselves or their patients in a position where they risk injury if the tool moves or fails in its function. In these unpredictable situations, by the time a person realizes they are likely to be caught under a shifting load, it can be too late.

Power rams have the least structural integrity when fully extended. When the plunger is stowed inside the body of the tool, there is maximum contact between the plunger and the ram cylinder. Extending the ram moves the plunger out from the body of the tool, diminishing contact between the plunger and the cylinder. Heavy loading or stressing of the ram during a long spread or push can deform the tool. Operating personnel should be constantly alert for long reaches or off-center loading that can cause undue stress and affect the integrity of the tool as it extends.

Rams are also vulnerable to destruction if they are improperly set up during ram pulling evolutions. To

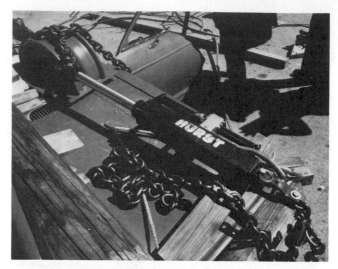

FIG. 6-17 Use of power rams for pulling operations can cause safety problems and tool damage when a load is applied unevenly to the ram, resulting in bending or twisting. Many rescue teams do not use power rams for pulling.

pull two objects closer together, the ram must first be extended, making it vulnerable to deforming. The base and plunger ends of the ram are then attached by chain or strap to the desired objects. As the ram retracts, its power is used to move one object toward the other. Destruction can occur if the ram is loaded and bends during this pull, such as when a ram placed on the hood of a vehicle is used to pull a steering column forward. If the end of the ram nearest the front of the vehicle is allowed to extend past the front of the hood area, this part of the ram may bend downward when the load is applied, damaging the plunger, O-rings, seals, and the tool's cylinder. Proper placement of blocking under the rams may control this deflection (Fig. 6-17).

Personnel using power rams for pulling operations must be sure that all loads applied to the ram run parallel to the tool. Having a completely solid base under the ram or having the ram suspended without any contact under it will ensure a safe, parallel pull. Some rescue crews unwilling to risk damaging their rams have adopted standard operating procedures that forbid power rams to be used for any pulling operations.

Ram manufacturers Kinman and H.K. Porter have designed their units to perform the pulling function while positioned perpendicular to the line of the pull rather than parallel to the pull. The Kinman ram, for example, pulls by use of a length of chain, the Kinman "stroke multiplier," and a roller adaptor accessory. A concern with this system is that the pull causes chain to pass around or over three separate rollers. Under a heavy pulling load, this path of travel can bend each individual link as it passes over the rollers. Close examination of the links of chain used with a Kinman ram will show evidence of this. With continued use, the links of chain will be weakened by being bent back and forth. The safe working capacity of a chain that has been subjected to this kind of abuse cannot be estimated. Personnel should exercise prudent judgment when deciding whether it is safe to employ rescue chain that has been bent and abused (Fig. 6-18).

Power rams are also vulnerable to damage while being used in the conventional pushing mode. Operating personnel must be certain that both the base and the plunger ends of the ram are properly positioned before any load is applied to the tool. Good solid anchor spots must be located on the surfaces being worked apart. Safe ram positioning when using Amkus rams *must* also include the use of the Amkus ram base plate accessory. On selected models of Amkus rams, the return hydraulic lines are located within the handle of the ram, flush with the base end of the tool. Most ram designs locate the grip handles and any hydraulic lines clear of the extreme ends of the tool. Without the Amkus ram base plate, it is possible for operating personnel to stress this grip handle, particularly when using the ram at an angle. This can fracture the handle bracket and the enclosed hydraulic lines. Amkus offers base plates for use at the bottom end of the ram to avert this damage. With this

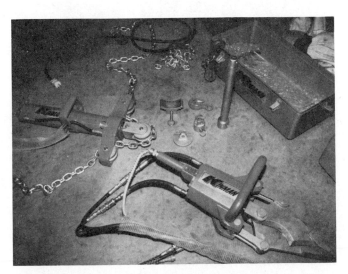

FIG. 6-18 Pulling with the Kinman ram requires an accessory roller adaptor to change the direction of pull as the chain is moved by the head of the ram.

large cast metal accessory in place, the load exerted on the ram is evenly distributed across the entire working area of the plate, eliminating the possibility of handle bracket damage.

Maintenance and Troubleshooting

Preventive maintenance of power rams includes visual inspection of all components of the tool after each use with particular attention given to any physical damage or evidence of oil leaks. All nuts, bolts, retainer rings, and screws should be in place and securely fastened. The control mechanism must operate freely and return to the neutral position easily. The base and plunger ends must be closely inspected for physical damage because these parts are most susceptible to wear and tear. With the plunger extended, the piston rod should be inspected for any scoring or bending and be cleaned of any accumulated dirt.

It is also recommended that the power spreader, cutter, and/or ram units be stored preconnected to the other components of the rescue system if possible (Fig. 6-19). Having the power rescue tools preconnected increases operational efficiency on the rescue scene and reduces the possibility of hook-up problems at an incident. Power rams should be stored with the plungers extended by ¼ to ½ inch to prevent their being overretracted into the body of the tool and creating excessive pressure on the tool's hydraulic system.

The pros and cons of simultaneous tool operations, which may be promoted heavily by vendors of rescue equipment, should be considered carefully. Simultaneous operations may reduce the overall operating time necessary to disentangle a trapped occupant, but rescue operations conducted on the same accident vehicle at the same time may also be detrimental. The operation of one piece of equipment may affect the work of another crew. Those using a cutting tool, for example, may be making it more difficult for a crew on the other side of the vehicle forcing entry on a door. Those pushing with a power ram may actually be crushing the very area where a second team must work to cut away portions of the vehicle. Simultaneous work with power rescue tools on the same vehicle can be a commander's nightmare. Personnel safety is jeopardized when the commander of the rescue operations is unable to effectively monitor two tasks at the same time; it may be better to quickly follow one task with another. The advantage of being able to couple two or more accessories together at one time to one power plant is that rescue personnel may be able to operate on two different vehicles at the

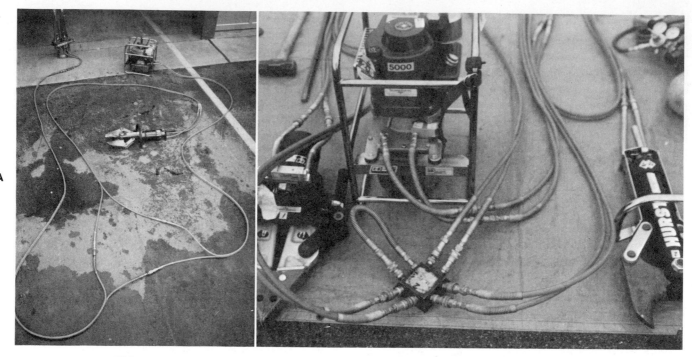

A   B

FIG. 6-19 Hooking spreader and cutter tool together requires a closed loop formed by **A,** hooking hoses together to establish a fluid flow or **B,** use of a manifold device such as an inline block. The latest generation of manifold blocks can be mounted at the power plant itself or inline and are equipped with pressure relief/dump values.

same time or perform one function on a vehicle with one tool and immediately follow it up with a second accessory on the same vehicle without a loss of time.

Hydraulic Jack Tool Family
PORTO-POWER RESCUE TOOL

A second family of rescue equipment, which also uses hydraulic fluid, is the hydraulic jack tool family. This family includes the standard hydraulic jack and the remote-controlled hydraulic jack, widely known as the porto-power rescue tool. Porto-Power is a registered trade name of the Blackhawk Co. The name has become so much a part of the language of rescue personnel during the past years that it is used throughout this text to indicate any remote-controlled hydraulic jack unit.

The earliest hydraulic rescue system was the standard hydraulic hand jack. The pumping section of this device creates pressure on hydraulic oil stored in a fluid reservoir. The oil moves into the cylinder of the tool to exert force upon a hydraulic plunger or piston. The plunger extends under pressure and retracts when the operator moves the relief valve, returning the fluid to the reservoir.

The standard hydraulic jack is available in capac-

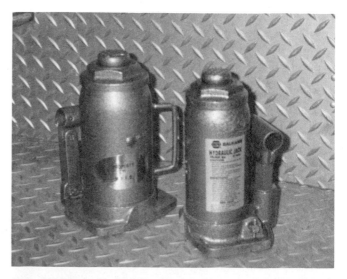

FIG. 6-20 Standard hydraulic jack units commonly found in rescue company inventories have 5- to 20-ton capacities; most also have the adjustable screw extension head feature.

ities ranging from 2 tons to over 500 tons for specialized industrial applications. In the field of vehicle rescue, common jack capacities include 5-ton to 20-ton capacity units. Better quality jacks also provide an adjustable screw extension feature (Fig. 6-20). This threaded rod extends from the top of the plunger to give the jack increased total extension height. The extension and retraction of the hydraulic plunger is the one simple function the tool is designed to accomplish. Rescue personnel can use this function to perform lifting, spreading, pushing, pulling, and stabilizing evolutions. Although all jacks function best when the plunger is vertical, certain models are designed to continue to function when held horizontally as long as the pump element is positioned below the cylinder. Still other models function while in any position.

Some 40 years ago, the pump and the jacking components of the hydraulic jack were separated. Encasing them as separate units and connecting them by means of a hydraulic hose produced the first remote-controlled hydraulic jack tools. This tool, now referred to as the *porto-power* by rescue personnel, was the premier rescue tool of its day and remained so until the introduction of the first power rescue tools in the early 1970s. Unfortunately, since the advent of power rescue equipment, what followed was diminished training and use of the porto-power among rescue personnel in North America. Some rescue companies have removed their kits from service, while others placed their porto-power in out-of-the-way locations in the belief that the unit was no longer as valuable. Progressive-minded rescue personnel, however, agree that the porto-power continues to have an important place in today's basic inventory of rescue equipment. At certain times and places, this tool can perform exceptionally well, and it is a valuable backup for primary rescue equipment should a primary tool failure occur. The porto-power in combination with other equipment plays an important role when similar rescue evolutions must be accomplished simultaneously at a multivehicle accident scene.

The porto-power was not developed to serve our rescue services. The tool was initially promoted as a body shop tool to be used for vehicle repair and restoration after a collision; this is still its largest application. The tool that the rescue service employs today was not specially designed for rescue. For the most part, our porto-power units are basic body shop kits with a new rescue label.

Many manufacturers now market these products. The two brands most widely used by rescue crews are the original Porto-Power tool manufactured by the Blackhawk Co. and the P-F Rescue tool manufactured by H.K. Porter, Inc. In recent years there has been an influx of inexpensive foreign-made units into

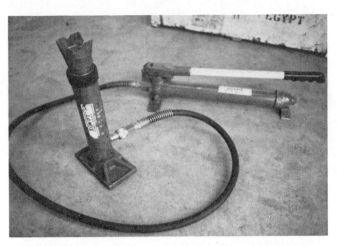

FIG. 6-21 Porto-power ram with 10-ton rating with single-stage pump unit of 10,000 psi capacity. The rating of hydraulic pressure that the pump creates must not be confused with the rated capacity of the ram.

the United States. These kits, many of which come from Taiwan, usually lack full system capabilities and are of barely minimum quality for rescue applications.

In discussing the basic porto-power system, it is important to identify and label its components. The terminology is the same for all porto-power systems.

Power to perform work with the porto-power is provided by operation of the hydraulic pump. Most pumps are the manual style, although some crews operate with an air-over-hydraulic unit. These pumps compress air to 100 psi, which in turn pressurizes the hydraulic fluid to the 10,000 psi necessary for tool operation. Manual porto-power pumps can be single-stage or two-stage units; the difference is in the method by which the pump creates pressure (Fig. 6-21). The first stage of a two-stage pump creates low pressure quickly when the tool is not under a load, working from 0 to 1400 psi, for example. The second stage of the pump functions as the load increases on the tool, building pressure up to the maximum pump rating.

Porto-power manual pumps have a pump handle, a fluid reservoir that makes up the body of the pump, an internal pump assembly, a manual relief valve, and an oil level dipstick. The manual relief valve is closed when the handle is pumped, to create pressure and opened to allow the fluid to return to the reservoir. This valve is threaded into the pump casing and should only be opened one to two full turns. Opening the valve more than that introduces the possibility that the stem may actually pop out of the pump.

Porto-power pump units should only be operated

when they are horizontal or when the hose end of the pump is held below horizontal. The P-F pumps from H.K. Porter Inc also require that the small air bleed knob located on the body of the pump be opened at least one-half turn to vent the pump. All porto-power systems use standard hydraulic jack oil. Most contain antifoaming and antisludge agents and include additives designed to inhibit rusting of interior metal components. Most standard hydraulic jack oils function to temperatures of –50° F. Brake fluid or any liquid with an alcohol base should not be used in any porto-power unit because they may destroy the various seals and 0-rings.

All pumps have a pressure rating expressed in pounds per square inch hydraulic fluid pressure. Small-size pumps typically have ratings of up to 10,000 psi, and the larger units are capable of achieving a maximum pressure of 20,000 psi. The pump pressure is *not* the power rating of a porto-power unit; it refers only to the ability of the pump to create pressure. A 10,000 psi (5-ton) pump, for example, may be used with a kit rated at 10-ton lifting capacity. Pounds per square inch is not the same as pounds of force exerted by the tool (see box).

The fluid leaves the pump, traveling through hydraulic hoses and couplings. The hydraulic hoses are rubber with ¼-inch or ⅜-inch inside diameters. The smaller hose is typically constructed with one internal wire braid and has a 12,000 psi bursting strength. The larger hoses have two-wire internal braiding and are rated at 20,000 psi bursting strength. Couplings attach to the hose with standard male and female pipe threads and use quick disconnect valve seats that permit disconnecting without significant oil loss.

The hydraulic ram or jack component of a porto-power kit is one of several items that can attach directly to the hydraulic hose coming from the pump. The ram and necessary attachments are required for most of the work that a porto-power accomplishes. Rams can be designed as push-only, pull-only, or combination push-pull units (Fig. 6-22). Push-only rams, the most common rescue ram style, or the less common pull-only rams are a single-acting design ram with spring or gravity return (Fig. 6-23). Combination push-pull rams are double-acting with extension and retraction of the plunger accomplished by hydraulic power similar to the power rescue system rams discussed earlier.

A basic 4-ton or 10-ton porto-power ram consists of a movable plunger, an external cylinder or body of the tool, and hydraulic hose female coupling. Both plunger and cylinder have male pipe threads at the top end. The cylinder may also have female threads at the bottom of the unit. A plastic or metal thread protector ring is provided to prevent damage to the

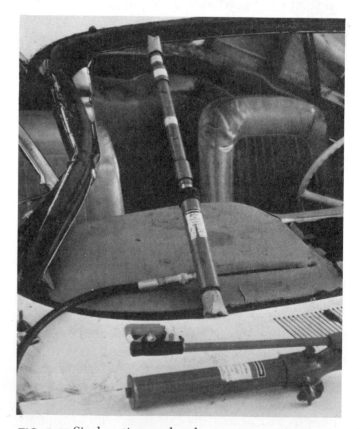

FIG. 6-22 Single-acting, push-only porto-power 4-ton capacity ram with accessories.

USEFUL HYDRAULIC FORMULAS

FORMULA A

Cylinder effective area (sq in)
X
Hydraulic working pressure (psi)
=
Cylinder force (lb)

FORMULA B

Cylinder effective area (sq in)
X
Cylinder stroke (in)
=
Cylinder oil capacity (cu/in)

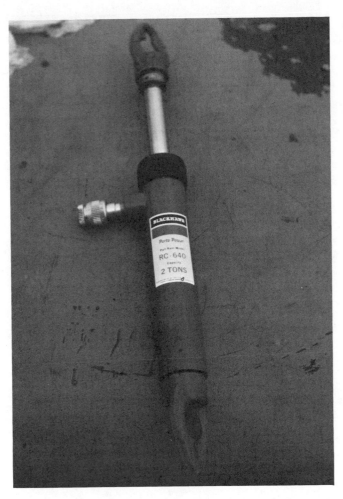

FIG. 6-23 Porto-power ram designed exclusively for pulling evolutions. This ram is a 2-ton capacity, single-acting, pull-only unit with special chain attachment heads.

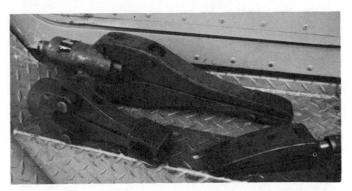

FIG. 6-24 *Left to right:* Duck bill, spreader, and wedgie accessories.

cylinder threads. This ring must be removed before attaching accessories to the cylinder threads. All attachments for the porto-power thread directly onto the ram at either the plunger threads, cylinder thread, or base end of the ram.

The rating of a porto-power ram and the rating of its kit are the same. If the kit is rated as a 10-ton outfit, the ram can deliver that work output. Contrary to what many rescue personnel believe, the ram is the only porto-power accessory that can achieve the full kit rating. All other accessories are rated at less than the full system rating.

The spreader, duck bill, and wedgie accessories are all designed for spreading and are three common components that can be attached directly to the hydraulic hose of the porto-power pump (Fig. 6-24). The smallest spreading attachment, the wedgie, has an upper arm and a lower arm that open a maximum of approximately 3 to 3½ inches. If the wedgie is designed with one flat and one curved arm, the curved arm should be placed against the object to be moved to operate most efficiently.

The large spreader has two arms of similar design. The unit has a typical tip opening of 12 inches. The intermediate-size duck bill spreader unit has a threaded collar with short, stubby mechanical arms and does not have its own hydraulic piston unit. The plunger of the porto-power ram is used to push the duck bill spreader arms apart. These units generally have a 6-inch maximum tip opening distance.

The most significant point to remember when working with the porto-power wedgie, duck bill, or spreader accessory is that these units *do not* have the same power rating as the porto-power ram; all are rated well below what is generally believed. These tools are designed as body shop tools and have been adapted for vehicle rescue by rescue personnel, not the manufacturers. In the body shop, they are used to spread wrinkled sheet metal on a damaged auto. The maximum ratings of these attachments vary by manufacturer and whether they were originally designed for body repair or industrial applications. The power ratings of body repair porto-power equipment tend to be lower than those of the similar industrial models preferred for fire service rescue applications.

The following ratings illustrate the light-duty capacities of many porto-power accessories. Generally speaking, wedgie tools have a *maximum* rating of 600 lb of lifting or spreading force. The duck bill and the spreader commonly have *maximum* ratings of 1200 lb of force. The rating of the Enerpac Company industrial model porto-power wedgie is either a 1500 or 2000 lb, their duck bill has a 2000 lb capacity rating, and their spreader is rated at 3000 lb. The Ausco

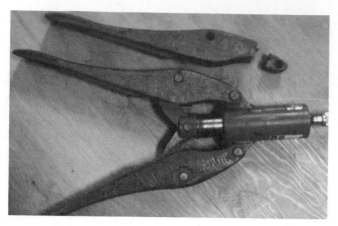

FIG. 6-25 Forcing porto-power spreader or wedgie to work beyond its rated capacity results in explosive failure. Failure points on the arms include the tips and hinge or pivot points.

company markets a uniquely design porto-power spreader rated at 1¾ tons.

Whatever the rating given a particular porto-power spreading attachment, it is not as powerful as the ram. All porto-power spreaders have less power than is needed to force open an automobile's Nader safety lock within a reasonable amount of time. Stress from a heavy load or from forcing a jammed door open can overpower the spreaders. Under conditions of misuse or improper application, the cast metal arms can fail violently (Fig. 6-25). The failure is explosive in nature. When a porto-power spreader arm breaks, the entire tool can fly out of its location, endangering anyone it its range.

To prevent overloading the light-duty wedgie, duck bill, and spreader accessory, personnel should always follow a very special safety procedure. To eliminate excessive pressure at the spreading tool, the operator of the hydraulic pump should be positioned with the pump in one hand and the handle in the other, holding the pump across the chest with the hose end pointed down (Fig. 6-26). Although this makes pumping the handle more difficult than it is when the pump is positioned flat on the ground, it reduces the possibility of overpressurizing the attached tool. The operator should only pump to the degree that can be achieved in this chest position. When the pump and handle can no longer be squeezed together, the capacity of the wedgie, duck bill, or spreader has been reached and the pumping should stop. To further increase safety, assisting personnel should retain a firm grasp on the spreading tool whenever it is being used. If the tool

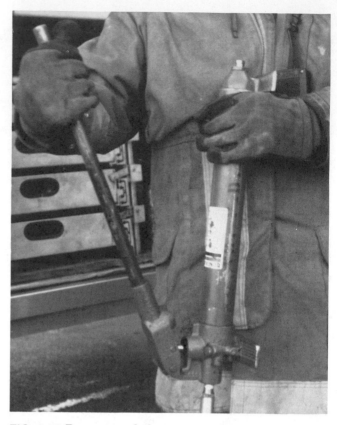

FIG. 6-26 Recommended operation of the pump across the chest minimizes overpressurizing. Pumping is halted when the operator encounters difficulty in moving the handle.

slips or fails, the crew member can restrain its movement.

Additional accessories also have lower capacities than the hydraulic ram, partly because of their less substantial construction. Most reputable manufacturers of porto-power equipment state that their accessories have a safe working capacity of only 50% of the power rating of the ram; some set this figure as low as 25%. It is vitally important for rescue personnel to be aware of this fact. A porto-power kit that is big and heavy and says "10-ton" on the box is not that powerful. Only the ram can achieve this maximum rating; the spreading accessories are relatively light-duty, and the attachments only perform up to 50% of this rating. Given the choice between buying a 4-ton porto-power or a 10-ton kit, rescue personnel would thus be smart to purchase the bigger unit.

Attachments are necessary to accomplish the three basic operations of lifting, spreading or pushing, and pulling with a porto-power tool. Spreading or pushing is actually a lifting function, accomplished horizontally. Typical porto-power accessories include several different items.

Heads

There are a variety of sizes and shapes of head attachments. A head functions to provide a contact point between the tool and an object. Heads are typically placed at the ends of a porto-power setup and at the plunger of the ram to protect exposed threads from physical damage (Fig. 6-27).

Terms used to describe heads reflect features such as their shape, design, or construction. Porto-power head attachments include the following:

- Smooth head: The cap has female threads and a smooth top.
- Serrated head: The cap has female threads and an uneven top surface. Head may have concentric rings, criss-crossed squares, or raised points. This type is appropriate for routine use in protecting plunger threads.
- Crowned head: The metal cap has female threads and a rounded top.
- Vee head: The cap has female threads and prominent raised points resembling a molar tooth. This head is the work horse of all porto-power head attachments and has superior strength and durability.
- Wedge head: The cap has female threads and a long, tapered, wedge-shaped top. Larger sizes resemble the roof of a house.
- Rubber head: This head resembles one half of a rubber ball with female threads located on flat side. Heads are described as 3-inch or 5-inch models according to diameter of the rubber ball. Head flexes or flattens under compression load, increasing the contact area with object.

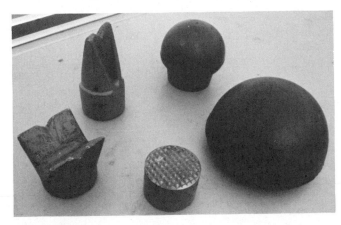

FIG. 6-27 Porto-power heads.

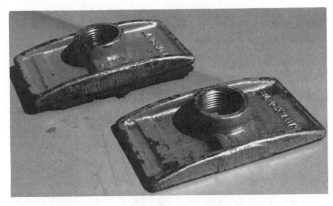

FIG. 6-28 Bottoms of porto-power base attachments are smooth metal, rubber covered, or metal cleated.

- Cleat head: The six-sided cap has male threads and a center cleat located on the side opposite the threads. This head is used when a solid anchor position is required.
- Wide-angle wedge head: The multipiece head has two or more flexible pads hinged to the head. The pads move to conform to the surface placed against it. The head provides a large contact area against objects being pushed.

Bases

The function of a base attachment is to increase the contact area between the working ends of a porto-power unit and an object (Fig. 6-28). Bases function much like the outrigger plates used by fire service personnel when setting up a piece of aerial fire apparatus. Terms for the bases also reflect their obvious features. Porto-power base attachments include the following:

- Flat base: This rectangular metal plate has a female threaded cup in center of top side and completely smooth bottom side. This is the standard base attachment.
- Flat base/rubber-faced: The standard flat base has a ¼-inch thick pad of rubber attached to the smooth bottom side. It is used to minimize slippage or travel of base during evolution.
- Cleated flat base: This standard flat base has multiple cleats protruding from the bottom side. This base is used when additional gripping is required.

Extension Tubes

As the name implies, extension tubes are used to increase the reaching capabilities of the basic porto-power ram. The tubing is provided in various lengths from the smallest piece, 1 inch in length, to the largest

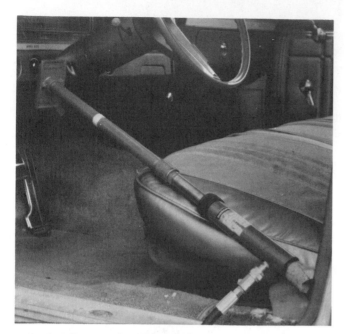

FIG. 6-29 Ram with vee head, flat base, threaded connector, and extension tubing in pushing application.

tubes, 30 inches in length (Fig. 6-29). The metal tubes in the better quality kits are of heavy-duty metal construction. The extrusion manufacturing process results in a finished extension tube with no seams or welds. Smaller porto-power kits use ¾-inch diameter pipe tubing, while the larger 10-ton outfits require 1¼-inch tubing.

Extension tubing generally has male pipe threaded ends with holes strategically located near each end. Longer length tubes may have a series of up to five holes placed near one end (required for one specific porto-power clamping setup that is described later). Kits designed only for basic pushing or spreading functions do not require threads or holes on the extension tubing.

Slip-Lock Extension

The more extensive porto-power outfits include a special extension piece that is adjustable in length. This slip-lock extension is used in conjunction with one of the longer-length standard extension tubes. It consists of a threaded rod with a large movable collar, a release button, and a male threaded cap. The collar has internal female threads. The slip-lock extension threaded rod is first inserted into one end of a standard extension tube. The collar is then threaded onto the tubing. By pressing the release button or turning the rod like a large screw, personnel can extend or retract the rod, making a tube assembly of various lengths

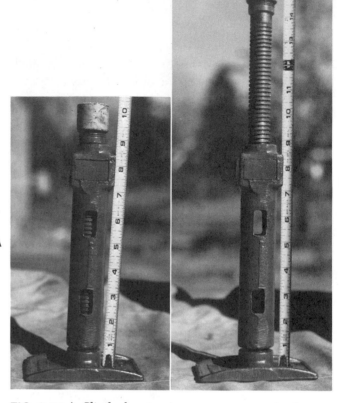

FIG. 6-30 A, Slip-lock extension accessory permits the tool to be adjusted. **B,** Slip-lock in extended position.

(Fig. 6-30). To maximize safety when working with the slip-lock extension piece, personnel should only extend the threaded rod to 80% of its total length. This limit enables the rod to maintain sufficient contact inside its threaded collar. The last 2 inches of the rod should be painted a bright, contrasting color to aid in maintaining this safety factor. During use, the rod is extended only up to the point at which the safety color becomes visible.

Connectors and Locking Pins

The extension tubes are connected together in several ways. The simplest method for use with threaded end tubing uses threaded male and female connectors (Fig. 6-31, *A*)). Better quality kits provide quick-connectors and locking pins. These connectors are short, solid metal pieces with a flush-mounted ball bearing and a hole in each half of the connector. A raised ridge identifies the center point of the connector (Fig. 6-31, *B*). The connectors are designed to be inserted into the open ends of the extension tubing and twisted until the holes in the tube and the connector align. A locking pin placed through the

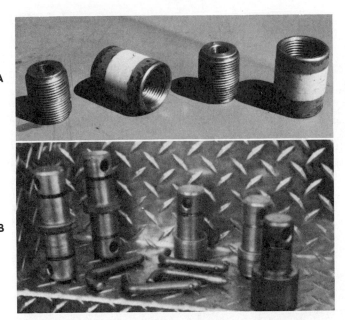

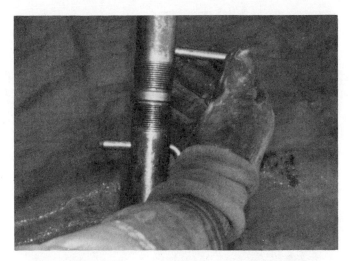

FIG. 6-32 Two locking pins must be used with each quick connector to safely secure the assembly.

FIG. 6-31 A, Threaded double-male and double-female connectors. **B,** Standard quick connectors, locking pins, and connector adapters with male and female threaded ends.

holes then secures the assembly in place (Fig. 6-32). H.K. Porter, Inc., manufacturer of the P-F porto-power, states that these connectors are twice as strong as threaded ones.

Tubing manufactured without threaded ends typically has a quick connector built into one end of each tube. This end simply slips into the open end of another tube to make a "push only" connection. The tubes can easily be pulled apart when different length porto-power setups are required.

Adaptors

Adaptors are attachments to make connections between ram, tubing, or other components. An adaptor accessory may have either male or female threads at one end and a quick-connector at the other. Adaptors are used to allow accessories to be attached to the ram at either the plunger or base end of the cylinder.

Cylinder Toe

This attachment resembles a shoe or foot in appearance. The main portion has a large threaded opening with a small toe area protruding to one side. The cylinder can be used in conjunction with the plunger toe or any flat base. During use, the cylinder toe is secured onto the cylinder threads of the ram with the toe facing away from the bottom of the ram.

Plunger Toe

This attachment is similar to its companion, the cylinder toe, except that it is smaller in size and has one flat side. The plunger toe threads onto the plunger of the ram (or extension tubing) with the protruding toe again facing away from the bottom of the ram.

The two toes allow the porto-power ram to operate in smaller areas for lifting or spreading evolutions (Fig. 6-33). With the cylinder toe and plunger toe properly installed, the ram is inverted for lifting. The plunger toe becomes the base, and the cylinder toe provides the lift as the ram extends. A flat base can be substituted for the plunger toe for most lifting evolutions. When used horizontally, the toes allow the porto-power to be used for spreading or pushing evolutions. The toes are subjected to severe shearing forces as they are used, and the metal protrusions can be overloaded to the point of failure. Most tool manufacturers rate their cylinder and plunger toe attachments at 50% of the rated capacity of the ram. With a 10-ton capacity ram, the toes enable rescue personnel to work with a 5-ton spreader, one that is lightweight, portable, and relatively small in size.

Clamp Head

The clamp head attachment is a one-piece unit resembling a figure eight. One loop has internal female threads, the other has a smooth inner surface. This attachment is used in conjunction with the clamp toe accessory for 10-ton units and works with the plunger toe on the smaller 4-ton kits.

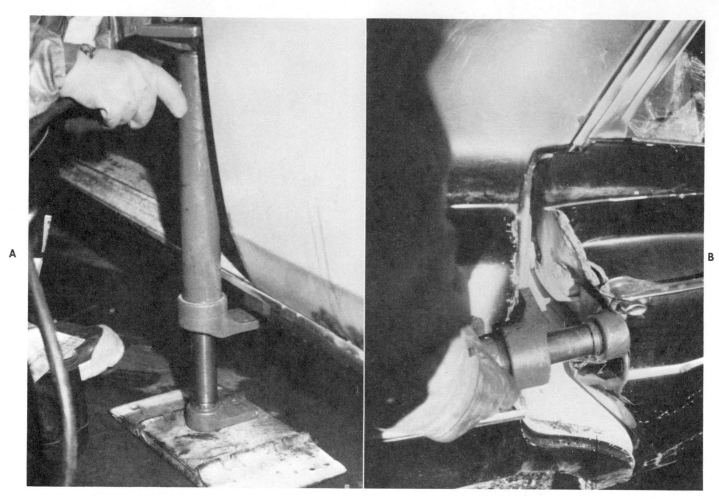

FIG. 6-33 Cylinder and plunger toe on inverted cylinder **A,** allow lifting, whereas toes on ram held horizontally **B,** permit spreading of door metal.

Clamp Toe

This attachment is only provided on units of 10-ton capacity. It is similar to the plunger toe although it is slightly larger and has no threads.

These accessories are used in the body shop to squeeze or clamp sheet metal. In the rescue environment the same clamp head and clamp toe are used for clamping, squeezing, or pulling evolutions.

To set up the 10-ton porto-power, personnel should attach the threaded opening of the clamp head to the cylinder threads of the ram. Lengths of extension tubing with a lengthwise series of holes are attached to the plunger. The holes are positioned furthest from the ram. The clamp toe is then slipped over the extension tubing and secured in place with a locking pin. The distance between the head on the plunger and the toe at the end of the setup can quickly be adjusted by locating the clamp toe at a different hole in the extension tube. There are two differences

in this clamping setup when working with the smaller 4-ton ram: the plunger toe is used instead of the clamp toe, and the long length tubing does not have a series of holes.

As the ram operates on either size porto-power unit, the plunger extends and moves toward the end of the tubing. Any object positioned between the head on the plunger and the toe at the end is clamped, squeezed, or pulled together. With this setup, it is possible to move objects such as seats, pedals, and shift levers and to perform simple pulling operations (Fig. 6-34).

It is important to remember, however, that regardless of the size of the ram being used, the clamp head, clamp toe, and plunger toe are generally rated at only 50% of the ram capacity. Caution must be exercised to minimize the chance of overloading this setup.

The P-F porto-power uses many accessories to accomplish the pulling or clamping assembly. The

P-F tool pulling setup is the most difficult and time consuming to assemble because it requires their pull arm attachment, pull arm guide, pull toe, adaptors, head, extension tubing, connectors, and locking pins.

The two-piece arm attachment incorporates a flexible elbow joint between its two pieces. The exposed male threads are attached to the thread portion at the bottom of the P-F ram. The pull arm guide has two holes in the shape of a figure eight. The smaller hole has a smooth inside edge, and the larger opening is threaded. This portion attaches to the cylinder threads on the ram. Extension tubing passes through the smooth opening of the pull arm guide and is secured to the threaded portion of the pull arm by use of an adaptor. A head is then attached to the plunger. The pull toe, a larger and longer version of the basic plunger toe, is threaded onto the end of the extension tubing by use of another adaptor. The flat side of the pull toe faces the plunger of the ram. In operation, the distance between the head on the plunger and the pull toe decreases, producing a clamping or pulling action.

There are several other methods of setting up a porto-power to accomplish pulling evolutions. Some of the methods use accessories specifically designed for pulling, other methods accomplish pulling in non-standard ways. Pulling accessories vary by size and manufacturer. All pulling setups are explained to facilitate their application to particular equipment. Although modified pulling arrangements, like many of the basic porto-power assemblies, cannot be described as quick or easy, knowledge of these optional tool assemblies broadens the rescuer's understanding of the porto-power and provides additional tools and techniques with which to accomplish given rescue evolutions.

Pulling with most 4-ton or 10-ton units can be accomplished by use of the porto-power chain pull plate accessory. This attachment resembles a large metal yoke: the center hole has female threads, and there are grooves and notches on the inside portions of the yoke. The chain pull plate requires the use of two individual lengths of chain provided with the kit. These chains are generally from 5 to 6 feet in length and have a grab hook at one end. In use, the large opening of the chain pull plate is threaded onto the cylinder of the ram with the flat side of the attachment facing the hose connection (Fig. 6-35). A head or flat base attachment is then positioned on the ram's plunger. The ram is positioned on the outside edge of one object while the chain lengths are maneuvered through the slotted area of the chain pull plate and locked into position. Using additional chain as necessary, the lengths are joined to form a loop around a second object. As the ram is operated, the distance between the plunger and the far side of the loop of chain diminishes, resulting in a pulling function.

This setup is typically rated at 50% or less of the capacity of the ram. The critical factor in this setup however, is the rating of the chain that is used. When a chain pull plate is used on a 10-ton capacity ram, the chain's working load rating must exceed the 5-ton rating of the pull. This pulling setup is simple to assemble and very effective when used. A more sophisticated pulling arrangement, which is available for porto-power kits rated at 10-ton or more, uses two

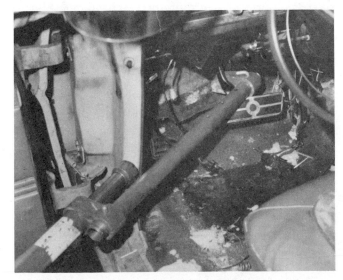

FIG. 6-34 Clamp head, clamp toe, and extension tubing allow 10-ton capacity porto-power to be used as a 5-ton capacity clamp to pull or bend brake pedal.

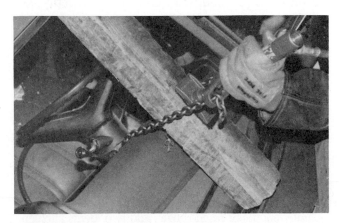

FIG. 6-35 Chain pull plate attachment with porto-power chain and wood cribbing block are used to lift the wheel and column away from a trapped driver.

identical attachments known as chain plates and the two lengths of porto-power chain. The chain plates resemble metal cloverleafs: two sides are slotted and the opposite two sides are open holes.

To set up the chain plates, personnel attach each chain plate to the ram at either the plunger or the base of the cylinder. One chain length locks into the slot of one chain plate, passes through the open holes of the chain plate at the opposite end of the ram, and returns to lock into the remaining slot of the first chain plate. The second chain is rigged in a similar fashion with its start being at the slot of the second chain plate. This chain passes through the open holes of the opposite chain plate and returns to the only remaining open slot. When assembled, the chain forms loops off each end of the ram. In operation, the ram extends and the chain lengths pass each other. In doing so, the distance between the loops of chain diminishes. This action accomplishes the pull. The chain plate pulling setup is rated at 50% or less of the ram capacity or the capacity of the chain used, whichever is less (Fig. 6-36).

The P-F unit is designed to pull by positioning the ram perpendicular to the line of pull. This is done by using the chain pull collar attachment, the chain provided with the kit, and a head specially designed to hold the links of the rescue chain. The collar resembles a small yoke with a threaded hole at its center and curved, slotted channels on each side. The bottom side of the collar is flat, and the top is curved toward the center hole. The chain head is a female-threaded cap with a head design that allows one link of the P-F rescue chain to lock into the head.

The collar threads onto the ram with its curved side positioned toward the hose connection of the ram. The chain head is then threaded onto the plunger of the ram. For personnel to complete the setup, the

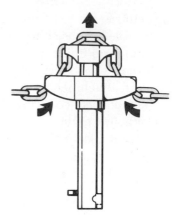

FIG. 6-37 Pulling setup for H.K. Porter unit uses chain head and chain pull collar.

open end of the P-F rescue chain is laced through the bottom side of the collar, over the chain head, and down through the remaining side of the collar. Each end of the chain is secured for the pull. As the plunger of the ram extends, the chain is pulled in through both slotted sides of the collar. One inch of ram travel will pull each side of rescue chain in the same distance. Therefore, 1 inch of ram travel can theoretically yield 2 inches of pull. This assembly is generally rated at 50% or less of the ram capacity or the capacity of the chain, whichever is less (Fig. 6-37).

Nonstandard porto-power pulling setups, those not using attachments specifically designed for pulling, work well under most situations. The simplest and most effective method of pulling involves the use of the basic porto-power ram, the vee head, a flat base, and a length of rescue chain. The vee head is attached to the plunger of the ram, and the flat base is secured to the bottom of the cylinder. The flat base of the ram is positioned on the outside of either a stationary object or a movable one. The chain is looped around the outside of both the vee head of the ram and the object at the opposite end of the setup, forming a loop. As the ram is operated, the vee head moves this entire loop of chain, reducing the distance between the fixed object and the stationary object and accomplishing a simple and effective pull (Fig. 6-38).

There are three important points to consider when comparing this "homemade" pulling arrangement with conventional pull setups. First, the ram is used at its 100% capacity rating. This makes the safe working capacity of the chain being used or the capacity of the ram the determining factors in the pulling power of this setup. Second, the only accessories used were a

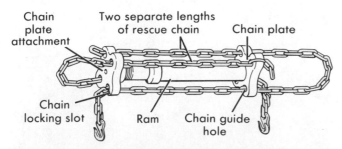

FIG. 6-36 Pulling with 10-ton porto-power ram, two separate lengths of rescue chain, and two identical chain plate attachments. Note that during tool setup, chain plates at each end of ram are rotated 90 degrees to each other to permit threading of chain.

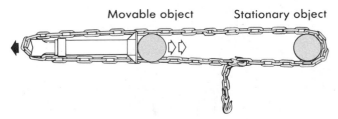

Movable object   Stationary object

FIG. 6-38 Placed against a movable object, the ram pushes objects closer together. Placed against a stationary object, the ram pulls the movable object.

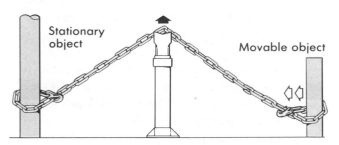

Stationary object   Movable object

FIG. 6-40 Ram with flat base and vee head attachment lifts the length of chain, pulling the moveable object inward.

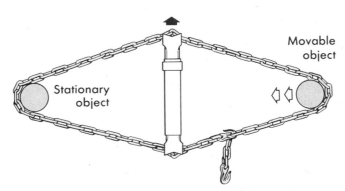

Movable object   Stationary object

FIG. 6-39 Porto-power ram with 2 vee heads can spread the chain, resulting in a pulling action.

vee head, a male threaded 1-inch adaptor, and the flat base. Most rescue crews carry the porto-power ram with these attachments already in place. This minimizes the time it takes to put the tool into this pulling operation at an actual incident. The third factor is the ease of resetting this pulling arrangement when the ram runs out of travel, which simply involves retracting the ram, pulling the slack out of the chain, and securing the grab hook back into the chain where appropriate.

The same porto-power ram and chain can be used in two other setups to pull objects closer together. These arrangements also have all of the above-mentioned advantages. If all work is to be done on a flat surface, one of the methods uses chain looped completely around the outside of a fixed object and a movable object. The ram is then placed at a perpendicular angle against the chain at a point halfway between the two objects. During its operation, the ram spreads the two lines of chain apart, which brings the movable object closer to the fixed one. If the rescue crew has a second vee head, it can be substi-

tuted for the flat base for improved stability (Fig. 6-39).

Another nonstandard pulling method uses the same accessories to place chain loops around both the fixed object and the movable one. A single line of chain is then run between the two objects. The ram is placed vertically under the center of this line of chain with the vee head pushing against the chain. As the ram operates, it lifts the center of the length of chain, moving the objects closer together and accomplishing the desired pull (Fig. 6-40).

Safety Considerations

As with all rescue equipment, full personal protective clothing for rescue personnel, including safety glasses or goggles, is necessary. Standard precautions are also necessary for medical personnel and injured patients.

The number one safety concern when working with the porto-power as a rescue tool is the capacity of each of the various accessories. Rescue personnel must be fully aware of the power ratings of their particular tool and its attachments. Depending on the make/model, these capacities are typical of most systems:

- Basic Ram: 100% rating (head or base attached)
- Wedgie: 600- to 2000-lb capacity
- Duck Bill: 600- to 2000-lb capacity
- Spreader: 1200- to 3000-lb capacity
- Attachments: 50% of ram capacity or less (If chain is used in setup, then 50% of ram capacity or safe working load of chain, whichever is less)

When long extension tube assemblies are used in any setup, personnel should anticipate flexing of tubing during load situations. This condition should be monitored, and if bending becomes excessive, the pumping should be stopped.

Personnel working with the porto-power ram must constantly guard against placing a load against the stiff metal female hose coupling on the cylinder of the ram. Sufficient clearances should be maintained as the tool moves during an evolution. Safe operations also require that all components of the kit be protected from excessive heat, which will melt the unit's seal, gaskets, and O-rings. In addition, solid particles that might contaminate the hydraulic system should be kept away from all hose connections and tool couplings. Any foreign matter that enters the hydraulic system can cause pump failure.

The equipment should not be carried by the hydraulic hoses because this unsafe procedure places undue strain on couplings and hydraulic fittings. During use, the hoses should be kept free of kinks or sharp bends to avoid restricting the free flow of oil to and from the pump.

It is also very important for rescue personnel to monitor the travel distance of the plunger as it is used. It is possible to overextend the plunger by pumping after the end of the plunger travel has been reached. Continuing to pump in this manner introduces the possibility of ram failure. It is possible to pump so hard that the plunger is pushed completely out of the top of the ram.

Because the porto-power originated as a body shop tool, several attachments that a rescue company might have in the porto-power outfit should be considered as "Do Not Use" tools for vehicle rescue applications. One such item is a large spreader accessory originally manufactured by H.K. Porter, the BUO750 spreader, which has been recalled by the manufacturer. This spreader was designed with long thin arms and a pad at the end of one arm that swiveled. Under rescue applications, the unit failed unpredictably (Fig. 6-41).

Any porto-power sheet metal clamp device, although well designed for vehicle repair, is unsafe to use for rescue operations. A small attachment known as the offset spreading toe is also unsafe when placed under heavy loads. This item has a female threaded cap and a wide flange located along one side of the top of the cap. The design causes severe off-center loading of the ram when used, making it possible for the ram to fail as it is extended.

None of the other body shop accessories designed specifically for body and frame repair should be used by rescue personnel for rescue applications.

If any porto-power attachment is damaged or fails, the item should only be replaced with genuine replacement parts from the tool's original manufacturer. Attempts to weld a broken piece together or to buy pipe at the hardware store to replace damaged

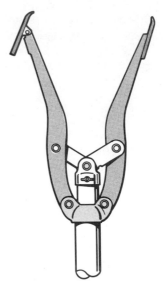

FIG. 6-41 This spreader from H.K. Porter should not be used for any rescue-related applications because it may fail unpredictably under load condition.

tubing should be forbidden. These makeshift repairs or replacements seriously reduce the degree of safety present when such equipment is used in real-world situations.

When seeking replacement chain for a porto-power, personnel should contact an authorized dealer for that particular brand of equipment. If this is unsuccessful, it must be understood that the replacement chain has to meet several important criteria. First, the chain must have equal or greater load ratings than the original chain. In addition, the shape of each individual link of chain and its diameter must be exactly the same as the original. Shape and diameter are critical when using slotted pulling attachments or special chain head accessories.

Efficiency

Several simple actions enable rescue personnel to get the most out of their porto-power equipment. One is to discard the large heavy carrying case that came with the tool and place all the parts of the system in carry trays. These homemade trays are constructed of wood or metal and can have specially designed cutouts placed in the bottom so that each component of the porto-power fits into its own notched-out place. This tray arrangement immediately accomplishes four very important improvements in the use of the porto-power.

First, having each item in its own slot prevents damage to the tools as they are transported in the

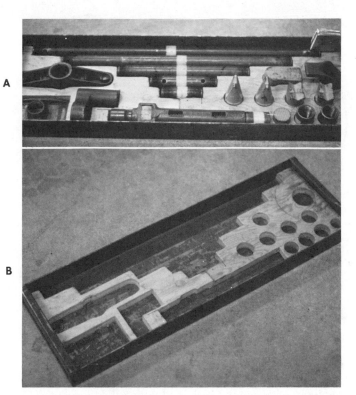

A

B

FIG. 6-42 A, Metal carrying tray with plywood insert protects tool accessories and allows a more efficient setup of the porto-power. B, Empty slots indicate components for which personnel must account.

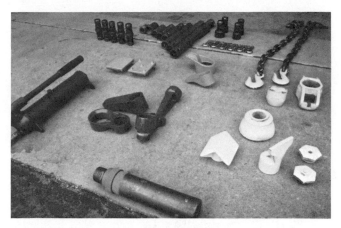

FIG. 6-43 Color-coded attachments allow efficient assembly of the tool.

rescue vehicle. In the large box provided by the manufacturer, the tools are piled one on top of the other. Second, placing a 10-ton outfit into two or more smaller carry trays makes the unit more portable. One person can now carry each tray from its location in the rescue vehicle to the work area. The original box, when fully loaded with a complete porto-power kit, takes a team of people to move it. The tool tray layout also makes the porto-power tool and its attachments more readily accessible when needed (Fig. 6-42). Personnel assembling the porto-power do not need to search through a pile of metal parts. Instead, all attachments are clearly visible and easily accessible. The tray also makes it easy to account for all accessories because any item that has not been properly stowed will be conspicuous by the shape of its empty slot in the tray.

Users of the porto-power soon learn that certain attachments work well together. The cylinder toe works well with the plunger toe, for example, and the chain pull plate works well with the chain. To increase the ease of using these attachments, rescue personnel should use paint to "color-code" the components according to their function with items designed to be

used together having the same color (Fig. 6-43). Personnel assembling the porto-power simply concentrate on the colors of the attachments when they assemble the necessary items.

Because of the many small parts of a typical porto-power outfit, personnel should assemble and disassemble the unit while in the rescue tool staging area. Placing a tarp beneath the work area makes it easy to locate dropped items that might otherwise quickly disappear in dirt, grass, mud, or snow.

To improve efficiency while working with the basic ram, personnel should measure several important tool distances and paint these on the ram itself. The side of the ram should have the height of the basic ram setup (base plate, ram, and vee head), the travel distance of the plunger, and the height of the ram with the plunger extended. Typical numbers might be 10, 7½, and 18 for a particular ram standing 10 inches tall when retracted, having 7½ inches of plunger travel, and standing 18 inches tall when fully extended. This information assists in estimating how best to place the tool in service at a rescue incident (Fig. 6-44).

Maintenance

Care and maintenance of the porto-power tool includes routine visual inspections of all components for loose items, missing parts, or physical damage. It is very important that proper oil levels be maintained in the pump unit. A proper oil level in the pump unit depends on two factors: the oil must be at the proper level, and all air must be removed from the system. If air is trapped, the oil level reading will not be accurate. Filling the pump to the proper oil level requires that the ram be connected to the pump with the plunger retracted. A check of the oil level is made following

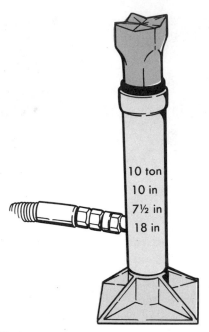

FIG. 6-44 Labeling the tool serves as a reminder when estimating tool placement and results of operation.

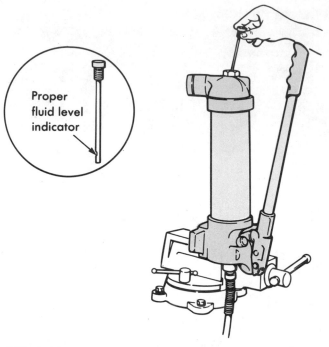

FIG. 6-45 Common procedures to check proper oil level require inverting pump, screwing dipstick into pump reservoir, withdrawing stick, and noting fluid level on dipstick. The porto-power hydraulic system must be purged of air before a fluid level check.

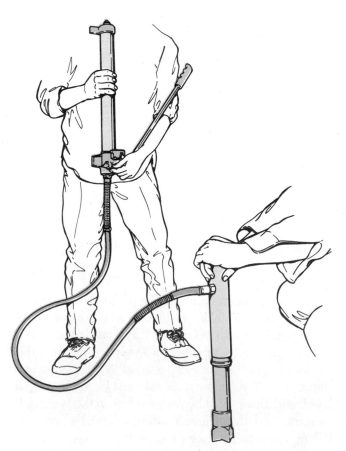

FIG. 6-46 As the inverted ram is retracted, air trapped within the system will be purged up the hose into the pump reservoir.

the manufacturer's instructions. This generally involves use of an oil level dipstick similar to that found on the engine of an automobile. Low oil levels means putting additional hydraulic jack oil into the reservoir. Personnel should *not* fill the pump beyond the oil level recommended by the manufacturer (Fig. 6-45). The oil should contain no impurities that could be introduced by use of a dirty oil can or one that previously contained other fluids.

Bleeding of the hydraulic ram, hose, and pump must follow this initial oil level work. To bleed the system, one of two crew members operates the pump, holding it as high as possible with its hose end pointed down. This person operates the pump until either the ram's piston is fully extended or the piston stops moving because of loss of oil or air trapped in the hydraulic system. The second crew member then inverts the ram and places it vertically on the floor. The operator of the pump then begins a slow opening of the pump relief valve while the other crew member pushes down on the inverted ram with a slow, steady effort (Fig. 6-46). As the ram retracts, any air trapped within the system will rise to the top end of the raised pump. The crew member holding the pump will be able to hear and feel the air bubbling into the reservoir of the pump. This process is repeated until no air is detected within the system. A second check is then made of the oil level, adding oil as necessary to maintain the proper level.

PNEUMATIC-POWERED RESCUE EQUIPMENT

Another important category of rescue equipment uses compressed air as its source of power. The pneumatic rescue tool family includes the air chisel, air gun, air impact wrench, air jacks, air bags, air cushions, and other specialized air-powered tools.

AIR CHISEL

Serving as an automated version of the basic hammer and cold chisel, the air chisel has been manufactured since the early 1930s. Air chisels are often referred to as air hammers because of their principle of operation. The air chisel was first used as a body shop vehicle repair tool. Even today, most of the components of a typical air chisel outfit are intended for body shop applications and are not specifically designed for vehicular rescue. The Superior Pneumatic and Manufacturing Co., a major producer of air-power equipment, clearly states in their air hammer safety rescue kit brochure that their rescue tool is the same one used by Sears, Goodyear, Firestone, and Western Auto in their service centers worldwide.

The basic air chisel has a long protruding metal chisel bit sticking out of the barrel and resembles a small handgun in appearance. The body of the tool, typically constructed of aluminum, contains the control trigger, a movable metal piston inside an air chamber or barrel, and a chisel bit retainer device. The barrel is produced from tool steel to increase its durability. The chisel bits, also produced from tool steel, are inserted into the open end of the barrel and secured in place. As the trigger is activated, compressed air flows into the tool and forces the solid metal piston in the barrel to slide forward. The piston, as large as ¾ inch by 2½ inches in size, impacts the end of the chisel bit inserted into the end of the barrel. The rapid piston movements against the chisel bit cause it to move back and forth, allowing the tool to cut through or into various materials (Fig. 6-47).

Once the piston inside the barrel has moved forward, the air that pushed it forward is exhausted out through ports built into the tool, completing one-half of the tool's cycle. Additional compressed air must then enter the tool, travel through a different internal pathway, and force the piston to return to its original

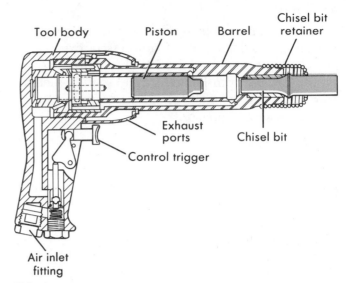

FIG. 6-47 Typical air chisel showing how a piston moves (reciprocates) inside steel barrel to strike end of chisel bit secured into retainer.

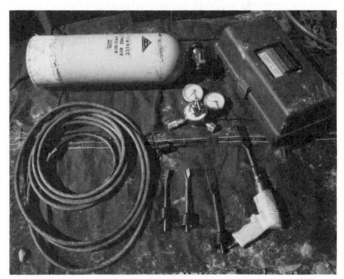

FIG. 6-48 Typical air chisel system with components detached.

position. This completes a full cycle of the air chisel, with each cycle considered as a stroke. If the control trigger remains in the open position, the piston continues to strike the chisel bit and return inside the tool.

A typical air chisel outfit consists of the following items (Fig. 6- 48):

- Air source
- Air regulator
- Air hose
- Air chisel tool
- Chisel bits
- Chisel bit retainer device

Air Source

It is vital that the source of power for the chisel tool be compressed air only. Compressed oxygen or acetylene gas must not be used. The compressed air supply can be from limited supply sources such as compressed air cylinders or constant supply sources such as an air compressor.

Air Regulator

The air regulator device serves to control the pressure of the air entering the tool. Variable pressures are necessary because the tool is used in different applications and on an assortment of materials. The regulator also incorporates a pressure relief device, designed to prevent excessive pressure from entering the tool during a regulator failure. A regulator with a maximum operating pressure setting of 300 psi would have a relief valve provided to activate at 400 psi, for example. A standard regulator is designed to accept incoming air at pressures of approximately 2216 psi and reduce this to a safe working tool pressure. Newer regulators on the market are designed to accept up to 6000 psi inlet pressures, making them compatible with 4500 psi self-contained breathing apparatus and cylinders.

A pneumatic hose is used to direct the air flow from the regulator into the tool. This hose is of typically double-braided construction with rubber or neoprene outer jackets. Hose considered for heavy-duty applications is generally of ⅜-inch inside diameter and a typical working pressure rating of 250 psi. Standard lengths of hose are from 15 to 25 feet with a maximum recommended length of 50 feet. Longer lengths reduce the ability of the air to flow through the hose, reducing the efficiency of the tool as it operates.

Air Chisel Body

The air chisel tool contains the pistol grip handle unit, the tool barrel, the piston, and the chisel bit retainer device. The trigger, which controls the operation of the tool and amount of air flow, is located in this pistol grip. The valve assemblies that direct the flow of air are located inside this housing of the tool. The air supply inlet coupling is secured to the bottom of the pistol grip handle. The barrel of the tool containing the piston threads into the housing of the pistol grip and usually has a set screw to secure it in place. A typical air chisel tool weighs approximately 5 lb.

Chisel Bits

The solid metal chisel bits are manufactured from tool steel and perform the actual work that is accomplished. Different size and shape chisel bits perform different operations ranging from cutting sheet metal to severing heavy-gauge stock to breaking rivets, nuts, and bolts. All bits have a working end, a shank, and the retainer end. Most chisel bits meet the design criteria of a .401 Parker Taper shank, the industry standard for air tools.

The more common types of chisel bits used for vehicle rescue evolutions and their general functions include the following:

- Flat chisel: This bit has a rounded shank end with a curved, half-moon-shaped cutting edge at the flat end (Fig. 6-49). It cuts heavy-gauge material and multiple layer material such as vehicle roof posts, firewalls, bolts, and nuts.
- Cold chisel: This bit has a rounded shank with a tapered, pinch point working end. It resembles a standard cold chisel in appearance. It cuts through solid stock materials such as rivets, bolts, and nuts.
- Single panel cutter: This has a rounded shank with a working end resembling a "T." The bottom of the "T" forms a sheet metal cutting tooth, with the top portion acting to control the depth of the bit as

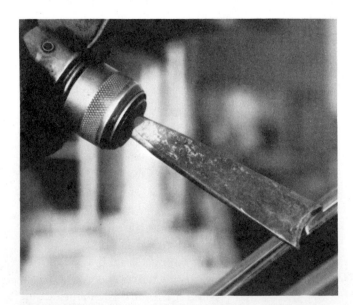

FIG. 6-49 Curved, sharpened, and half-moon shaped chisel, called a *flat chisel*.

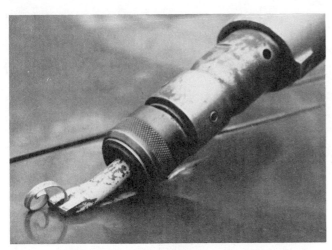

FIG. 6-50 Chisel bit with one protruding tooth, called a *single panel cutter*.

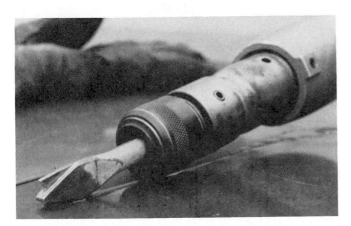

FIG. 6-51 Double panel cutter. The newest generation has a protruding point at the forward point of the bit to make a starter hole for the cutting evolution.

it moves along the surface of the metal being cut (Fig. 6-50). It cuts light-gauge material up to 12-gauge thickness.

- Double panel cutter: This bit has a rounded shank with a wide flare at the working end. Each corner of the flared end forms a small metal cutting tooth. One tooth cuts sheetmetal, guided by the thicker center portion of bit. Second tooth remains pointed away from the cutting area, serving as a backup in the event of tooth failure (Fig. 6-51). It cuts light-gauge material up to 12-gauge thickness. The advantage of double tooth features is that the spare tooth is immediately available if the primary tooth fails.

- Double panel cutter with bull point: This bit is exactly the same as the standard double cutter except for the addition of an extended point on the working end of the bit between the two cutting teeth. It cuts light-gauge sheet metal with tooth. Bull point feature allows operator to readily make small puncture holes in metal to aid in starting the cutting process.

Other chisel bits are designed for specific applications. For vehicle rescue operations, examples of specialized bits that are available include a rivet cutter, a straight bull point piercing bit, a one- or two-piece windshield removal bit, a combination padlock breaker and sheetmetal cutter bit, and a rubber plug and driver bit for use during hazardous materials incidents. The minimum inventory of chisel bits for vehicle rescue should include two each of the standard flat chisel and the panel cutter bit. The recommended style panel cutter bit is the double panel cutter with the bull point feature. With these two basic types of chisel bits, all basic air chisel operations at a motor vehicle accident can be accomplished. Although chisel bits range in length from 6 to 18 inches, the 10-inch length seems most effective.

There are four different methods of retaining the chisel bit in the open end of the barrel of a air chisel (Fig. 6-52). These retainer methods include the following:

- A coiled spring on the shank of the chisel bit
- A threaded collar on the shank of the chisel bit
- A quarter-turn collar on the air chisel barrel
- A pull-back swivel collar on the air chisel barrel

The original method uses threads on the end of the air chisel barrel and a coiled spring that fits onto the shank of the chisel bit. The coiled spring looks much like a small beehive. The use of this spring for holding the chisel bit is the most unsafe of all methods. It is possible for the chisel bit to unexpectedly fly out of the tool if the spring stretches or breaks during use. A second retainer method also uses a threaded tool barrel but adds a large metal collar assembled around the shank of each chisel bit instead of the coiled spring. The bit is inserted into the tool, and the retainer collar is threaded onto the barrel to hold the bit in place.

The quarter-turn collar, a third retainer style, is an integral part of the barrel of the tool. This permanent collar uses internal ball bearings to hold the bit in place. The knurled collar is rotated to release or hold the chisel bit. The newest method of holding the bit in place is the pull-back swivel collar, referred to as the

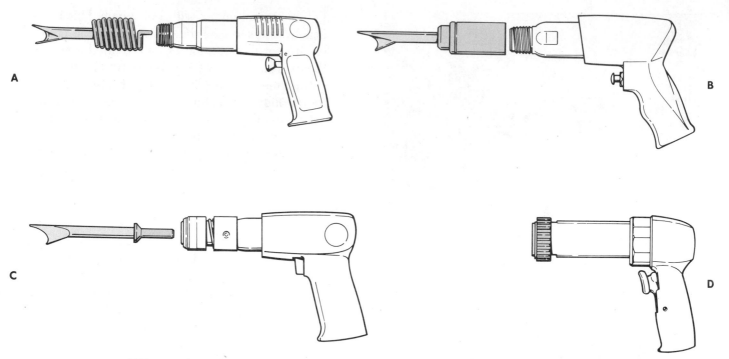

FIG. 6-52 A, Beehive coiled spring retainer. **B,** Threaded collar on the shank retainer. **C,** Pull-back swivel collar retainer. **D,** Quarter-turn collar retainer.

safety retainer. This assembly uses ball bearings and a spring inside the collar of the retainer, giving it the ability to swivel. To release or insert a chisel bit, personnel should pull the collar toward the pistol grip. With the collar in its forward position, the chisel bit is secured inside the barrel of the gun.

Occupational Safety and Health Administration (OSHA) regulations, currently applicable in many states for fire service personnel, have stringent requirements for retention of the .401 Parker Taper shank. The older, coiled spring, beehive-style retainer system *does not* meet the safety requirements of this standard. A pull-back swivel collar retainer is now available for retrofitting from a noncompliant retainer to an approved safety retainer.

The retainer style also influences the action of the chisel bit once it is inserted into the barrel. In place, the chisel bit can either rotate a full 360 degrees freely or be locked into a horizontal or vertical position depending on the retainer. The coiled spring and the threaded collar system allow the bit to rotate freely when secured into the barrel. These are *turn* retainers. The rotating collar method that holds the bit in a fixed position is a *nonturn* retainer. The shanks of the nonturn chisel bits have special slots on their sides for the ball bearings inside the retainer to secure into. The pull-back swivel collar can be either turn or nonturn.

Most air chisel outfits work with variable pressure regulators. The advantages of having variable operating air pressure units are that the speed of the stroke per minute and the tool's air consumption rate can be controlled to best advantage. High operating pressure yields a faster stroke rate and greater air consumption.

Consumption Rate

The consumption of an air tool is measured in cubic feet per minute (cfm). Typical air chisel consumption rates of 7 cfm are common. The length of time that a given tool can operate off a limited air source such as an air cylinder is determined by the cubic footage of air contained in the cylinder (Table 6-3).

The length of time that an air chisel will operate can be estimated by dividing the total cubic foot capacity of the cylinder by the consumption rate of the tool. At 90 psi tool operating pressure, for example, a typical air chisel supplied off a fully charged breathing apparatus air cylinder will give approximately 4 minutes of operating time. As the unit nears the 4-minute mark, the efficiency of the tool decreases.

Air can quickly drain from compressed air cylinders. The lower the operating pressure, the lower the air consumption rate of the tool. It is therefore essential to operate the air tool at the correct pressure for a given task so that maximum efficiency and operating time can be achieved. Recommended tool "flowing"

TABLE 6-3 Cubic Foot Capacity of Air Cylinders

Cylinder	Maximum Pressure (psi)	Capacity (cu/ft)
SCBA	2216	45
Scuba	2250	70–72
Air Cascade (K cylinder)	2400	300

pressures for cutting material such as automobile vehicle body panels range from 90 to 110 psi. The Superior Pneumatic Co. recommends that its model of rescue air chisels be operated at 130 to 150 psi flowing pressure. The air gauge needle on the regulator may need to be set higher when there is air pressure on the system and the tool is not being used. This higher reading will then yield the correct flowing pressure as the air is consumed. Cutting heavier gauge metal requires increased flowing pressures of 200+ psi. Most air tool manufacturers do not recommend prolonged use at pressures higher than 110 psi because of possible damage to the tool.

The most popular air source for air chisel tools is the fire service 45 cubic foot capacity breathing apparatus cylinder. Many fire departments are using old 1980 psi steel SCBA cylinders, no longer acceptable for structural fire suppression use as the air supply for their pneumatic rescue tools (Fig. 6-53). The cylinders can be painted a different color from the standard SCBA cylinders and carried in the rescue tool inventory. Other sources of air include constant supply portable air compressor units and vehicle air brake systems (Fig. 6-54). With these systems, there is virtually no limit to the supply of air, although the compressor cfm must be adequate to supply the demands of the air tool. With vehicle air brake systems, an additional reserve air tank is usually needed to maintain an adequate supply of air to the tool. A moisture trap must also be provided in-line to limit moisture from reaching the air tool where it will cause internal rusting of metal parts.

Air Chisel Tool Operation

When personnel are getting the components of the air chisel ready for service, it is important that the entire system be hooked together before pressurizing it with air. The initial step in connecting the hardware together is to attach the regulator to the proper air source. This thread connection needs to be applied only hand-tight to be sufficient. Tightening further with a wrench is unnecessary and may actually dam-

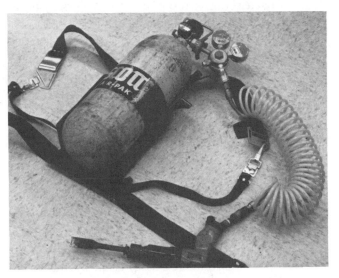

FIG. 6-53 Older 1980 psi steel air cylinders, no longer permitted for structural firefighting, may be effectively used to supply rescue tools, providing that the cylinder is inspected and maintained with a current hydrostatic test date.

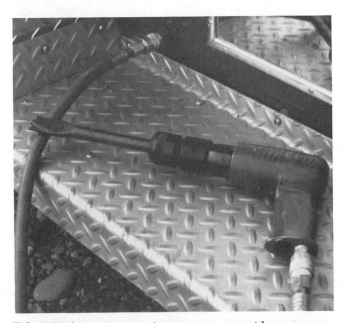

FIG. 6-54 An apparatus air system can provide a constant supply for air-powered tools. Precautions should be taken to ensure adequate air compressor ratings, sufficient system storage tanks, and moisture-free airflow.

age the air connection. Next, several drops of a light-weight lubricating oil recommended by the air chisel manufacturer should be dropped into the air inlet at the bottom of the handle of the air chisel. This small quantity of lubricating oil, added at the beginning of each use, will ensure that the tool and all its moving parts remain adequately lubricated and functional. Next, the air hose is connected between the regulator and the air chisel tool.

The final assembly step places the necessary chisel bit into the open end of the barrel of the tool and secures it in place. This effort also requires a firm and definite tug and twist on the chisel bit to confirm that it is in place and securely fastened. With all connections made, a quick safety check is made of the system. A final visual check of the connections, with a gentle tug on each, is especially important for the tool operator's safety. If all items are in order, the air system can then be pressurized. From this point on, the air chisel is to be held, carried, and used as if it were a *loaded* gun. When it is not actually working, the barrel end of the tool must always be positioned toward the ground and away from personnel who may be nearby.

As the air source is turned on, a visual check of the pressure readings of the regulator gauges is made. It is best if the setting on the regulator at this time is lower than the anticipated operating pressure of the tool. When it becomes necessary to make adjustments to the regulator pressure control knob, having an initially low setting means that the adjustment knob must be turned in the "increase" direction. This action brings the needle up to the correct pressure for the operation to be undertaken. Having to adjust the regulator down from a initially high pressure setting with no air flowing through the system can give a false pressure reading on the regulator gauge.

To begin the actual tool operation, personnel place the chisel bit against the object to be cut. If a single panel cutter bit is to be used in cutting across sheet metal, the bottom point or "tooth" must be pressed into the material to make a starter hole. With a double panel cutter, either the center bull point or one of the two cutting teeth can perform this function. When the starter hole is sufficient, the tool is maneuvered into a position parallel to the work surface. If an object such as a vehicle roof post is to be cut through, the operator can use the corner of the flat chisel to start a puncture hole in the first layer of the post. The chisel bit is then pressed into the surface of the material, taking care to "attack" the object from all possible sides. Maintaining one position and attempting to drive the flat chisel into the material will usually only succeed in jam-

ming the chisel bit deeper into the metal. If this happens, it is best to leave the jammed bit in place, bleed off the air pressure in the system, remove the tool, insert a second chisel bit, and use it to attempt to cut the first one free of the material. Any decorative trim material, such as vinyl roof covering, side door trim strips, or plastic molding, should be removed as much as possible before cutting any material with the air chisel.

Proper body position for the tool operator requires a stance that is balanced and not overextended. The operator should not force the tool, but rather learn to work with it without overexerting themselves or over-extending their reach. This makes it possible to maintain proper footing and body balance at all times. Cutting work should be performed below eye level to minimize the chances of debris falling onto the tool operator.

Proper hand placement requires at least one strong hand on the pistol grip of the tool. One finger of this hand squeezes the trigger of the tool. The trigger control enables the operator to regulate the speed of the hammer-like blows by controlling the degree the trigger is depressed. Light pressure starts the piston moving inside the tool at a slow rate, causing light blows to the chisel bit. Full impact power and full speed are reached when the trigger is fully depressed. The operator's other hand can best be placed on the shank of the chisel bit to effectively guide the tool as it works. This second hand can also be placed on the barrel of the tool if that position is more convenient to the operator. The chisel bit must be firmly guided into the material being cut and held tight to the surface. The body of the tool should be maneuvered to place the tool into the best position for completing the assignment.

During transport, handling, and use, the tool should not be held or carried by its hose or regulator. The hose should be protected from physical damage resulting from cuts, crushing, abrasion, or heat.

Shutting down the air chisel system requires one important safety precaution. All pressure should be removed from the entire system before any item is disconnected. Even though the source of compressed air is initially shut down, pressure remains within the system. To disconnect a hose at that point could trigger an explosive disconnect, causing injury or tool damage. The bit of the tool should be placed against an object and the trigger activated until the piston no longer cycles within the tool. The pressure has then been removed from all parts of the system, and it is safe to disconnect.

Safety

Damage to the air chisel barrel and bit retainer can occur in two ways. If personnel continually pressurize and operate the trigger of the tool without having a chisel bit inserted, the rapid blows of the piston against the end of the barrel, averaging over 2000 impacts per minute, will begin to distort the internal portions of the barrel. Second, operating the tool without the bit being placed against a load will result in the same damage. Whenever the trigger is operated, there must be a chisel bit in place and the bit must be "loaded" against an object.

Protection for personnel in the work area when an air chisel is in operation includes standard protective clothing with a special emphasis on total eye protection. Hearing protection should also be provided for key operating personnel. For those inside a vehicle while work is being performed on it with an air chisel, that tool is the noisiest rescue tool that can be used. For the trapped and conscious patient, the noise is frightening. The patient not only hears the tool operate but also *feels* the tool work as it vibrates through the entire structure of the vehicle. If you do not believe this can be a problem, have someone cut into a roof post on one side of a vehicle with an air chisel while you position yourself inside the auto at a training exercise. Place your head, shoulder, or leg against the solid part of a door or roof post on the opposite side from the chisel. The noise and vibrations are intensified as your body increases its contact with the vehicle.

It is therefore recommended that approved hearing protection, either ear plugs or ear muffs, be available for medical personnel inside the vehicle and for patients if their condition permits. Unnecessary personnel should be removed from the work area.

The noise of an air chisel also influences the operation of the tool at an incident. When medical personnel inside a vehicle need something quickly for the patient or when an important direction needs to be given to other personnel, the noise of the tool can prohibit this vital communication. During tool operation, communication in close proximity to the tool is virtually impossible. It is therefore mandatory that the tool operator operate the air chisel with a series of frequent pauses to allow necessary communication to take place.

A standardized procedure for quickly stopping the operation of the air chisel must be developed. Trying to communicate verbally with the tool operator during a cutting job is senseless. The recommended procedure for halting this noisy work must involve a predetermined action such as a firm grip on the operator's back or shoulder or a tap on the helmet. This physical contact can be understood regardless of noise level.

Efficiency

Several important improvements can be made to an air chisel outfit that are both inexpensive and effective in improving its use. One such modification involves replacing the standard-length air hose with "recoil" hose. A typical length of this hose will stretch up to a 25-foot distance and then recoil into a convenient 24-inch length. This minimizes kinks and hose damage and reduces the amount of storage space needed.

For ease in making the air connection to a compressed air cylinder, a large hand wheel available from air tool manufacturers can be installed directly on the air coupling nut. This wheel dramatically improves the ease and efficiency of connecting the coupling to the threaded stem of a cylinder.

As a means of making the entire chisel outfit portable, many organizations that use SCBA cylinders as their air source are securing the cylinder to an extra breathing apparatus backpack harness (Fig. 6-55). With this system tool operators can actually wear the cylinder on their back, leaving both hands free when moving around the work area.

If running out of air is a problem, a manifolded air

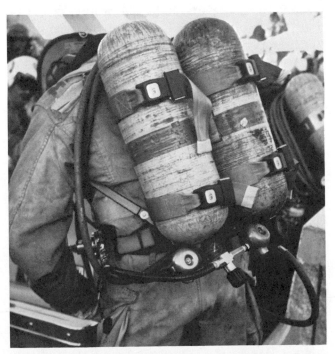

FIG. 6-55 SCBA backpack harness assembly used with dual compressed air cylinders and low-pressure warning bells allows increased mobility and operation of air chisel.

bottle system similar to that designed for use with the Gator power rescue tool is recommended. With the dual bottles, one can be exchanged for a fully charged cylinder while the tool continues to operate off the second manifolded cylinder.

A means of providing an audible warning of low air pressure in any cylinder supplying the air chisel is possible by adapting the low pressure warning bell from older style fire service breathing apparatus units. The bell unit is installed between the cylinder and the air chisel regulator and activates when the cylinder pressure approaches 500 psi. Although the tool will continue to function at this pressure, if continued operations are needed, a bottle change can be anticipated.

Another improvement that can be made to an air chisel outfit is preconnecting the individual components of the system and storing them in this manner. This step reduces the time needed to place the tool in service at an accident, minimizes incorrect setups, and reduces the chances of lost or misplaced components. Everything is assembled and ready to go when needed.

Preventive Maintenance

The single most important preventive maintenance aspect of working with an air chisel is proper tool lubrication. Lubrication of the piston and all critical internal components is necessary to reduce the normal wearing of these parts. Initial lubrication should be done before operating a brand new tool, and subsequent lubrication should be done after each use or once for every hour of operation. Lubrication is accomplished by simply turning the pistol grip handle of the tool so that it points upward and adding three to four drops of a light pneumatic tool oil or light machine oil such as SAE No. 5 to SAE No. 10 viscosity into the air inlet fitting. The tool should next be operated under a load to allow excess oil to blow out the exhaust ports. The residue is then wiped off, and the tool is ready for service. Constant and continual attention to lubrication of all internal components of the tool is vital to the "health" of the air chisel.

Tool vibrations continually loosen components of the tool. Preventive maintenance involves tightening any loose parts, with special attention given to the set screw that secures the barrel into the handle of the tool.

The tool and all parts of the system must be cleaned and inspected after each use and at regular intervals, making sure that no dirt or foreign matter can be found at air inlets, exhausts, or between portions of the tool. Any surface moisture should be removed, and the metal barrel lightly oiled.

Maintenance of the air chisel bits requires periodic sharpening by holding the cutting edge at a 45-degree angle to a grinding wheel or belt sander. Caution must be taken to be sure that the blade is not "burned." Overheating the blade during grinding will burn and discolor the edge of the metal and seriously weaken the strength and integrity of the blade. The flared portion of the shank of each air chisel may also become worn. Any burrs or depressions should be removed by gentle grinding. An adequate supply of each required style of chisel bit should be maintained in a tool inventory because not all blade problems can be corrected by grinding. A problem such as a broken corner of a blade or a fractured cutting tooth will require total replacement. Once properly maintained, the tool and all its components should be stored in a dry location to minimize rusting.

AIR GUN

Problems can develop when rescue personnel work with air chisel units despite the best preventive maintenance measures. Even when an air chisel is operating properly, there is no assurance that it will be able to accomplish all that is necessary. Cutting through the heavy-gauge metal of a school bus or the structural frame areas of a truck or train can be too much for a light-duty air chisel. The heavy-gauge metal simply overwhelms the limited power of the tool. These heavy-duty materials need a larger, more powerful tool, one designed to stand up to the uses and abuses put to it by fire service and rescue personnel. An air-powered tool that can accomplish both routine vehicle rescue evolutions and tougher, heavy-duty rescue problems can quickly become a valuable addition to any organization's rescue tool inventory.

In 1984, Paratech Incorporated, an Illinois rescue equipment manufacturer and supplier, pioneered the development of an air-powered rescue and forcible entry tool that represents a new generation of pneumatic equipment. This tool, like those that are sure to follow in its footsteps, is designed to go beyond the capabilities of any of the conventional air chisel tools currently available. The product, the Airgun 40, was so named because its appearance suggests that it can "gun through" many obstacles encountered by rescue personnel.

The Airgun 40, with its black aluminum alloy body, resembles a submachine gun and weighs approxi-

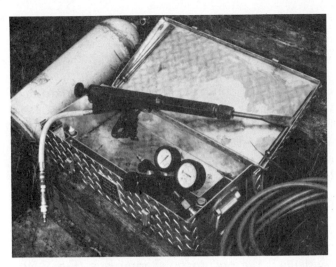

FIG. 6-56 The Airgun 40 rescue tool system from Paratech, Inc., has a lower cubic-foot-per-minute air consumption rate than smaller air chisels.

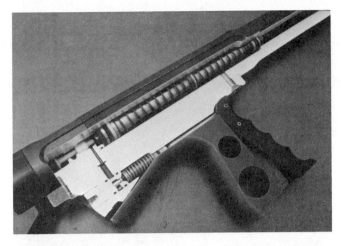

FIG. 6-57 Cutaway view of the Airgun 40 reveals a heavy-duty air piston inside the tool barrel wrapped with two large, coiled steel springs.

mately 6 pounds. Its size makes it the largest air-powered cutting tool available for rescue applications. It is unique in that it is specifically designed to be operated at pressures up to 250 psi yet maintains a low air consumption rate while in operation (Fig. 6-56).

The low air consumption rate is made possible by an interesting addition inside the tool. The Airgun 40's long barrel, similar to those found on conventional air chisels, contains a solid metal piston rod. The barrel also contains two alloy steel springs positioned between the piston and the forward end of the barrel. When the trigger in the pistol grip is depressed, air enters the tool, travels through internal valve assemblies, and forces the piston forward. This action hammers the piston against the end of the chisel bit inserted into the tool. At that point the air in the barrel is exhausted through ports in the gun. Unlike conventional air chisels in which more air is used to return the piston to its starting position inside the barrel, air stops flowing into the tool. The steel springs, which have been compressed by the piston, push the piston back into its starting position. Continuing to depress the trigger repeats the "air down, spring return" cycle (Fig. 6-57).

The Airgun 40 operates with a very distinctive cycling sound, like the rat-a-tat-tat of a miniature jack hammer. The estimated 600 blows per minute are powerful impacts that allow the tool to cut thicker and more solid materials than possible with conventional air chisel tools. According to Paratech, the air consumption rate of their tool is less than one-half the rate of many other air chisel tools. This means fewer air

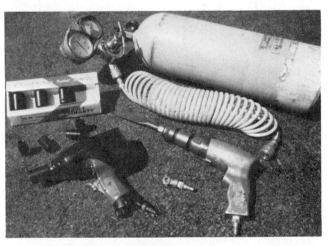

FIG. 6-58 Industrial-quality air impact wrench. Note air tire chuck for use off air regulator.

cylinder changes at a rescue incident, more operating time per cylinder, and better performance while the air is being consumed.

PNEUMATIC IMPACT WRENCH

An air impact wrench tool also makes a fine addition to a rescue tool inventory. Again, this tool is adapted for rescue use from the vehicle repair industry (Fig. 6-58). Compressed air provides the turning motion necessary to drive a socket. When fitted with case-hardened sockets and controlled by a skilled operator, the tool functions well in disassembly work. It may be possible to remove an automobile door with an air impact wrench by unbolting the door hinges. In the case of a stubborn bolt or one that has rusted in

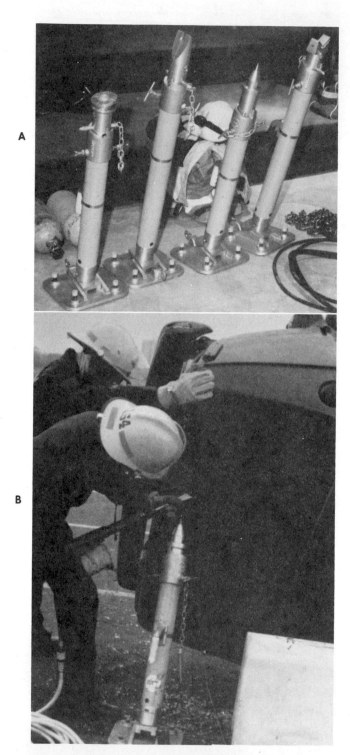

FIG. 6-59 A, Telescoping air jack with locking pins, accessory base plates, and attachment heads compose a pneumatic shoring jack tool system. **B,** Cutting an anchor-point hole in a vehicle with an Airgun 40 allows placement of the air jack in this vehicle stabilization evolution.

place, a true, heavy-duty impact wrench of good quality can still accomplish the task by vibrating the bolt loose or fracturing the head completely off the bolt simply by the torque that it can produce. It is crucial to have complete sets of both standard and metric size sockets available along with extension pieces and universal swivel connectors. If the sockets are to withstand the rigors presented by typical rescue applications, only the case-hardened variety should be purchased.

PNEUMATIC SHORING JACK

Another air-powered rescue tool that was designed originally for below-grade or confined-space rescue incidents is the pneumatic shoring jack (Fig. 6-59). Known by trade names such as Jimme-Jak or Air-shore, the equipment is finding additional applications in the vehicle rescue field. The jack unit itself is a two-piece assembly of metal tubes with an air-powered piston inside. Assembled, the unit resembles a military mortar gun of the kind used by infantry units. The smaller diameter end of the jack tube telescopes inside the larger base section, with the jack being extended manually or by compressed air. The unit is locked at any position by inserting large pins through holes in the tubes.

Because the tool is designed to serve as an adjustable length unit, it can be applied to below-grade rescue situations with several jacks bridging the distance from one side of a trench to the other for safe shoring of the trench walls. It can also be used to stabilize portions of a collapsed building during rescue operations. Because the jack can be fitted with an assortment of special purpose ends and large base plates, rescue personnel can adapt the tool to fit many rescue situations.

The full scope of the jacks in performing vehicle rescue evolutions is not yet known. The tool is still relatively young; it has only been available since the early 1980s. Its most successful vehicle rescue application to date has been as a manual stabilization tool. When used with an appropriate end attachment and base plate, the jack can secure an unstable vehicle. An automobile that has rolled onto its side or is totally resting on its roof surface, for example, can quickly be stabilized with wood blocking and Jimme-Jaks placed at strategic locations.

AIR BAGS

The principle of compressing air inside a flexible rubber container to lift or support great amounts of

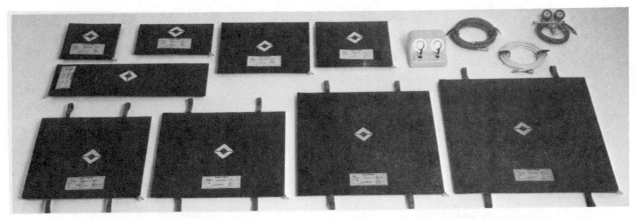

FIG. 6-60 High-pressure air bag systems have individual bag lifting capacities from 1 to over 70 tons and inflation heights up to 21 inches. (Courtesy Vetter Systems, Pittsburgh, Pa.)

weight is certainly not unique to the field of rescue. This same concept allows a pressurized automobile tire weighing only several pounds to support its share of the total weight of an automobile. Air bags and air cushions, although far more sophisticated than tires, use the same laws of physics. Air-lifting bags, developed by Manfred Vetter in the mid 1960s, were approved first by the German government and eventually introduced to the North American rescue service in the 1970s. There are two categories of air-lifting systems, each with important similarities and differences in design and operation. The most popular style of air bag resembles a rubber pillow when inflated to a pressure of between 116 and 145 psi of air. The various size bags expand to different heights, exerting tremendous forces (Fig. 6-60). This action allows the air bags to lift, spread, bend, or pry objects.

The second type of air-lifting tool is the air cushion. Although similar to the air bag in that it is constructed of a rubber material and filled with air, the cushion is considerably lighter in design and construction (Fig. 6-61). Air cushion systems can be either medium-pressure or low-pressure types. Medium-pressure air cushion systems operate at approximately 15 psi air pressure, while the low pressure cushions function at 7 psi.

Air bags are the more rugged of the two types of air-lifting systems. A typical bag is manufactured by either a "hot" vulcanization process or a heat and molding process to form the tops and sides. The bags have multilayered sides built in a sandwich design of neoprene/nitrile rubber outer layers and either Kevlar fiber or steel wire inner layers. (Butyl rubber is used to construct the MatJack brand air bags.) Neoprene rubber, a product of the DuPont company, is resistant to more than 800 chemicals. If steel wire side reinforcement is used in the bag's construction process, the strands of wire are neoprene coated. When completed, each side of an air bag has a minimum of three layers of mesh wire or mesh Kevlar fibers; the total thickness of a finished air bag is approximately 1 inch. This internal reinforcement material does not, however, extend as three full layers over and around the edges of the bags (Fig. 6-62).

The outer rubber surfaces have a design molded into them to minimize slippage of the air bag during use. Paratech, Inc., one air bag manufacturer, bonds bright yellow rubber strips in an "X" design into the outer surface of its units as an aid in centering the bag during use. Holmatro, Inc., another air bag manufacturer, places a red dot at the center. One corner of each air bag has an air inlet/discharge tube permanently bonded into it.

A high-pressure air bag generally functions at 116 to 118 psi internal air pressure, although the Lampe-Lifter air bags from Zumro, Inc. operate at 145 psi, and the MFC Series L air bags from Kinman operate at only 90 psi. Depending on the manufacturer, air bags generally have a minimum burst pressure of four times their operating pressure, and a continuous service operating temperature range of -15° F to 150° F. Quality control measures for air bags also vary by manufacturer; most companies proof test each finished unit at twice its normal operating pressure before approving the unit (Table 6-4).

An air bag system consists of four basic components (Fig. 6-63). The *source of pressurized air* is the first component of the system. For most rescue applications, this supply typically comes from SCBA compressed air cylinders. Other supply sources include

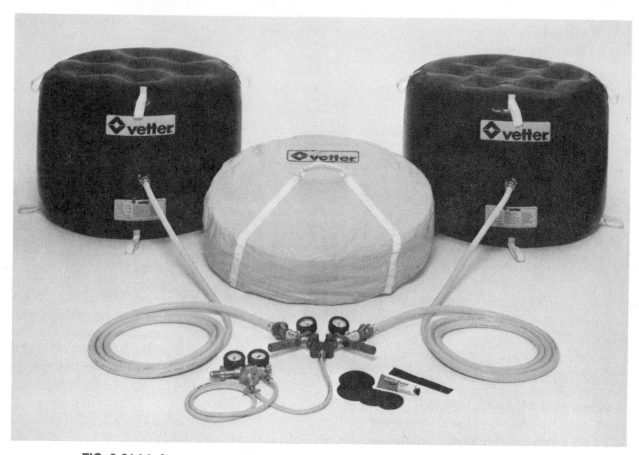

FIG. 6-61 Medium-pressure or low-pressure air cushions offer higher inflation heights than air bags but do not have the lifting capacities or durability of the high-pressure bags. (Courtesy Vetter Systems, Pittsburgh, Pa.)

TABLE 6-4 High-Pressure Air Bags

Type	Internal Air Pressure (psi)	Burst Pressure (psi)	Proof Pressure (psi)
Paratech	118	700	236
Vetter	116	696	232
Lampe-Lifter	145	500	–
Holmatro	116	464	232
MatJack	120	–	–
MFC Series L	90	350	250

Dash (–) signifies information not available.

compressors, manual pumps, or even vehicle air brake systems. With the proper type of pressure regulator, supply pressures as high as 4500 psi can be reduced to the particular system's operating pressure. Air bags consume air each time they inflate. The more resistance against the bag as it inflates, the more air is consumed. Small bags may contain 1 or 2 cubic feet of air in volume when fully inflated; larger bags can require as much as 42 cubic feet of air volume.

The *controller*, the second component, is the piece of equipment responsible for air bag system operation. The controller allows air to be directed into or

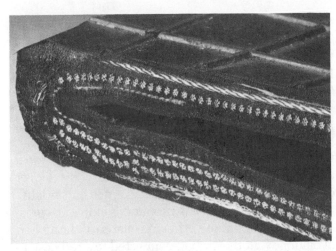

FIG. 6-62 Cutaway of a high-pressure air bag with neoprene rubber outer walls and steel mesh interior reinforcement. The new generation of air bags has a synthetic Kevlar reinforcement instead of the heavier steel. (Courtesy Vetter Systems, Pittsburgh, Pa.)

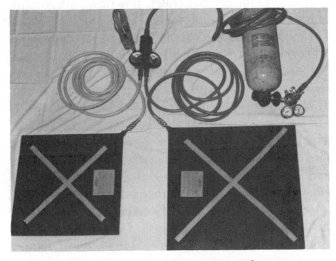

FIG. 6-63 Components of high-pressure air bag system include the air source, regulator, hoses, controller unit, and air bag. Line splitters and individual shutoff valves are also available.

out of two individual air bags and contains gauges to monitor the internal pressure within each bag. Built-in safety relief valves monitor the pressure in each air bag supply line and act to limit any excessive pressure. One problem with the original style "pipe-fitting" controller units is that the valve directing air to the bags can be moved to the open or flow position and remain in that position by itself. In 1980 the Vetter Systems company first introduced the *deadman controller*, which revolutionized air bag controller units;

all manufacturers now offer this type. The deadman controller requires constant human intervention to flow air to the bags. As soon as operators remove their hand from the flow control, the valve returns to the neutral or closed position, stopping the flow of air. All rescue crews operating with air bag systems would be well advised to use only the safe deadman style controllers with their systems.

A third air bag system component, the *air hose*, is responsible for air delivery within the system. Hose sections are generally between 16 and 32 feet in length, are of different colors, and have either a male or female coupling at each end. Most air bag hoses have a working pressure rating of 250 psi and a minimum burst pressure of 550 to 1000 psi depending on the manufacturer. Vetter Systems intentionally designs its air hoses to burst at between 525 and 550 psi, making the hose the weakest component of the air delivery system. If a sudden surge of excess air pressure goes toward the air bag, the hose will rupture first, protecting the integrity of the bag. The synthetic air hoses have a useable temperature operating range of -15° F to 150° F.

All hose couplings are designed with some means of preventing accidental disconnection; the industry standard is a slide-back female collar securing to a single rib on the male nipple. Paratech, Inc.'s air hose couplings have an additional safety lock ring located behind the female collar. The ring can be screwed forward to hold the release collar in position. Vetter Systems uses a double rib design on the male coupling as their safety device. The double-locking coupling requires the female collar to be forced forward to release the first lock and then held and pulled backward to release completely from the male nipple. This design affords the highest degree of operating safety and minimizes accidental hose disconnections.

A variety of adaptors and attachments are available for use with air bag systems. The most important accessory is the in-line shutoff relief valve, which enables operating personnel to maintain pressure in more than two air bags at the same time. These shutoff devices also have a pressure relief device incorporated into their design. When rescue personnel work with these shutoffs, safety must be maintained. The shutoff device should always be in place before pressurizing the system. It is also crucial that the valve only be attached directly to the discharge outlet of the controller unit. The in-line shutoff valve *should not* be attached directly to the air bag as is so often done. This practice places the rescuer in a potentially dangerous position when opening or closing the shutoff valve. There should be a separate hose with its own distinctive color for every air bag to permit isolating each bag individually. The inflated bag, the section of hose, and the shutoff remain intact as the crew uses additional hose sections and shutoffs for other bags.

The *air bag* is the component of the system that exerts forces measured in pounds. Capacities of the various bags range from 2000 lb (1 ton) to 150,000 lb (75 ton). Sizes range from 6 in x 6 in up to 36 in x 36 in. Each bag has a fitting molded into one corner that accepts a replaceable brass thread-on style nipple. The internal diameter of this air bag coupling is generally a 7 mm bore. This size opening is chosen specifically to control the escape of air through the nipple at a relatively slow rate. A larger diameter opening would allow the bag to collapse very rapidly, possibly endangering operating personnel. The slow, controlled descent through the small air fitting allows for controlled deflation of the bag.

Various manufacturers subject their products to endurance and abuse tests to demonstrate their versatility and durability. Vetter Systems periodically conducts several air bag endurance tests; in one, a single air bag performed 25,000 repetitive lifts without failure. In a second test, one Vetter air bag remained inflated at 700 psi for 5000 hours at a temperature of 176° F.

The steps necessary to place an air bag in service resemble those required for setting up an air chisel or an air gun tool. A pressure regulator must be attached to an air source. Hand-tightened connections should be sufficient if the fittings are properly maintained. Next, an air supply hose is connected between the regulator and the controller unit. Hoses are then run between the discharge outlets of the controller and the inlet fittings of the air bags themselves. It is crucial that each individual hose section used with an air bag system be of a different color. No duplication of hose colors should ever be tolerated within any one system because the rescue officer relies on the colors of these hoses when directing the operation of the system.

The in-line control valve, located at the pressure regulator, and the air control valves located at the controller unit, should be closed before turning on the air supply. This reduces the possibility of uncontrolled bag inflation. A final check should be made to ensure that the pressure regulator is at the lowest pressure setting. When all valves are closed, the air supply source can be opened. The high-pressure air supply source should always be opened slowly; failure to do

so may damage the regulator's internal diaphragm.

The pressure gauges on the regulator unit should display incoming air supply pressure and the current pressure setting of the regulator. The small flow valve on the regulator is then opened, allowing pressurized air to flow to the inlet of the controller unit. The air pressure regulator can be adjusted at this point to a pressure setting several pounds higher than the operating pressure of the particular system. As an individual air bag is to be inflated, the appropriate control lever on the controller unit is operated. As each bag inflates, the controller operator can monitor its individual pressure gauge. Should the officer in charge of the air bag evolution want the air bag connected to a red hose to be inflated, the command, "Up on red," would be given. The order, "Halt!", would stop the action. If that same bag were to be deflated, the command, "Down on red," would be given. Controller operators should repeat each command back to the officer to confirm what they have heard and notify assisting personnel of the action being taken. Rescue personnel must discipline themselves to work by the color of the air hose attached to the bag and not by the bag's location or position. If two hoses of the same color are in use in the same system, one hose should either be replaced with a different color hose or be clearly and distinctly marked with a different color tape or tag.

When personnel are shutting down the air bag system, the air supply should be shut off first. The bags should then be deflated at the controller by using the deflation control valves. When all pressure gauges indicate no pressure within the system, the hoses supplying the air bags can be disconnected at the bags. The control levers should then be momentarily moved into the inflate or open position, with the deflation valves still in the deflate or dump position. This action will ensure that all remaining pressure within the system has been relieved. The system components can be disconnected at this point, although the system should be left as preconnected as possible to reduce the time needed to place the air bags in service and ensure that the necessary components are present in one place when they are needed.

Capabilities

Rescue personnel that place an air bag system in service must understand several basic laws of physics and how these laws relate to the use of air bags. An air bag is able to perform its basic functions of lifting, spreading, pushing, or pulling because of the air pressure being exerted within the air bag itself. Air pressure is just one of the factors that determines an individual air bag's lifting capacity and the maximum height that it can achieve. There is a direct relationship between the bag's lifting capacity and its inflation height.

All high-pressure air bags have ratings for both the maximum force in pounds that they can exert and the maximum height they can achieve when fully inflated. For example, a particular air bag could have a rating of 73 tons *and* a maximum lifting height of 20 inches. Air bags, however, *cannot* achieve both ratings simultaneously. Because of basic laws of physics, high-pressure air bags can either exert their maximum force in pounds or achieve their maximum inflation height in inches. They *cannot* do both at the same time.

To fully understand this crucial fact, personnel must consider the method used to determine the lifting capacity of an air bag. This rating, expressed in pounds of force, is obtained by multiplying the working length of the bag by the bag's width and multiplying the result (square inches of bag surface) by the bag's internal air pressure. Length times width times the internal psi air pressure yields the maximum force output of that bag. A bag with a working area of 30 in x 30 in has 900 square inches of working surface area. If 118 psi air pressure is provided inside the bag, the total air bag force can then be calculated at 106,200 lb (118 psi multiplied by the 900 square inch surface area). This particular bag would be rated by the manufacturer as a 53-ton capacity bag (Fig. 6-64).

The same bag would also carry a height rating, probably 18 inches maximum. As the inflation height

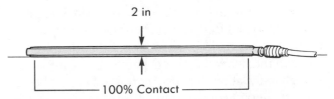

FIG. 6-65 A high-pressure air bag maintains its theoretical 100% capacity only until the center is approximately 2 inches in height. Further inflation diminishes the capacity.

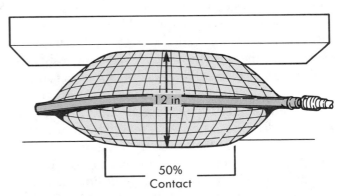

FIG. 6-66 Higher inflation means lower capacity. Maximum height yields one-half maximum capacity.

increases, however, the lifting capacity diminishes dramatically. This is not due to a defect in the air bag but to a reduction in the bag's total working contact area. For the maximum lifting capacity, it must be remembered that 100% of the bag's working surface is counted. As the bag inflates, the four edges of the bag lift off the surface below them. As the bag is further inflated, the center of the bag continues to rise, lifting the edges even higher (Fig. 6-65). The contact area also decreases when the working surface of an air bag is placed against a narrow object such as a frame rail or an I-beam.

As a rule, an air bag will exert its maximum-rated capacity until the center of the bag has lifted 2 inches. As the bag continues to expand, the contact surface area begins to diminish, thereby reducing the total lifting capacity to the point that at full inflation height the bag generally has only 50% of its original working surface area still in contact with the surface below. Achieving maximum air bag height usually means that only one half of the lifting capacity of the bag is available — the bag rated at the 53-ton capacity and 18-inch inflation height, when inflated to its maximum height, is capable of only lifting approximately 27 to 28 tons of weight (Fig. 6-66). When working a rescue

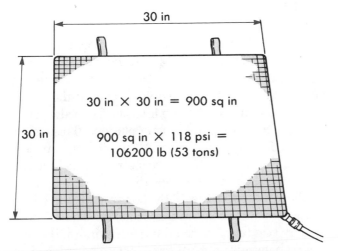

FIG. 6-64 For this air bag, the theoretical lifting capacity is the bag's length (30 inches) times the bag's width (30 inches) times the system's maximum pressure (118 psi), which equals 53 tons.

evolution, if there is some doubt about the weight of the object to be lifted, crews should attempt to use as large a bag as possible. This ensures that the bag will still have the needed lifting capacity as it approaches its higher inflation heights. Efforts should also be made to maximize the contact area of the top and bottom of the bag with the objects it touches.

Lifting an object with air bags can be accomplished in a single-point lift or in a multiple-point lift. In a single-point lift, one bag alone or two bags stacked together are placed under an object at only one point and inflated. This single-point lift also becomes a tilting lift. Tilting a load serves to lighten the total weight that the air bags must lift, reducing resistance to the bag as it works. This phenomenon of a changing load is especially true when lifting one portion of a vehicle containing a fluid cargo product such as fuel oil, mixed cement, or water. The lifting action causes the product in the tank to settle to the lowest level, which changes the load that the air bag is lifting. A multiple-point lift, where two bags lift simultaneously at two different locations on the same object, may or may not lighten the load as the lift is accomplished (Fig. 6-67). The important difference here is that although the lifting capacities of each air bag depend on their inflation heights, the useable capacities of both bags can be added together to estimate the total lifting capacity of the multiple bag setup.

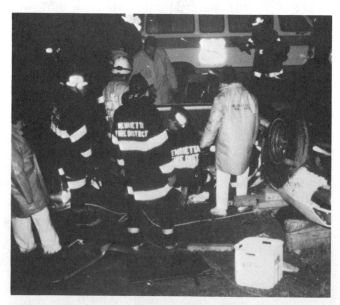

FIG. 6-67 Rescuers use high-pressure air bags at two different lifting points along the passenger side of the accident vehicle to accomplish a two-point tilting lift. The rescue effort was successful in freeing the occupant of the vehicle.

Safety

As with any rescue tool, safety for operating personnel, other emergency service providers, and patients must remain the top priority. Standard protective clothing and equipment must be required for all operating personnel. Clearing the work area of all unnecessary persons is extremely important when working with air bags. Even in the most carefully planned and controlled air bag evolution, bags can suddenly kick out of position. Command personnel have to anticipate any possible bag movement, and act to prevent it. If a bag does kick out, the path that it takes (its strike zone) can be predicted. The leaning direction of a bag and the shifting of a load can indicate the possible path of travel. This strike zone should be cleared of *all* persons for a distance in excess of 25 feet from the bags.

The rescue crew member working the controller unit should seek a position for themselves that also allows them to be within eyesight of at least one of the working air bags. This allows the operator to visually monitor the progress of that portion of the evolution. The controller should not be too close to the action; this would decrease operator safety and limit perspective of the overall air bag operation. The control operator should only accept directions or commands from *one* individual. Too many directions from too many people can lead to unsuccessful and unsafe operations. All commands should refer to the color of the appropriate air hose connected to each air bag. Command personnel must not get in the habit of asking for more air in the "bottom" bag or the "bag on the left." Standardized commands such as "Up on red!" or "Down on yellow!" will result in the safest and most effective evolutions.

It is acceptable to place one air bag on top of another for increased total lifting height. The larger bag should be placed as the bottom bag for maximum stability. Stacking bags can quickly change the center of balance of the load being lifted and can also result in some very effective lifting evolutions. This higher lift, however, also means that the air bags are less stable and more susceptible to shifting or kicking out of position. Stacking air bags does not allow you to add the lifting capacities of the bags together to get an estimate of their total lifting capacity. The smallest capacity bag that is inflated is the maximum that the stacked bags will lift. A 10-ton capacity bag placed on top of a 26-ton capacity bag can still only lift a maximum of 10 tons or less. Depending on which bag is inflated, this stacked bag arrangement could lift either

10 tons of weight or 26 tons. Greater weights, up to the sum of the two lifting bags, could be lifted if these bags were positioned in two separate locations and inflated simultaneously.

It is always advisable to stack air bags if at all possible to do so. If only one bag is needed to accomplish the task, having the second bag in the stack does no harm. If, however, the single bag cannot move the object as far or as high as necessary, the second bag is already in position to continue with the evolution. In stacking, only one bag should ever be placed on top of another; personnel should never stack more than two bags. The larger air bag should be on the bottom and be inflated first, but only partially. Once the bottom bag begins to form a base of stability, it can hold its position, and the upper bag should be partially inflated. The evolution continues as the two bags are alternately inflated, little by little, until either the desired result is achieved or the maximum safe total lift is obtained (Fig. 6-68).

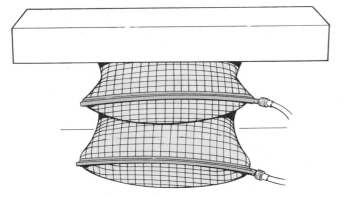

FIG. 6-68 Two bags properly stacked.

The safe total lift with stacked bags is a rescue officer's judgment call based on the circumstances of each actual situation. This limit is achieved when the contact area between the two bags is diminished to the point at which the stacked bags could become unstable. If both stacked bags were to be inflated fully, it would be like trying to balance one basketball on top of another. The hard, crowned surfaces of the bags actually become like wheels, allowing the load to roll or shift. Full inflation of stacked bags makes "kick out" very possible. Maintaining the bags at less than full inflation pressure and height allows the surfaces of the two bags to bond themselves together, thereby increasing stacking stability.

In all rescue work the use of wood blocking plays an important role in maintaining scene safety. Wood blocking is particularly important when lifting evolutions are being performed. With these evolutions, rescue personnel must be able to safely and effectively build "box crib" arrangements of wood to secure the object in its position. A box crib is a crisscross pattern of equal-size wood pieces arranged as a column to support the weight of the object. The box crib, by design, has a hollow center. While this is acceptable for cribbing supporting an object, it is totally unacceptable for use under an air bag. Whenever wood is used in contact with an air bag, it *must* be a *solid* layer of wood. If a box crib is necessary to lift an air bag closer to an object, the crib can be hollow, but the top layer must be solid (Fig. 6-69). Without a complete layer of wood under an air bag, the pillow-like shape of the bag will push the wood outward when inflated. This action has produced some serious injuries to

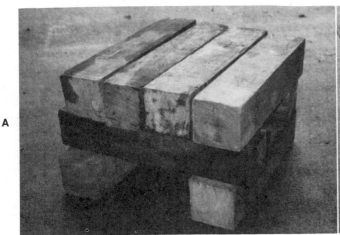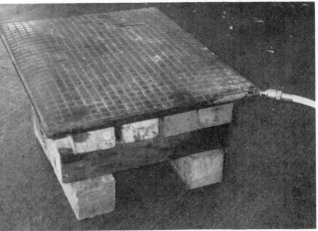

FIG. 6-69 A, When wood is used under air bags to support a lifting evolution, it must be a solid layer **B,** to minimize slippage and box crib movement.

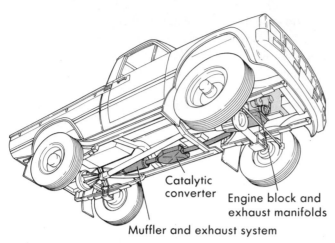

Catalytic converter

Engine block and exhaust manifolds

Muffler and exhaust system

FIG. 6-70 When placing air bags, personnel should avoid heat sources such as the engine block, exhaust system, and catalytic converter.

rescue personnel in actual cribbing failure incidents. To further ensure safety, personnel should avoid placing wood on the top and the bottom of the same air bag. The top surface of the bag functions most effectively when it is placed directly in contact with the surface of the object being lifted or spread and allowed to mold itself to the shape of that object.

Air bag placement at rescue incidents should be intended to maintain the safety of the bag itself. Exposure to chemicals or heat sources can quickly destroy the integrity of the tool (Fig. 6-70). The neoprene rubber outer surface of an air bag will permanently scorch and lose strength when exposed to temperatures of 220° F or more. When an object is at least this hot, water sprayed onto its surface turns to steam. The rubber air bag actually begins to melt at 330° F. The bags should also be protected from sharp objects like bolts or nails and small working surfaces such as I-beams or sharp metal edges. Although air bags are resistant to punctures, scrapes, and cuts, they are not indestructible. Protection from such damage can be provided by relocating the bag or placing old mud flaps, leather or rubber pads, heavy canvas material, or even plywood sheeting over the damaging object. Air bag protection accessories marketed under the names Monster Mesh or Bag Mate which are specifically designed for this purpose, are also available. Protection is also crucial for the nylon ratchet strap accessory that can be purchased with the air bag systems. Holmatro, Inc., for example, manufactures their synthetic air bag ratchet strapping with a protective shroud installed over the strap. Rescue personnel should heed Holmatro's suggestion and

slide short lengths of old fire hose over any brand of nylon strapping for this purpose. When new, these ratchet straps are rated at a given working capacity. This rating, which ranges from 5000 pounds to 11,000 pounds of pull depending on the manufacturer, is for a pull in a straight line only, using a single strap. Physical damage can reduce this rating, as can sharp bends, twists, or knots in the strapping.

When personnel are operating air bags in an environment of high humidity and low air temperature, components such as the regulator or controller unit may become ice coated or freeze. In these circumstances, it is permissible to warm the unit or use a commercially available automobile de-icer spray to remove the frost or ice.

Preventive Maintenance

Preventive maintenance and safety inspections of air bag systems should be performed at regular intervals by rescue personnel. Such routine inspections are relatively easy to perform and can detect minor problems before they become serious. In conducting a typical maintenance inspection, personnel assemble the system and closely examine each component for any physical damage or abuse, as well as for loose or missing parts. As each portion of the system is pressurized, it should be checked for potential air leaks. Each individual air bag should be inflated to 50% of its operating pressure (30 psi maximum for unrestrained air bag if following the recommendations of Paratech Inc. for their Maxiforce air bag product). Potential air leakage areas include the supply hose itself, all couplings, and the brass nipple of each bag.

Next, the exterior surface of the partially inflated bag should be examined. Small nicks, cuts, and abrasions on the bag are of minor concern unless the inner steel or fabric cords are exposed. Deep cuts or slices through the outer rubber layers that expose the steel wire inside the bag can cause the steel to rust, seriously weakening the integrity of the bag at that point. A minor cut or slice can be filled in with a pliable filler compound such as rubber cement. Serious cuts require returning the damaged bag to the manufacturer for a hot vulcanization repair or total bag replacement. The bag surface must also be inspected for any swelling or bulges. A leak test of the bag can be performed by submerging the partially inflated bag in water and looking for bubbles to appear.

Vetter Systems advises users of their product to routinely test the operation of their system's pressure relief valve. To do this, install a shutoff valve after the control unit and leave it in the closed position. Allow air to flow thorough the system up to the closed valve. As the air pressure is gradually increased to the controller unit, the system's maximum safe operating pressure is reached. At this point the pressure relief valve within the controller unit should function. The pressure when the relief valve opens should be within 5% of the red line setting on the face of the pressure gauge. If the relief valve on an older unit fails to function properly, it may be sticking because of the relief valve being stored in a tightly closed position. Unnecessary pressure actually bonds the relief valve to the brass seat of the valve, delaying or preventing the valve from opening. If the relief valve activates prematurely, particles of dirt may have fallen into the valve seat. To dislodge this dirt, open the relief valve and flow air through it. Dual controller units actually have two separate relief devices, each of which monitor pressure in one discharge line. It is important that the relief valve operation test be performed for both halves of the controller unit.

Crews working with the original fitting style of controller units should also check to see that any factory-installed lead seals are still intact on the ends of the relief valve. The relief valve is the heart of the safety system for the air bags. It is important to keep these valves properly adjusted to factory specifications.

System Storage

Air bag system components should be stored on the rescue vehicle to protect from damage or abuse. The pressure regulator is particularly vulnerable to physical damage. The regulator adjustment knob should be near the 0 pressure setting to relax the tension on its internal components. Relief valves on the fitting controller units should not be so tightly closed that the valve is damaged. Vetter Systems suggest that their original fitting dual controller be stored with the manual flow valves slightly open to prevent the internal washers from becoming bonded to their valve seats.

Storage of the system should also afford protection to the air hoses, which are susceptible to damage from cuts, abrasion, heat, and heavy loads. If the air bags themselves are stored on edge, the brass air nipple should be facing up. Small nipple caps or short pieces of rubber hose can be placed over the nipple to further protect it from damage. If the air bags are to be stored in the flat position, the air nipples should always face the rescue crew member loading or unloading them.

In this manner, the operator is aware of the location of the nipple and can protect it.

System Cleaning

Routine cleaning of the air bags involves washing them with a mild soap and water solution. Dirt and grime can be scrubbed off with a stiff bristled brush. Rubber preservatives, black rubber tire paint, or other coatings should never be applied to an air bag, because these substances would make the working surface of the bag very slippery. After cleaning, the bags can be air dried but should not be placed in direct sunlight. The remaining components of the system should be wiped clean. A light application of silicone spray can be added to each air coupling to ensure that the female portion remains free and functional.

AIR CUSHIONS

The theory behind air cushions is simply to provide a vertical lift over a large surface area. Originally designed during World War II to salvage airplanes and large pieces of equipment, the cushions were first adapted commercially for truck and equipment salvage and recovery operations. They perform especially well when thin-skinned, light-walled vehicles such as aluminum truck trailers, tanker vehicles, buses, or aircraft require lifting or moving. Current fire service rescue applications of air cushions include vehicle rescue evolutions and hazardous material leak and spill control.

Air cushions and air bags are constructed of different materials. Their methods of construction also differ, as do their operating pressures, working capacities, and lifting heights. High-pressure air bags may not perform well in situations perfectly suited to low-pressure air cushions, and an air cushion may be ineffective in the very situation where a high-pressure air bag performs well. One kind of system does not replace the other; they complement each other. The most widely used system in the North American fire service is the high-pressure air bag system.

Air cushions are manufactured by several major companies, many of whom also produce air bags. Most air cushion manufacturers are based in Germany or England. All cushions are basically constructed in the same manner, which differs greatly from the construction of a high-pressure air bag (Fig. 6-71). A strong, reinforced fabric material (up to 7-ply) forms the top and bottom "plates" of the cushion. This can be a simple canvas or an Aramid/Kevlar-impregnated material bonded to neoprene. Kevlar fibers are known

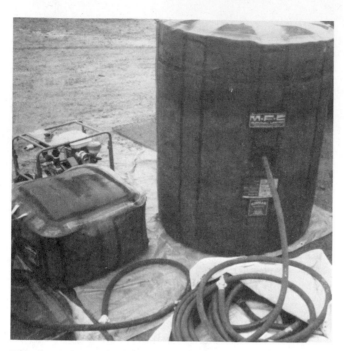

FIG. 6-71 Air cushions consist of thin-walled materials assembled in a cold vulcanization process.

to be the strongest man-made material in the world. The collapsible sides of the cushion are neoprene. The cushion may be reinforced internally by nylon strapping supports to maintain a correct inflated shape. These ties hold the top and bottom plate together, minimizing ballooning and maintaining flat working surfaces.

All air cushion materials are cut from large sheets and assembled in a cold vulcanization process. This involves placing the sheets together and gluing them with an epoxy cement. When inflated, the completed cushion resembles a pillow, large cube, or cylinder. This manufacturing process offers advantages and disadvantages. In comparison with high-pressure air bags, air cushions are more vulnerable to physical damage during rescue evolutions. Their relatively thin surfaces make them easier to cut or puncture than an air bag. The cold vulcanization process, however, permits quick and effective repairs without having to return the cushion to the manufacturer.

System Components

The components of an air cushion system resemble those of an air bag system in their basic functions. An air source supplies the compressed air through a regulator, then through hoses, into a controller unit. The controller can be a single or dual unit design and has safety relief valves to prevent overinflation of the cushion. The compressed air leaves the controller and is directed into the individual cushions through additional air hoses. It must be noted that the air supply hoses used in this system are much larger in diameter than air bag system hoses and typically have a built-in metal spiral to reduce kinks or sharp bends. Air fittings are usually twist type of metal units with an interlocking claw feature. The large outlet connection molded into the air cushion makes for rapid deflation of the cushion if a hose disconnects while the cushion is under a load. This loss of air and operating height cannot be stopped or controlled as easily as with the high-pressure air bags. For this reason, all air cushion manufacturers are very emphatic in directing that air cushions always be used in pairs.

Air cushions available in North America are designed as either medium-pressure or low-pressure systems. A medium-pressure system works at approximately 15 psi operating pressure, although most work can usually be accomplished as the cushion works at between 8 and 12 psi. The 15 psi working pressure cushions have bursting pressures of 58 to 100 psi, depending on manufacturer, size, and style.

Low-pressure air cushion systems function at 7 psi working pressure. These systems may have slightly thinner side surfaces than the medium-pressure cushions. The lower operating pressure means lower psi surface pressure within the cushion. This allows the cushion to easily mold itself around uneven surfaces or objects placed in contact with it.

Air cushion capacities range from 3 to 18 tons. Specialized vehicle recovery cushions are designed with lifting capacities up to 30 tons. These units, however, are not used by fire and rescue service personnel. Air consumption can range from 2 cubic feet of air in small cushions to 25 cubic feet or more in larger cushions. If a portable air compressor is being used as the air supply source, a rating of 30 cfm is recommended.

Air cushions can produce greater lifting heights than high-pressure air bag systems. Deflated cushions are generally 1 to 3 inches thick, depending on capacity, and extend to fully inflated heights of 24 to 60 inches. Unlike air bags, the cube or cylinder-shaped cushions do not lose their surface contact area at these increased heights and achieve maximum capacities only when fully inflated.

Safety

For safety it is imperative that rescue personnel always use two air cushions of equal size and capacity simultaneously when working with these systems. This safety procedure is recommended by *all* air cushion manufacturers because of the possibility that one cushion can slip out of position or fail.

When working with air cushions on slippery or wet ground or in mud, ice, or snow, personnel should place a sand or gravel material under the cushion for increased adhesion.

Personnel operating with air cushions must also be extremely conscious of the vulnerability of the cushion to physical damage. Cushions can be damaged in may ways at an auto accident. Protruding metal screws or bolts, sharp edges of sheet metal, or broken glass from windows, mirrors, or headlights can quickly puncture or tear the cushion, as can pieces of hard plastic from the damaged vehicles. Due to their rubber construction, air cushions are vulnerable to scorching and melting on contact with a heat source such as a vehicle exhaust system, catalytic converter, or hot metal that has been involved in a fire. Chemical contamination should also be avoided when working with the cushions.

System Maintenance

Preventive maintenance of air cushion systems can easily be carried out by following several basic procedures. Cushions should be cleaned after each use to remove any grease, oil, or dirt accumulations. The most effective cleaning procedure is to inflate the cushion to 50% of its working pressure, wash it with a mild soap solution, and rinse it with water. While the cushion surface is wet, all areas should be inspected for small bubble leaks. Any tears, cuts, or bad scrapes should be noted and repaired as necessary. While the cushion is inflated, all remaining hoses, couplings, regulators, controllers, gauges, and valves should be inspected for loose or missing parts or for damage. A hose that has been damaged internally may bulge noticeably when pressurized. The operation of the relief valve device should also be checked, noting the pressure at which it operates.

Splits, small tears, or minor cuts can be repaired by the use of a patch kit supplied by the air cushion manufacturer. Minor repairs are cold patched and secured with adhesive much as bicycle or car tire inner tubes are. Any cushion that has been field repaired should be tested at 50% of its system operating pressure for a 5-minute period after the patch has properly dried. During this test, the cushion should not lose any pressure. Vetter Systems recommends returning their air cushions to them for inspection

once every 5 years, at which time they issue certificates of factory inspection.

ELECTRIC-POWERED RESCUE TOOLS

Electricity is a major source of power for operating rescue equipment. Electricity can be AC or DC and can be 12, 110, or 220 volts (Fig. 6-72). Electricity is most commonly used at vehicle rescue incidents to provide artificial lighting of the scene and the individual work areas inside a vehicle. In addition, the capability to generate electricity at an accident gives rescue crews a choice of power for hydraulic equipment and a wide selection of smaller electric tools for their inventory of equipment. In recent years, electricity has become increasingly popular for power plants operating power rescue tools. The electric units are much quieter than their gasoline counterparts and provide a reliable source of power for the rescue systems.

The disadvantages of electric power plants are slight and evident only at those times when the power rescue tools are being operated. The reaction of a power spreader, for example, is different when it is operated off an electric power plant. Personnel must realize that their spreader will probably react to the trigger controls a bit more slowly, move more slowly as it opens or closes, and generally *not* develop as

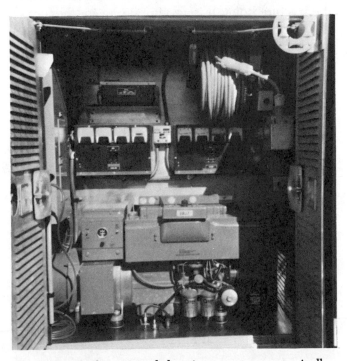

FIG. 6-72 Vehicle-mounted electric generators are typically powered by gasoline or diesel engines or operate off a hydraulic power take-off unit.

much power at its peak as when it operates off a gasoline power unit.

The electric reciprocating saw, a small tool powered by electricity and better known by the trade name Sawzall, is a valuable addition to a rescue tool inventory. This small, hand-held saw is not to be confused with the larger rotary power saw, which is not recommended for use in vehicle rescue operations. In the hands of a skilled operator, the reciprocating saw can safely and effectively remove many portions of a vehicle trapping an occupant. When equipped with a 6-inch saw blade, for example, it can saw through vehicle roof posts, steering wheel rings, or steering columns, as well as through such smaller components as gear selector levers, bolts, metal or plastic bracing, and brake or clutch pedals (Fig. 6-73).

It is important for rescue personnel to understand the function of the part of the saw located along the side of the blade where the blade secures into the saw itself. This component, called the foot, assists in guiding the saw blade as it cuts. More important, the foot helps the operator control the motion of the tool as it moves along the surface of the metal. To work properly, this foot must be in contact with the surface of the object being cut at all times. Inexperienced operators of reciprocating saws tend to lift the foot off the surface, virtually eliminating the efficiency of the blade's reciprocating action and stressing the blade to the fracture point. It is also important for the foot of the saw to move along the surface being cut with a gentle rocking action of the entire saw. This pivoting

back and forth enables the saw to yield its greatest efficiency.

The recommended reciprocating saw has a variable speed trigger and is equipped with break-resistant saw blades. These bimetal composite blades will take severe abuse and are more resistant to the problem of fracturing than standard saw blades. The Hackmaster 614R or 618R blade by Lenox Manufacturing Co. is an example of the best quality "shatterproof" blades. Although not truly unbreakable, it is extremely rugged and durable. Rescue personnel should always lubricate the blade during its cutting action. The back and forth movement of the blade against the metal creates intense heat that quickly damages the blade and makes cutting more difficult. Lubricants clean the loose particles out of the cut, cool the saw blade by reducing friction between it and the metal object, and minimize the likelihood of sparks being produced during cutting.

Lubrication requires a fluid of some sort, which does not necessarily mean a wet liquid. Liquids such as soapy water or light-grade lubricating oils, applied from spray or squeeze-type bottles like those used for household detergents, work well for blade lubrication (Fig. 6-74). Even compressed air can be used for lubrication in an emergency. Air is a fluid medium

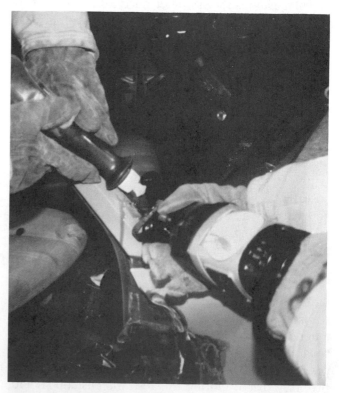

FIG. 6-74 Applying lubrication to the reciprocating saw during operation.

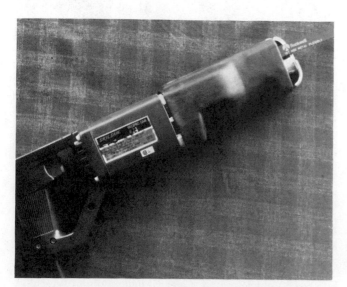

FIG. 6-73 An electric reciprocating saw should have a heavy-duty industrial design with a variable-speed trigger.

that lubricates as well as liquids do. The important point is to keep a lubricating agent applied to the saw blade during all cutting.

Other recommended electric-powered tools for rescue operations include electric drills and impact wrenches. A drill with a ¼-inch bit may be used by rescue personnel if it is their standard operating procedure to "vent" the hydraulic piston unit of an energy absorbing bumper.

VEHICLE-MOUNTED TOOL FAMILY

Vehicle-mounted tools that may be present in a rescue tool inventory are those tools permanently mounted to and powered solely by the vehicle to which they are attached. A vehicle-mounted winch and an A-frame apparatus are two tools that fit into this family.

HAND TOOLS FOR VEHICLE RESCUE

Some rescue tools used at accident scenes never run out of air, electricity, or gas. Instead, it is the operators of these tools who usually run out of "steam." The next category of rescue equipment to be discussed in this tool overview is the versatile family of hand tools, which are the most basic rescue tools of all. To be classified as a hand tool, a piece of equipment must receive its power by simple, mechanical means directly from the tool operator. A hand tool uses no electricity, hydraulic fluid, compressed gas, or fuels of any type.

Hand tools can be grouped according to their prime function. These groupings include cribbing blocks, forcible entry tools, cutting tools, pulling tools, safety control equipment, and basic medical equipment.

The recommended cribbing blocks must meet several important criteria to function safely and successfully as a rescue tool (Fig. 6-75).

CRIBBING BLOCKS

Hard maple, ash, or oak are the most acceptable woods for use as blocking. Softer woods such as pine will not only produce problems when the blocks are stressed during an evolution but also can become an unnecessary safety hazard in certain situations. Soft wood blocks are very susceptible to fracturing during use. The wood can splinter, crack, or com-

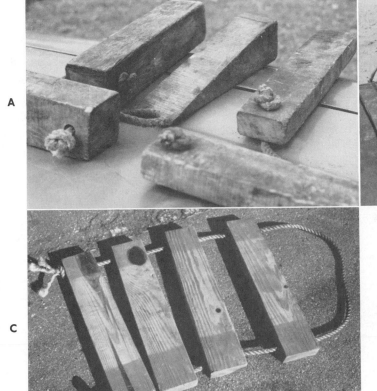

FIG. 6-75 Rescue cribbing includes **A,** wedges and 18-in blocks, **B,** 4 in x 4 in x 48 in block supporting the spreader during column-pulling evolution, **C,** ladder cribbing assembly.

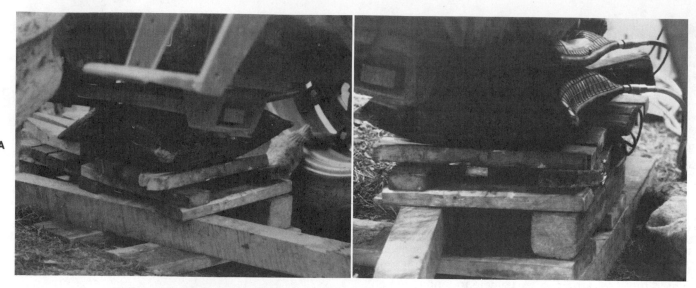

FIG. 6-76 A, Failure of soft pine wood blocking under a farm tractor. Note the splitting of the top layer 2 in x 4 in block and **B,** total failure of the pine block on the right side of the fifth layer of wood. All oak blocking functioned properly.

pletely disintegrate under actual conditions. What happens when a block fails depends on each individual situation.

In a demonstration evolution conducted as part of a farm rescue training program, a heavy farm tractor was being lifted with air bags. The stacked bags were placed on wood blocking, with a solid layer of wood directly under the bags. The terrain around the tractor was dirt and gravel, and an overnight rain had made the soil damp. Unbeknown to the instructor, several pieces of 2 in x 4 in blocking used to construct the box crib wood formation were actually soft pine. Because the wood blocks were dirty, their presence went undetected among the other oak blocking.

At the conclusion of the tractor lift, almost as though there had been an invisible signal, several pine blocks suddenly snapped in two with a loud crack (Fig. 6-76). Because the rescue students had placed safety cribbing at two other points on the chassis of the tractor, the machine's downward movement was minimal. A later review of the incident, however, showed that had the soft wood failed before placement of the final safety cribbing was accomplished or had the failure occurred at an actual incident, the situation would have been far more serious. All rescue blocking except specially designed step chocks should be hardwood only. It is not worth the risk to use anything else.

The blocking should also be cut into different sizes and be in standard dimensions. Recommended di-

mensions for the thickness or height of rescue blocks are 1 inch for the plates or planking wood, and 2-inch and 4-inch thicknesses for the remaining blocking. Thicker blocks are bulky to use and require unnecessarily large amounts of space on the rescue truck for storage. The recommended length that is most popular among rescue companies for wood blocking is 18 inches (Fig. 6-77). This length wood will not, however, serve every purpose at a rescue scene.

Several longer length blocks are needed at a rescue scene to support certain basic evolutions. The most popular dimension for longer blocks is 4 in x 4 in x 48 in. These *four-footers* are ideal for spanning across the crushed front end of an automobile where conventional 18-inch blocks only crush deeper into the wreckage as a load is applied across them. The four-footers also work well when stabilizing a vehicle on its edge or lifting an object. Although 4-foot lengths are handy to have at a scene, many busy rescue companies also include additional 4 in x 4 in blocks up to 8 feet in length if they have the space on their rescue vehicles. A special situation may require just such an item for a successful rescue.

To place blocking into very small openings, personnel must have wedge-shaped blocks included in the rescue inventory. These blocks are made by cutting a 4 in x 4 in x 18 in oak block on the diagonal. The strongest wedge blocks are constructed by cutting from one corner of the block to a point 1 inch from the

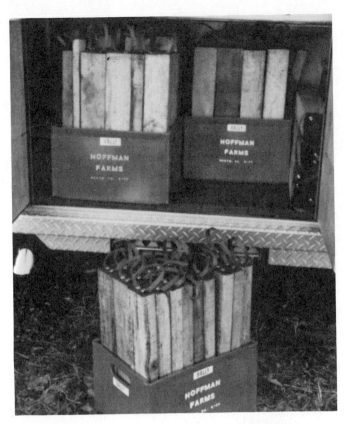

FIG. 6-77 Storage of cribbing in crates allows efficient storage and transport from vehicle to tool staging area. At accident scene, crate makes blocks readily accessible to rescuer deploying them.

exact opposite corner. This cut leaves a solid 4 in x 4 in x 1 in butt end at the large portion of the block, which strengthens the wedge and minimizes the chances of fracturing under a load condition.

Standard building material wood is rarely suitable for use as rescue blocking because it is often soft pine and its surfaces have generally been planed or sanded smooth. This destroys the ability of the block to grip under a load. For this same reason, pressure-treated wood or wood such as railroad ties that has been soaked or penetrated with an additive should not be used for rescue blocking. Under load conditions, the additive in the wood's outer surface can prevent the block from holding or gripping. Like droplets of water on a freshly waxed automobile, one block can "float" above the surface of another, making for an unsafe situation.

It is vital for the wood surface to remain in its natural state. Varnish, shellac, or paint should never be applied to the wood. If it is necessary to paint a block to identify the crew that owns the wood, it should only

be stenciled or painted at the very ends of the wood. The working surface of the wood must be kept free of any coatings.

The wood should be assembled so that transportation from the rescue vehicle to the work area at an emergency scene can be accomplished quickly and efficiently. Handles secured to the ends of the blocks, ropes strung between two blocks, or plastic open-mesh crates of blocking allow for the expeditious handling of the wood.

The recommended tool inventory (see box on pp. 214-216) outlines the basic quantity of wood blocking that should be immediately available at an accident scene. This wood does not have to be carried to the scene by one emergency vehicle, although that is the ideal situation. The total inventory of wood includes the wood carried by several vehicles responding on the first rescue assignment. Exceeding this basic starting quantity is highly recommended. You will never have too much blocking at a scene, only too little. Additional quantities of wood should be accessible either at the rescue station or through mutual assistance calls to other rescue companies. It is important for the rescue command officer to know the quantities of blocking and the locations of additional supplies.

FORCIBLE ENTRY TOOLS

Forcible entry hand tools get their name from the fire service application of the tools to gain access to buildings. In vehicle rescue, these same tools are used for prying, chopping, hammering, cutting, or spreading. The tool inventory lists only a basic minimum quantity of these hand tools, although additional quantities of each are highly recommended (Fig. 6-78).

The hand tools listed as cutting and disassembly hand tools are basic in their operation and require simple maintenance (Fig. 6-79). A minimum of four hacksaw tools is recommended so that when a blade breaks during use, time need not be wasted changing a blade. When several complete saws are available and one saw blade breaks, the crew member simply changes to another hacksaw. Rescue work should never come to a halt just because of a broken blade.

Rescue personnel must provide break-resistant hacksaw blades for their hacksaws. The preferred blade is 12 inches in length. There must also be spare blades available at the rescue scene to place into frames as necessary. Hacksaw frame and blade

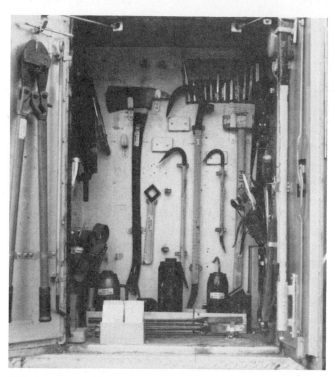

FIG. 6-78 Efficient and functional storage of hand tools in compartment in rescue vehicle.

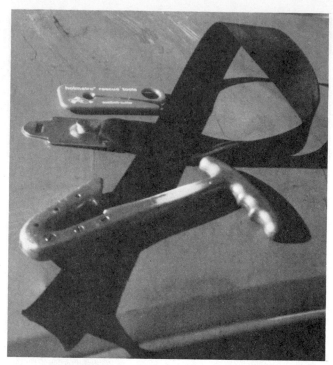

FIG. 6-80 Because of the increased use of seat belts, it is important that seat belt cutting tools be readily available. Military-specification, all-metal type of seatbelt cutter is recommended.

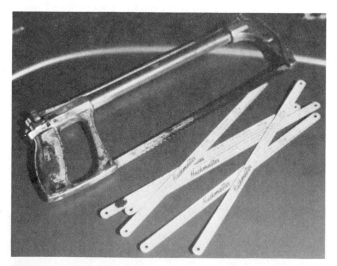

FIG. 6-79 Rescue hacksaws should be heavy-duty, one-piece frames and be equipped with break-resistant, 12-in metal cutting blades.

manufacturers all recommend that the blade be placed into the saw frame with the slant of its cutting teeth facing forward. In this manner, cutting is done on the pushing stroke, and the pulling action serves to "clean out" the cut. On certain styles of hacksaw frames, it is possible to install two blades simultaneously on the one frame. A "double-bladed" hacksaw would therefore have one blade with the teeth facing forward and one with its teeth facing rearward. With this setup, the tool operator cuts metal on both the push and the pull stroke. The two blades also make a wider cut, minimizing the binding or pinching of the saw blades in the cut. For personnel to make double-bladed hacksaws work most effectively, the blades must be replaced often and be fully tensioned in a heavy-duty, top-quality hacksaw frame.

The only acceptable hacksaw frame for rescue applications is a one-piece frame of heavy-duty construction with a good blade tension adjustment feature. The typical multipiece, hardware store hacksaw frame, adjustable to accept 8-, 10-, or 12-inch blades, is *not acceptable* for vehicle rescue work. When the blade breaks or works loose from the frame, the entire frame collapses. The small metal piece that holds the saw blade into the frame at the end opposite the handle readily dislodges itself when blade tension is lost. If this piece flies out of the frame, it can easily be lost, rendering the remaining portion of the frame useless. The better quality, one-piece frames available from tool suppliers and reputable hardware stores offer the safest and most efficient method of securing the blade in the saw.

One modification that can be made to a hacksaw frame is to add a second handle at the opposite end of the frame. Working in tandem, as with an old-fashioned, two-person buck saw, two rescue crew members with the modified frame can quickly saw through material at an incident.

The most important aspect of hacksaw operations is blade lubrication during the cutting action, preferably with soapy water or an acceptable lubricating oil. With a good saw frame, break-resistant blades, lubrication, and a skilled operator, the hacksaw becomes a valuable vehicle rescue hand tool.

Other hand tools for cutting include metal-cutting can opener type of tools, tin snips, serrated-edge scissors, utility knives, and seat belt cutters (Fig. 6-80). An additional cutting tool that may be found in the inventory of a rescue company is the hand bow saw, used for cutting away wood, brush, bushes, limbs, or small trees at an accident scene. Another cutting tool (although not a hand tool) that can be extremely effective in just such special situations is the gasoline or electric powered chain saw. The addition of a carbide tooth chain to the unit makes it possible to cut away wood or brush quickly and efficiently.

PULLING TOOLS

In the category of hand tools for pulling, the most widely known is the come-along tool, properly referred to as a hand winch. Come-along tools are available with chain, steel cable, nylon strapping, or nylon rope attached to the core of the tool. The most popular choices for vehicle rescue work are the chain and the steel cable units. A steering column pulling evolution or a rearward pull of a front seat with a come-along tool requires a force of approximately 2 tons to accomplish. The tool inventory therefore lists the 1½-ton or 2-ton capacity units as the minimum for vehicle rescue work. Most 1½-ton come-alongs will actually develop 2¼ tons of pulling power.

Come-alongs of these sizes are relatively small and easy to store, carry, and operate. The chain come-along units are preferred over the cable come-alongs because of their durability, high degree of reliability, and simple method of operation (Fig. 6-81). A chain unit with large control knobs or levers is recommended because it is easily operated while rescuers are wearing gloves. Many inexpensive come-alongs, not designed for rescue applications, have small, intricate control levers that can only be operated with bare hands. These poor-quality tools should *not* be used for vehicle rescue work.

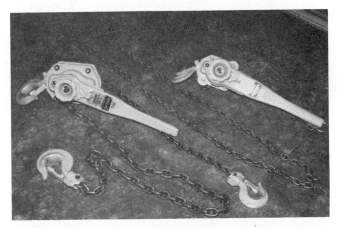

FIG. 6-81 Chain come-along should have a minimum rating of 1½ ton and have large controls that can be operated by personnel wearing gloves.

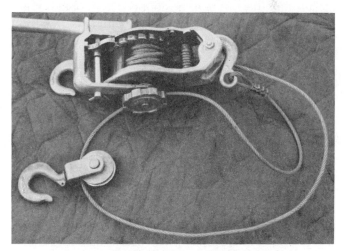

FIG. 6-82 Cable come-along for vehicle rescue work should be rated at minimum 1½ ton capacity, have heavy-duty construction and approximately 22 feet of aircraft specification stranded cable, and be equipped with a floating hook and pulley for double rigging.

The most common brands of cable come-alongs used for vehicle rescue work have 22 feet of cable and a floating hook and pulley assembly on the cable itself (Fig. 6-82). These cable come-alongs may be used as either single-rigged or double-rigged units. In the single-rigged mode a single line of cable is run from the spool on the body of the tool to a chain secured around an object. This allows for a tool rating of 1 ton to be exerted over the total length of the cable. If personnel attach the hook at the end of the cable directly to the body of the tool, the unit is double rigged. Double-rigged cable come-alongs double the working capacity of the unit, making the 1-ton, single-rigged come-along into a 2-ton tool. The only loss is that the tool has only half of its cable length to use because of the doubling of the lines, and the speed of the cable and pulley is half that of the single line set up (Fig. 6-83).

Cable come-alongs must be treated with extra caution to prevent tool damage. The cable of the tool consists of many small-diameter wire strands twisted to form the cable itself. If a cable becomes twisted (Fig. 6-84), is pulled across sharp edges, crushed, or exposed to heat, a loss of strength occurs, reducing the tool's overall safety margin. Care should always be taken to protect the cable from physical damage. Cable that has been damaged must be replaced with rated strength cable.

Come-along tools perform one basic function. They work in a straight line to move two lengths of chain closer together. When positioned horizontally between a stationary object and a movable one, the tool pulls. When positioned vertically, the come-along

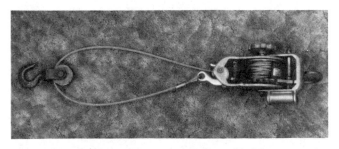

FIG. 6-83 Double rigging a come-along doubles its single-line pulling or lifting capacity and cuts its operating cable length and cable travel speed in half.

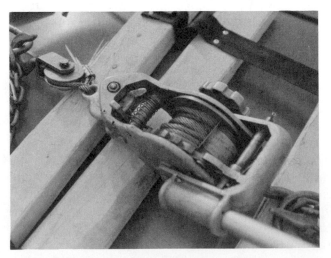

FIG. 6-84 Improper setup and careless operation of cable come-along results in a twisted and damaged cable and a jammed machine.

causes a lifting action. The cable or chain of the tool should *never* be secured directly around the stationary or movable objects. Instead, separate lengths of rescue chain must be secured to these objects, and the two hooks of the come-along attached to these assisting chains. Attempting to pass the cable or chain of a come-along around a sharp corner of an object is usually not only unsuccessful but also unsafe. The friction of the chain or cable of the come-along moving over the object reduces the effective operation of the tool and will more than likely damage the chain or cable. Damaged wire cable looks like hair that has split ends. The individual strands of the wire cable fracture and fray outward, weakening the cable, which then requires replacement.

The tool must be positioned in as straight a line as possible between the stationary and movable objects. This means that in most applications involving pulling with the come-along at a motor vehicle accident, the body of the tool should be on the top of the hood or on the trunk area of the vehicle. Chains are secured to a low point on the undercarriage and also attached directly to the movable object (steering column, dashboard, pedals, doors, or seats as required).

A household electrical circuit contains a fuse designed as the weak component of the system. When the circuit is overloaded, the fuse "blows" to protect the other components of the system. A come-along also has a fuse designed into it. Reputable come-along manufacturers design a weak spot into the tool handle or include an internal shear pin that will fail before the tool is overloaded. This component fails *before* the maximum capacity of the cable or chain is achieved. It is therefore vital for safe operation of the come-along to replace a failed handle or pin with an exact factory replacement part. Homemade replacements — of solid pipe handles instead of factory handles or heavy-duty bolts instead of shear pins — eliminate this most important safety feature.

Two lengths of either rescue chain or strapping must be used with every come-along to put the tool in service. The rescue chain listed in the tool inventory is chosen for a working strength rating that provides adequate safety margins to operating personnel. It is also maneuverable and of sufficient length to accomplish routine vehicle rescue evolutions (Fig. 6-85). All rescue chain should have grab hooks at each end. These narrow throat hooks grab across the links of the chain, allowing rescue crew members to form loops of chain of a fixed size. Slip hooks, the large open-throat hooks, should be present only on tools like the

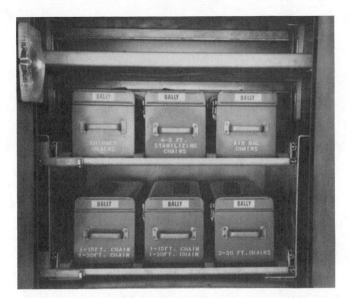

FIG. 6-85 This storage system for rescue chains uses metal tool boxes with labels to indicate the contents and function of chain lengths.

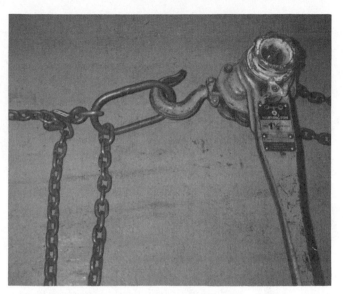

FIG. 6-86 All rescue chains should have grab hooks on one or both ends. The slip hook should be on the come-aling tool itself.

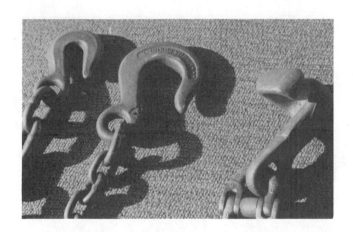

FIG. 6-87 Grab hook *(left)* designed to lock across a link of chain. Chain *(center)* equipped with a slip hook and designed to slide along chain. European style of grab hook *(right)*.

come-along (Fig. 6-86). These hooks allow the working chain to slide through the throat of the sliphook, forming a "noose" in the chain (Fig. 6-87). The small-length chain listed as a chain shortener is recommended for a multitude of practical applications (Fig. 6-88). The shortener can join two chains together or shorten a length of long chain, among other uses.

It is imperative that all rescue chain be of the highest quality material. Of the various grades of chain, the top quality choice is generally an alloy composition (Fig. 6-89). It has the highest strength rating for its size and offers personnel working with the chain the greatest degree of safety. Departments purchasing rescue chain should also request that the vendor provide tagged and certified lengths of chain. This process requires factory load testing and certification and tagged identification of the particular chain lengths. Certification tagging of chain or strap assemblies is a standard practice in industrial applications to ensure that the best quality material is being used.

Another hand tool, listed in the manual lifting group, is worthy of note. The tool is a 7000-lb capacity steel, mechanical jack known by the tradenames Hi-Lift or Handyman Jack (Fig. 6-90). Manufactured by the same company, these jacks have a long history in the agricultural field. In the past 10 years, they have gained in popularity as versatile rescue tools. The mechanical jacks range in height from 36 to 48 inches and can be purchased for under $50 at agricultural supply stores or quality hardware stores. Rescue

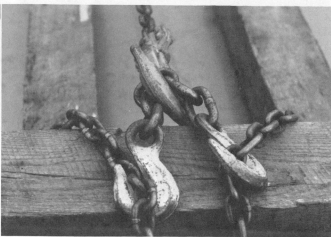

FIG. 6-88 **A,** Top and bottom chains are chain shorteners, and item at center is vehicle tie-down chain used by new-car transport companies to secure vehicles to the tractor trailer. **B,** Chain shortener shortens one length of chain or joins two lengths of chain.

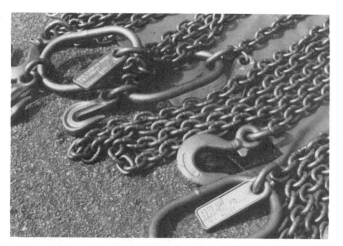

FIG. 6-89 Approved type of rescue chains are high-quality alloy metal, with alloy-quality hooks and clevis links.

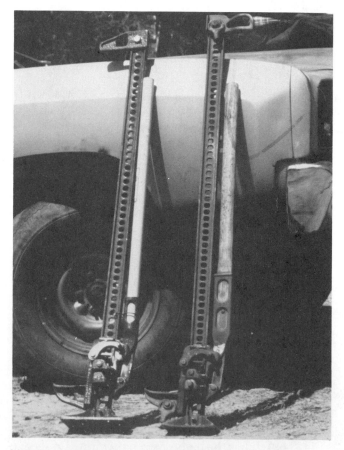

FIG. 6-90 Handyman and Hi-Lift brand units. The tool was so well designed and is so rugged in construction that the 1990 model tool *(left)* is very similar to the original 1954 Handyman jack *(right).*

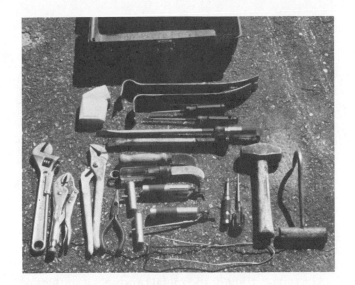

FIG. 6-91 Small hand tools used by a rescue company as their glass entry kit are stored and carried in a small tool box.

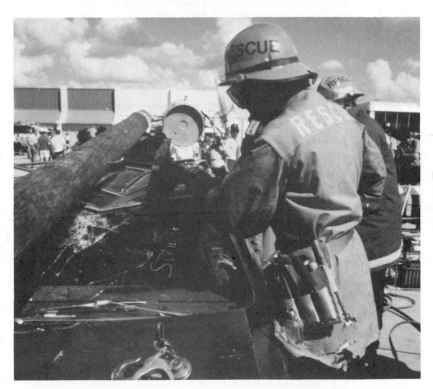

FIG. 6-92 Arranging small hand tools such as seat belt cutter, pliers, center punch, and screwdrivers in a tool pouch makes them immediately available at the rescue scene.

personnel can perform vehicle stabilization, lifting, pulling, spreading, squeezing, or clamping functions with the mechanical jack. The tool has a 7000-lb lifting capacity, a 5000-lb pull capacity, and a 750-lb squeeze or clamp rating. The uses of the mechanical Handyman or Hi-Lift jack are discussed in Chapter 7.

The inventory also recommends many small hand tools for vehicle rescue work. Rescue personnel need to obtain these tools and become knowledgeable in their use and operation. Once in the inventory, these items must be stored and maintained properly. Small

hand tools are frequently carried in a large tool box (Fig. 6-91). While this arrangement does allow the rescuer to quickly transport all the tools at once, time is lost searching for an item buried under all the other tools. Keeping track of the exact contents of a tool box is also difficult, requiring a complete unloading of the contents to take an accurate inventory.

Alternatives to the tool box include placing the smallest tools in an electrician's tool pouch or a carpenter's tool belt (Fig. 6-92). Carried in this manner, these little items can be accounted for quickly. Storage ideas for larger hand tools include tool boards or racks, brackets or hangers, and tool pouches made of soft material. Anything is better than having these important rescue tools simply tossed into a compartment or tangled in a tool box.

SAFETY CONTROL EQUIPMENT

The motor vehicle accident safety and hazard control equipment listed in the tool inventory is *not* intended to make emergency service personnel into hazardous material handlers or sanitation workers for the Public Works Department. The inventory is designed to allow for basic activities when emergency service personnel are confronted with numerous safety hazards routinely found at an accident scene. The golf tees, cone-shaped plugs, absorbent materials, sealant compound, shovels, and brooms are intended to allow for first response control of debris hazards, liquid leaks, and spills of vehicle fuels or oils.

The recommended lighting equipment is listed to ensure that consideration is given to providing at least a minimum level of portable handlights and general scene floodlighting. The smoke ejector is recommended when it is necessary to move fresh air into a vehicle's interior. This may be required if high heat, stale air, or noxious fumes have accumulated inside the vehicle. The smoke ejector can have other applications as well. For example, at a motor vehicle accident during summer's high temperature and humidity conditions, rescue activities to free the trapped occupants can take a physical toll on the operating personnel. In a shaded area designated for rehabilitation of beleaguered medical and rescue personnel, a smoke ejector that is set up to blow fresh air across the area can leave the personnel more rested and refreshed.

BASIC MEDICAL EQUIPMENT

Emergency medical response equipment is intended to supplement the equipment carried by the basic and advanced life support emergency medical crews. It should be considered additional support equipment for personnel that have received proper training in its use.

Deciding which rescue or EMS tools are proper for a particular department to own — and in what quantities — is a difficult task. The answers lie in part in a basic understanding of the rescue service goals of the emergency organization itself and the peculiarities of the locality being served.

HAZARDOUS TOOLS

Certain tools that fire service and rescue personnel are familiar with are unusually dangerous for vehicle rescue work. Their particular methods of operation create safety hazards at the emergency scene. One of these, as mentioned earlier, is the rotary power saw (Fig. 6-93). This saw, usually powered by a small, self-contained gasoline engine, can be equipped with an assortment of blades designed to cut various materials. The "abrasive" blade, used for cutting metal, cuts by wearing away the metal through its abrasive action. Although it does an effective job of cutting even heavy-gauge materials, the risks associated with its use are not worth the end result.

Abrasive cutting of the metal produces a shower of molten metal sparks that can readily ignite flammable vapors or combustible materials. An abrasive blade that has been contaminated by oil or gasoline can also disintegrate under the stresses of cutting, producing shrapnel-like pieces of flying debris. Research following a fatal accident in Phoenix, Arizona, where the use of a rotary saw in a metal cutting operation ignited flammable vapors, has confirmed that even applying a spray of water on the blade at the point of the cut is not adequate to eliminate the spark ignition potential. Rotary cutting saws should *not* be used on damaged vehicles as a means of freeing trapped occupants.

Another tool that may be in the inventory of a rescue company is a cutting torch (Fig. 6-94). Most units use compressed oxygen and acetylene gas mixed together and ignited to produce an extremely hot flame. Newer units, such as the Slice Pack from the Arcair Co, burn special rods to produce an exothermic reaction that gives the tool its cutting action. When used properly, this tool can sever through relatively thick metal, structural steel, and even porous material such as cement blocks. As with the rotary saw, however, operation of this cutting tool presents an unacceptable safety hazard at automobile accidents. Its burning action can easily ignite flammable vapors or combustible material. Also, with either the oxy-acetylene torch or the Slice Pack, if the oxygen regulator becomes contaminated with a hydrocarbon material such as oil, fuel, or grease, a violent explosion instantly occurs.

The appropriate situation for personnel to use a rotary saw, cutting torch, or Slice Pack is at a special rescue incident such as an agricultural accident, industrial emergency, or building collapse and not at a motor vehicle accident.

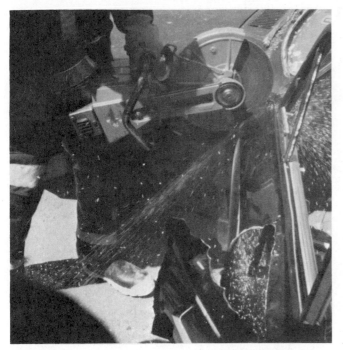

FIG. 6-93 Outer edge of a rotary power saw operating at full rpm travels at the same velocity as a .22 caliber bullet shot from a gun. Note the tremendous generation of sparks, even to the area between the door panels as they are cut.

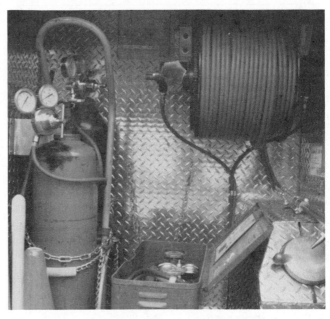

FIG. 6-94 Compartment contents include vehicle-mounted oxy-acetylene cutting torch with hose reel, wheeled unit, and small cutting torch in metal carry box.

BASIC RESCUE TOOL INVENTORY

All emergency service units must have tools and equipment available for immediate use at emergency incidents. A tool is simply a means of extending the capabilities of an emergency service worker. A tool allows an individual or team to accomplish a task in a safe and efficient manner. The tool can be a simple pry bar, a specially constructed ladder crib block assembly (Fig. 6-95), or a sophisticated hydraulic rescue tool system. The nature of the service that the emergency vehicle and arriving crew members intend to provide at an accident scene will determine the type and quantities of equipment needed.

The basic equipment inventory should be available for *all* vehicular incidents. Crews with vehicles dedicated to more extensive rescue emergencies and those responding more frequently to rescue incident should exceed the minimum tool inventory as necessary for their particular response problems and past experiences.

Basic extrication equipment that should be available at the scene of a motor vehicle accident and minimum recommended quantities of each tool are listed on pp. 214–216.

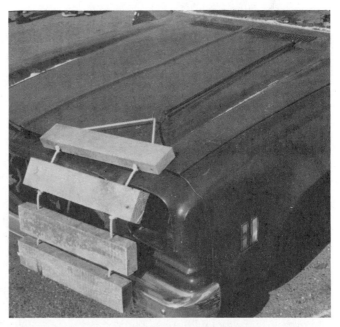

FIG. 6-95 Applications for ladder crib blocking include use over the front or rear of the vehicle during pulling operations or between the ground and bottom air bag during lifting evolutions. Note the use of the bungie strap to hold the ladder crib in the proper position during tool setup.

TOOL INVENTORY

REMOTE-CONTROLLED HYDRAULIC JACK TOOLS

Equipment	Quantity
Hydraulic pump	2
Hydraulic ram (10 in, 10-ton capacity unit)	2
Hydraulic jack oil supply with a pour funnel or spout (quart)	1
Extension tube (5 in)	1
Extension tube (10 in)	1
Extension tube (18 in)	1
Extension tube (30 in)	1
Double male threaded adaptor	2
Double female threaded adaptor	2
Lock-on connector	5
Locking pin	9
Adjustable (slip-lock) extension piece	1
Serrated head	2
Vee head	2
Wedge head	2
Rubber (flex) head	2
Flat base	2
Plunger toe	1
Cylinder toe	1
Clamp head	1
Clamp toe (if provided as separate accessory for unit)	1
Chain pull plate	1
Chain with grab hook (8 ft x ⅜ in)	2
Shortener (10 ft x ⅜ in)	1

CRIBBING BLOCKS

Equipment	Quantity
Hardwood block (2 in x 4 in x 18 in)	18
Hardwood block (4 in x 4 in x 18 in)	18
Hardwood block (4 in x 4 in x 48 in)	10
Wedge block (4 in x 18 in)	10
Ladder crib block assembly	2
Step chock wood block assembly (soft wood permitted)	6
*Hardwood cribbing block (4 in x 4 in x 18 in)	40
*Hardwood cribbing block (4 in x 4 in x 48 in)	18

MANUAL FORCIBLE ENTRY TOOLS

Equipment	Quantity
Flat head axe (6 lb, 36 in handle)	1
Pick head axe (6 lb, 36 in handle)	1
Halligan forcible entry bar (36 in)	2
Forcible entry tool with metal cutting claw (pry axe)	1
Pry bar with nail puller	2

*Recommended extra inventory for safe air bag systems operations.

Equipment	Quantity
Carpenter wrecking bar with claw and pinch point ends (24 in)	1
Metal pry bar with flat and pinch point ends (66 in)	1
Sledgehammer (8 lb)	1
Heavy-duty dent puller with spare screws and thread-on collar	1

CUTTING AND DISASSEMBLY TOOLS

Equipment	Quantity
Hacksaw (12-in, one-piece frame with break-resistant blades)	4
Replacement hacksaw blade	12
Squirt or spray containers with saw blade lubricating solution (soapy water or oil)	2
Tin snips	1
Stainless steel scissors with serrated blades	2
Bolt cutter (36 in; ratchet preferred)	1
Air chisel or air gun tool	1
Double panel cutting chisel bit	2
Flat chisel bits (8 to 12 in)	2
Air impact wrench (½-in drive) with case-hardened socket sets for standard and metric applications	1
Air cylinder or air supply source (45 cu/ft at 2216 psi)	4
Electric-powered reciprocating saw tool	1
Break-resistant reciprocating saw blade (6 in)	12
Manual sheet metal cutting tool	2
Hand carpentry saw (26 in)	1
Box saw with wood cutting blade and blade protector	1
Medium-duty chain saw with spare wood-cutting chain, carbide-toothed chain, fuel, and oil	1
Electric drill (½ in) with drill bit set	1

MANUAL PULLING TOOLS

Equipment	Quantity
Hand winch (come-along, minimum 2-ton rating)	2
Chain length ⁹⁄₃₂- or ⅜-in diameter, 12 to 15 ft	4
Chain shortener (10 in)	2
Snatch block device	1

Working Load Ratings for Chains

Alloy-grade chain (⁹⁄₃₂ in): 4100 lb
Alloy-grade chain (⅜ in): 7300 lb
Alloy-grade chain (½ in): 12000 lb

MANUAL LIFTING EQUIPMENT

Equipment	Quantity
Mechanical jack (3½-ton capacity)	3
Hydraulic jack (12-ton capacity)	1
Hydraulic jack (20-ton capacity)	1

ROPE RESCUE

Equipment	Quantity
Static kernmantle rope and rope bag (½ in x 20 ft, 9000 lb tensile strength)	2
Static kernmantle rope and rope bag (½ in x 300 ft, 9000 lb tensile strength)	2

Rope Rescue Support Components

Equipment should support the tactical requirements of deploying a 4-firefighter team to access and stabilize a patient and accomplish a basic low-angle evacuation. Equipment for a rescue raising or lowering system with a three to one mechanical advantage is also necessary and should include safety belay lines, carabiners, a figure eight with ears, tubular web strapping, life support harnesses, and pulleys.

BASIC HAND TOOLS AND EQUIPMENT

Equipment	Quantity
Utility knives	2
Open-end wrench (12 in, adjustable)	1
Open-end wrench (8 in, adjustable)	1
Standard socket set (½-in drive)	1
Metric socket set (½-in drive)	1
Flat-bladed screwdriver (6 in x ¼ in)	1
Flat-bladed screwdriver (8 in x 5⁄16 in)	1
Flat-bladed screwdriver (12 in x ⅜ in)	1
Phillips screwdriver (#2)	1
Phillips screwdriver (#3)	1
Standard slip-joint pliers	1
Arc-joint (channel lock) pliers	1
Locking grip (vise grip) pliers with wire cutter	1
Needle-nosed pliers	1
Wire cutter pliers	1
Pipe wrench	1
Adjustable (crescent) wrench	1
Set of box-end/open-end wrenches (standard and metric)	1
Automatic, spring-loaded center punch with adjustable tension	2
Solid center punch	1
Cold chisel set (1-, ¾-, ½-, ⅜-in blade, 12-in shank)	4
Tape measure with lock (12 ft x 1 in)	1
Standard mallet (3 lb, nonsparking head)	2
Claw hammer (20 oz)	1
Ball peen hammer (32 oz)	1
Collapsible straight ladder (8 ft)	1
Fiberglass pike pole (8′ ft)	1

Equipment	Quantity
Closet hook pike pole (36 in)	1
Hay hooks (baling hooks)	2
Leather tool pouch with waist belt	1

SAFETY AND HAZARD CONTROL TOOLS

Equipment	Quantity
Electric generator (5000 watt, 120-volt AC with grounding device)	1
Floodlight units with electrical cable and junction boxes (500 watt)	4
Hand-held sealed beam flashlight with carrying handle or strap	2
Electric-powered smoke ejector fan unit with electric cable	1
Industrial-quality ear protective devices	4
Set of golf tee fuel-line plugs	2
Granular absorbent material (5 lb)	1
Absorbent pad (⅜ in x 18 in)	100
Leak-sealing plugs (rubber or soft wood)	6
Duct sealant (1 lb)	1
ABC Multipurpose dry-chemical fire extinguisher (10 lb)	3
Pair of vehicle wheel chocks	2
Positive-pressure SCBA	4
Compressed air cylinders for SCBA	8
PVC traffic control cones (flourescent orange)	8
Crowd-control line banner (100 ft)	2
Road warning flares without metal spikes (30-min duration)	12
Adhesive duct tape (2 in x 60 ft)	2
Fire safety blanket (62 in x 84 in)	2
Salvage tarp cover (12 ft x 20 ft)	2
Stiff bristle push broom (24 in)	2
Scoop shovel	1
Round shovel	1

EMERGENCY MEDICAL RESPONSE EQUIPMENT

Emergency	Quantity
First Responder trauma kit	1
Flexible patient immobilization device	2
Immobilization collars (large, medium, small, and pediatric)	2
Shortboard device (18 in x 32 in)	2
Longboard device (18 in x 72 in)	2
Skinny board (8 in x 30 in)	1
Immobilization straps with buckles (2 in x 9 ft)	8
Orthopedic stretcher	1
Rescue basket with 4-point sling harness	1
Cravat cloths	12
Padded board splints (3 in x 15 in)	4
Padded board splints (3 in x 36 in)	4

Continued.

TOOL INVENTORY — cont'd

POWER RESCUE TOOL SYSTEM†

Equipment	Quantity
Power spreader unit with tips and attachment pins	1
Pair of spare attachment pins	1
Pair of spare automotive tips (for training)	1
Chain with grab hooks (12 ft x ½ in, alloy grade) with clevis link/shackle unit with attachment pins or nylon ratchet straps with attachment shackles	2
Power cutter unit	1
Power plant with hydraulic hose	1
Gasoline safety can (2-gal capacity)	1
Funnel	1
Spark plug and changing wrench tool	1
Spark plug feeler gauge	1
Hydraulic fluid (quart)	1

Equipment	Quantity
Spare power plant recoiler unit with rope	1
Oil additive for piston lubrication (2 oz, 2-cycle power plant engine only)	24
Motor oil (quart, 4-cycle power plant engine only)	2

AIR BAG OR AIR CUSHION RESCUE SYSTEM†

Equipment	Quantity
Air bag (20-, 30-, and 40-ton capacity) or air cushion	1
Control regulator	1
Dual air bag controller unit with deadman feature and pressure relief valves	1
‡In-line shutoff and relief valve	1
‡Air supply hoses	1
Air bag protective mat (36 in x 36 in)	2
Compressed air cylinder (45 cu/ft)	5

†This additional equipment is recommended for districts providing increased levels of rescue service.

‡Quantity required per bag.

SUMMARY

A department responding on high traffic volume expressways or a department making almost daily motor vehicle responses may require different types and amounts of rescue tools for their operations. A small department that responds to a minimal number of rescue calls in a year may provide itself with only basic extrication tools, relying on the automatic response of a neighboring community's fully equipped rescue vehicle. A rural department with limited funds must consider purchasing and maintaining equipment that will serve several functions for the variety of rescue problems that its district may present.

To determine what is proper and sufficient, the department should plan for possible scenarios of multiple vehicle collisions where each vehicle has at least one occupant trapped or multiple accidents occurring in the same district at the same time. Organizations that respond without the primary vehicle rescue apparatus (out of the district on fire or rescue calls to assist other organizations) must consider what is left behind when their primary vehicle is gone. Minimum levels of rescue tools and equipment should be maintained within the community while the rescue vehicle is involved in these mutual-assistance incidents.

It is important that each responding rescue organization have the capability of using different methods and different rescue equipment for each evolution it may have to accomplish. In the event of a tool failure at an incident, alternate equipment must be readily available to complete the task. Do not discard the basic tools just because you have the more sophisticated ones. Do not be caught overrelying on only a certain few tools.

Most important, what you can do with the tools that you have is the true measure of the ability of a rescue crew. Tools do not work by themselves. They all take trained personnel to make them function. Adequate, well-maintained tools and properly trained personnel constitute the best inventory possible.

7

Vehicle Rescue Evolutions

OBJECTIVES

At the end of this chapter, you will be able to:

- Correctly describe a realistic scenario in which a given rescue evolution would be necessary.
- Accurately describe and fully explain the objective of the rescue evolution based on a realistic scenario.
- Fully explain all safety procedures that must be fulfilled to accomplish the evolution without further injury to yourself or others present.
- Correctly describe the estimated total time frame in which the individual rescue evolution should be accomplished.
- Correctly and completely describe a primary tool and disentanglement technique for the rescue evolution.
- Correctly and completely describe a backup tool and disentanglement technique for the rescue evolution.
- Given a damaged vehicle, simulated patients trapped by the vehicle, appropriate rescue personnel, and necessary rescue tools and supporting equipment, demonstrate the accomplishment of the given disentanglement assignment within the prescribed time period.

Chapter 7 presents specific information on the how-to procedures and techniques necessary to accomplish a variety of basic vehicle rescue evolutions. Because a picture is worth ten thousand words, there are photos and sketches to illustrate the reality of each evolution. Specific titles or names are given to describe either the intent of the evolution or the action that takes place during the assignment.

The evolutions are arranged in sequence, from the simple to the complex. This sequence is *not* intended to imply a specific sequence of rescue evolutions to be accomplished at an actual incident. Strategy decisions and specific tactical rescue evolutions are the responsibility of the IC at the scene of the rescue emergency.

Evolutions are grouped into several general categories to facilitate locating specific techniques. These categories and their specific evolutions include the following:

- *Vehicle stabilization evolutions:* Includes stabilization of vehicles on four wheels, side, or roof.
- *Vehicle glass evolutions:* Includes tempered or laminated glass removal and evolutions for victim impaled in windshield.
- *Vehicle door evolutions:* Includes evolutions to open locked vehicle door, deactivate vehicle safety lock mechanism, open jammed door, widen door opening, remove vehicle door, access through closed vehicle door, widen "B" posts, and remove "B" posts. Also includes three-door, four-door, and five-door evolutions.
- *Vehicle steering wheel and column evolutions:* Includes evolutions to cut steering wheel and/or spokes, move steering column, and remove steering column.
- *Interior component evolutions:* Includes evolutions to accomplish pedal access opening from exterior, move brake pedal, remove brake pedal, move dashboard, and remove dashboard.
- *Vehicle roof evolutions:* Includes evolutions to raise portion of collapsed roof, make three-sided sunroof opening, complete flip-top-box roof opening, make A-B-C roof opening, and accomplish total roof removal.
- *Vehicle seat evolutions:* Includes evolutions to move one side of bench seat forward or rearward, move both sides of bench seat simultaneously forward or rearward, and remove vehicle seat.
- *Specialized vehicle access evolutions:* Includes undercarriage opening and trunk evolutions.

• *Hazard control and safety evolutions:* Includes evolutions to open vehicle hood, open vehicle tailgate, plug leaking fuel system, and remove vehicle fuel tank.
• *Miscellaneous evolutions:* Includes jacking and shoring of vehicle.

VEHICLE STABILIZATION EVOLUTIONS

Unstabilized vehicles are unsafe vehicles. They are hazardous to the trapped and injured patient and to all emergency service personnel working at the scene. All accident or fire-involved vehicles, regardless of size, shape, condition, or position, must always be promptly stabilized in the position first found. There are *no* exceptions. A vehicle can roll forward or rearward, suddenly drop lower to the ground, or sway from side to side while emergency service personnel are working around, on, or inside the vehicle. Any unexpected vehicle movement can aggravate existing patient injuries and cause injury to emergency service personnel working at the scene.

When confronted with a vehicle that has been involved in a fire or vehicle accident emergency and using available vehicle rescue stabilization equipment, the rescuer should be able to do the following:

• Recognize that an unstable vehicle presents an unsafe working environment at the accident scene for all emergency service personnel.
• Determine to what degree the vehicle requires stabilization.
• Determine whether any potential safety problems or hazards exist or are likely to arise during the fulfillment of the vehicle stabilization evolution.
• Determine the most appropriate stabilization tools, equipment, and techniques necessary for accomplishing vehicle stabilization.
• Safely and efficiently render a given vehicle stable in the position as found upon arrival of emergency personnel at the accident scene within a 2-minute elapsed time period, to prevent undesired movement of the vehicle throughout all disentanglement evolutions and patient extrication activities at the accident scene.

Vehicle stabilization is one rescue evolution necessary at *all* motor vehicle accidents or fire emergencies. Stabilization at routine incidents (those considered relatively minor) may be the most neglected and misunderstood vehicle rescue evolution discussed in this text. Stabilization, along with various hazard control activities, serves to render a safer working environment at and around the emergency scene (Fig. 7-1).

For personnel to understand the potential movements of a vehicle and their consequences, it is useful to imagine a series of lines drawn through a vehicle (Fig. 7-2). All of the lines pass through an imaginary point that approximates the center point of the passenger compartment. (This invisible center point differs with each make and model of vehicle.)

Each of the imaginary lines represents an axis, a straight line about which the entire structure of the vehicle will rotate or can be expected to rotate. These basic axis lines include the following:

• *Longitudinal (horizontal) axis line:* A horizontal line drawn from the rearmost point of the vehicle toward the front that runs parallel to its sides and passes through the imaginary center point of the passenger compartment.

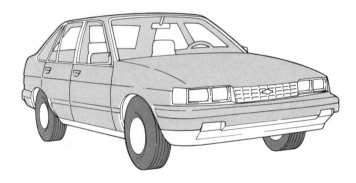

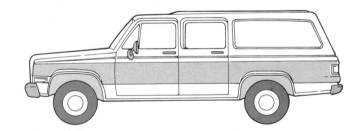

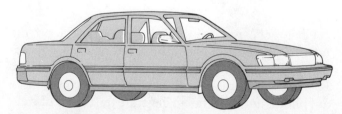

FIG. 7-1 Stabilization of an accident vehicle resting on its four wheels on a level surface is always necessary. The lack of stabilization of a seemingly innocent-looking vehicle is probably the most neglected and misunderstood rescue evolution.

- *Vertical axis line:* A vertical line drawn from a point above the roof of the vehicle that passes through the imaginary center point of the passenger compartment and terminates at ground level below the undercarriage area.
- *Lateral axis line:* A horizontal line drawn from a point outside the passenger's side of the vehicle to a point outside the driver's side that runs parallel to the front and rear of the vehicle and passes through the imaginary center point of the passenger compartment.

Using these three axis lines as a point of reference, personnel can see that an unstabilized vehicle can move in five basic directions (Fig. 7-3):

- Horizontal movement: A vehicle moves forward or rearward on its longitudinal axis or moves horizontally along its lateral axis.

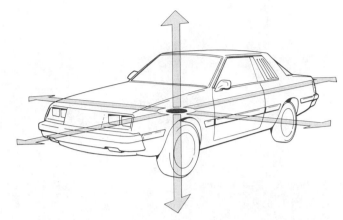

FIG. 7-2 Imaginary lines drawn through a center point inside a car represent potential directions that an unstabilized vehicle can move.

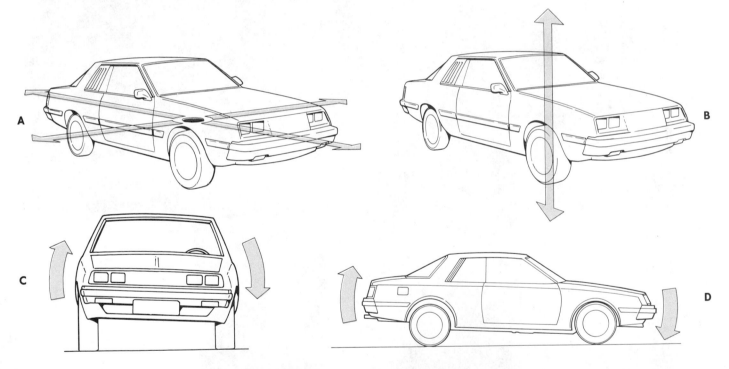

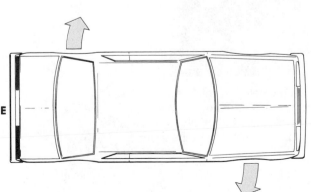

FIG. 7-3 A, Horizontal movement can include an accident vehicle rolling forward or backward. **B,** Vertical movement of an unstabilized vehicle is of special concern to rescue personnel who must operate on or under a vehicle. **C,** Roll movement of an unstabilized vehicle can cause further injury to patients as they are tossed from side to side. **D,** Pitch movement of an unstabilized vehicle can occur whenever a weight or load is applied over the rear or front areas of the vehicle. **E,** Yaw movement is a possibility, especially when an unstabilized vehicle is on snow or icy terrain.

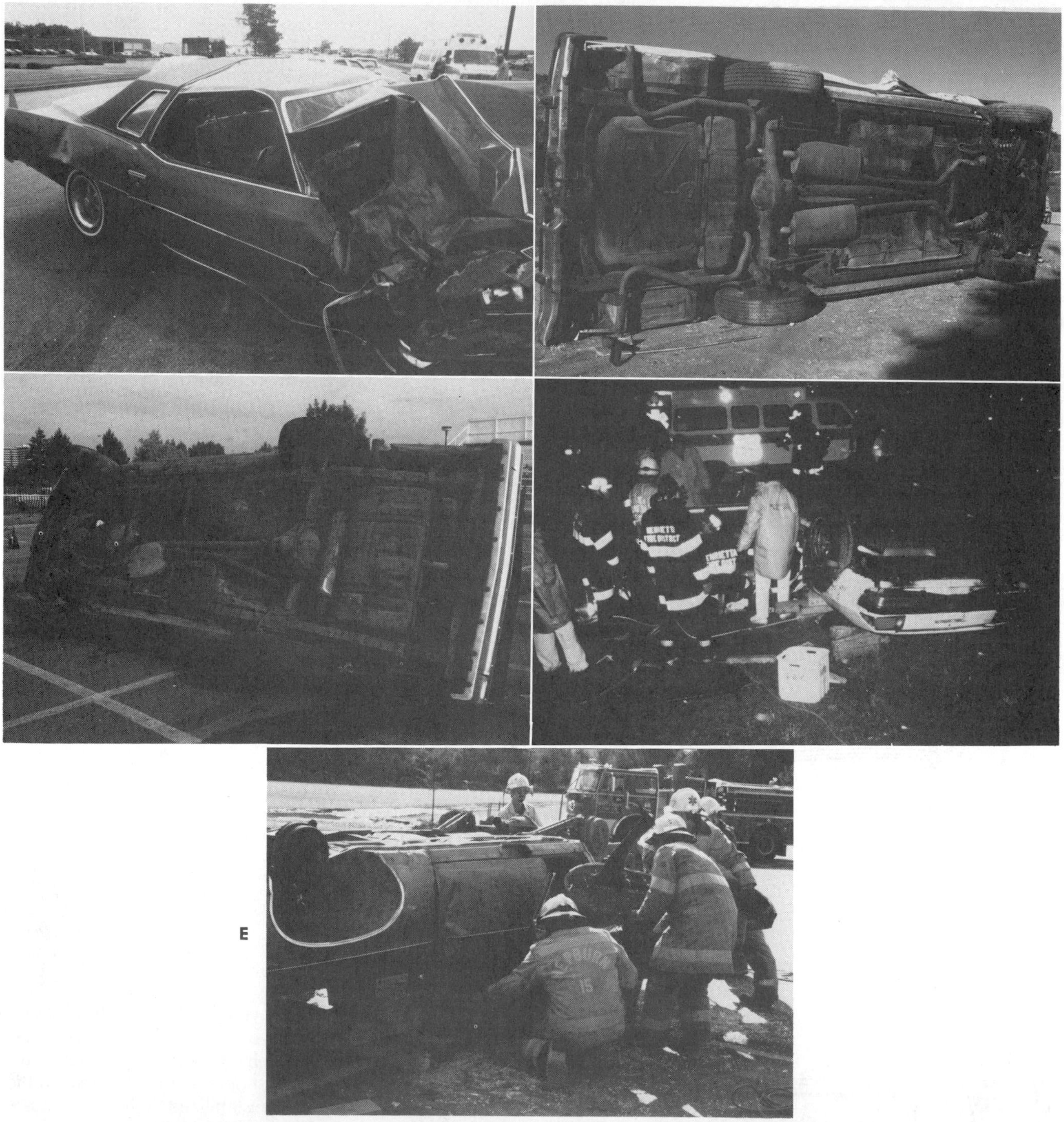

FIG. 7-4 Basic vehicle positions requiring stabilization include vehicle **A,** on inflated and deflated tires, **B,** on side with tires in contact with the ground, **C,** on side with roof edge in contact with the ground, **D,** on roof with the hood or trunk in contact with the ground, and **E,** on roof with no hood or trunk contact with the ground.

- Vertical movement: A vehicle moves up or down in relation to the ground while moving along its vertical axis.
- Roll movement: A vehicle rocks side to side while rotating about its longitudinal axis and remaining horizontal in orientation.
- Pitch movement: A vehicle moves up and down about its lateral axis causing the vehicle's front portion to rise or fall in relation to its rear portion.
- Yaw movement: A vehicle twists or turns about its vertical axis causing the vehicle's front and rear portions to move left or right in relation to their original position.

Any effort to stabilize a vehicle must adequately prevent movement in every one of these possible axis directions. The vehicle must therefore be secured in position as it is found. Unstable vehicles have some degree of contact with the ground that can be measured in square inches of contact area. Proper vehicle stabilization activities increase this ground contact area and relieve the existing vehicle suspension system of its load or tension, thereby minimizing unwanted vehicle movement. Although a damaged vehicle may be found in many positions after a motor vehicle accident, the basic stabilization evolutions (Fig. 7-4) most commonly required include the following:

- Stabilization of a vehicle resting on inflated or deflated tires on a horizontal or inclined surface with a functional suspension system.
- Stabilization of a vehicle on its side with the inflated tires in contact with the ground.
- Stabilization of a vehicle on its side with the roofline in contact with the ground.
- Stabilization of a vehicle on its roof with the front hood or trunk area in contact with the ground.
- Stabilization of a vehicle on the roof with the hood and trunk areas not in contact with the ground.

Commonly used stabilization equipment listed in the recommended tool inventory in Chapter 6 includes cribbing blocks, come-along tools, rescue chains, rescue ropes, mechanical jacks, hydraulic jacks, and a porto-power tool. Other equipment for vehicle stabilization evolutions includes power rescue spreaders or rams, air bags, air cushions, vehicle-mounted winch units, and tow truck cable.

For a vehicle resting on inflated tires, at least one wheel must be completely chocked or blocked to immediately prevent horizontal movement in a forward or rearward direction. This will prevent any unwanted movement that might complicate injuries or entrapment conditions. This is a simple, basic task that must be accomplished at all accident scenes.

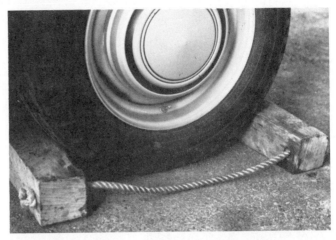

FIG. 7-5 Basic stabilization of vehicle resting on inflated tires requires initial chocking of tires to prevent horizontal movement.

Wood blocking at least 4 inches high or manufactured wheel chock devices are best suited for this task. The front and rear of the tire must be chocked to prevent horizontal vehicle movement (Fig. 7-5). Wedge-shaped rescue blocking should *not* be used as makeshift wheel chocks. Stabilization equipment must be fitted into the space between the underside of the vehicle and the ground at several points to prevent a vertical dropping movement and any roll or pitch of the vehicle. Wood blocking arranged as a box crib will quickly and efficiently stabilize the vehicle when placed under the rocker panel and "B" post areas on each side of the vehicle. Preassembled step chock stabilization blocks can also be effective.

Once positioned properly, the blocking should be fitted snugly against the vehicle to take the load off the suspension system. Once the blocking is positioned under the vehicle, there are several ways to relieve the load on the suspension system. One method involves releasing the air from the tires of the vehicle. Without air in the tires, the entire vehicle settles down onto the stabilization blocking. However, this deflation technique raises several concerns. If a rescue organization insists on accomplishing vehicle stabilization by deflating the tires, crew members must consider the following points:

- The vehicle must be raised after the rescue to recover the blocking placed underneath it.
- The damaged vehicle cannot be readily moved at the accident scene and is more difficult to tow.
- Deflating the tires is only an effective stabilization technique for vehicles resting on flat ground. When used on inclined or uneven surfaces, the procedure may be ineffective.

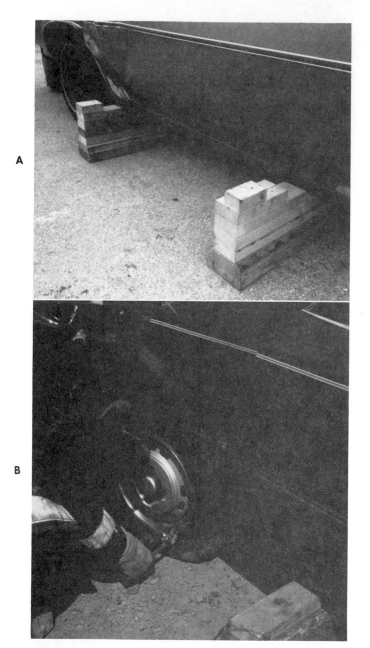

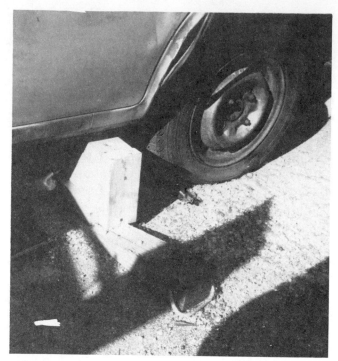

FIG. 7-7 Alternative to stabilization by deflating tires requires raising the blocking by adding wedge blocks. Advantages are that vehicle movement is minimal, blocking can be retrieved easily at termination, and the vehicle can be removed from accident scene more efficiently by a tow agency.

FIG. 7-6 A, Step chocks must be placed at strong support points along rocker panel area of vehicle. **B,** Air can be released from inflated tires once blocking has been strategically located under vehicle. Rescuer uses pliers to pry valve stem from wheel.

With step chock blocking, rescue personnel must realize that the blocks work best when the vehicle is resting on a flat, even surface and that alternative procedures should be considered (Fig. 7-6). Rather than lower the vehicle to the blocks as is commonly advocated with step chocks, it may be more effective to raise the blocking up to contact the underside of the vehicle (Fig. 7-7). This can be accomplished simply and effectively by inserting wedge-shaped blocks

under the step chock to ensure firm vehicle contact. After the incident the wedge can be removed quickly, allowing the step chock to be easily removed. The mechanical automobile scissors jack or basic hydraulic jack are other tools that can be positioned and operated to contact the vehicle firmly, relieving the load on its suspension and effectively stabilizing it. Any of these techniques make it easy to move the vehicle at the scene or remove it completely upon conclusion of the extrication.

When a vehicle remains on its tires but comes to rest on an inclined surface, the danger of downhill movement increases. Initial stabilization accomplished with these blocking or jacking procedures must be accompanied by additional procedures designed to prevent this movement. By employing kernmantle rope or rated rescue chain along with a winch line, tow truck cable, or come-along tool, rescuers can effectively hold the vehicle in the position found (Fig. 7-8). The attachment points at the vehicle must be structurally strong points, capable of holding the total weight of the vehicle. Emergency service personnel should not enter vehicles on steep inclines until they are fully stabilized.

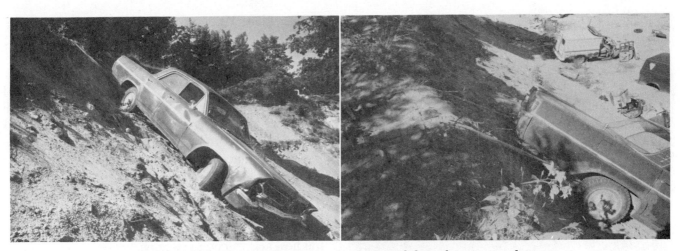

FIG. 7-8 A, A vehicle on an incline presents many possibilities for unwanted movement. **B,** Initial stabilization efforts include strapping, winch, or tow lines secured to rear structural areas of the vehicle.

A vehicle on its side or edge usually comes to rest in one of two ways. The most common scenario finds the vehicle on its side with inflated tires in contact with the ground. Less frequently, a vehicle on its side continues to roll toward its roof until the roofline contacts the ground and the wheels and tires are off the ground. This position is dangerous and requires more complex stabilization procedures. All stabilization efforts are intended to increase contact with the ground and widen the base of stability. Unless stabilized, the vehicle can roll onto its roof or fall back onto its wheels. Safety hazards such as fluid leakage may also be present at the scene. Depending on the vehicle and the rollover position, there may be a 20-gallon or more fuel leak and spill at the scene, along with hot engine oil or antifreeze spills and leakage of battery acid.

Stabilization of a vehicle on its side can be accomplished with wood blocking (18 and 48 inches in length), mechanical or hydraulic jacks, rescue chains used with a winch, a tow truck cable, a come-along tool, or any combination of these tools (Fig. 7-9). The blocking and the jacking tools must be located along both sides of the vehicle to maintain it on its side effectively. Along the undercarriage side, personnel must avoid high heat-yielding areas such as the catalytic converters, muffler, or exhaust pipe. Wood blocks placed along the ground contact area should be parallel to the length of the vehicle to maximize surface contact. Running the blocking lengthwise instead of placing its 4-inch width in contact with the vehicle maximizes the use of the block.

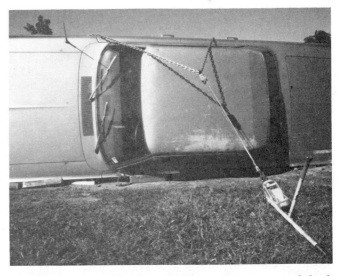

FIG. 7-9 Stabilization of a vehicle on edge is accomplished with blocking placed at ground contact areas and rescue chains and cable come-along tool secured to anchor point at ground level.

When a vehicle rolls onto its roof during a collision, two possible scenarios can confront rescue personnel. Typically, the overturned vehicle will come to rest in a nose-down configuration with its front hood and bumper area in contact with the ground (Fig. 7-10). This suspends the rear of the vehicle off the ground. It is also possible for the vehicle to rest entirely on its roof, with neither the hood nor the trunk areas in contact with the ground. Any vehicle perched solely on its roof is extremely unstable (Fig. 7-11). Simply opening a door of the vehicle may cause the vehicle to slide or

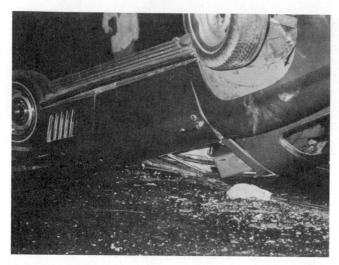

FIG. 7-10 Rollover accident involving a Corvette Stingray resulted in an unstable nose-down position for the automobile.

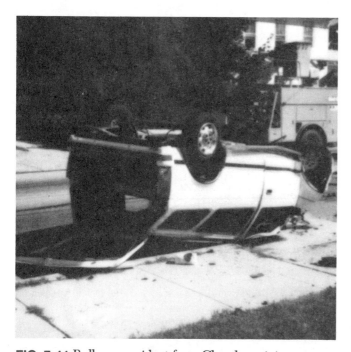

FIG. 7-11 Rollover accident for a Chrysler mini van ended with the vehicle resting entirely on its roof. Note the extreme distortion of all roof and door posts on both sides of the van.

the roof to collapse. As with the vehicle on its side, spill or leak safety hazards may also be present.

In a vehicle rollover scenario, efforts must be initiated to span the distance between the vehicle and the ground, immediately increasing ground contact and preventing unwanted horizontal, vertical, or lateral movement. The rollover vehicle is also particularly

susceptible to sliding forward or rearward, or spinning about its vertical axis. Action must be taken to prevent this from occurring.

The stabilization equipment chosen for the assignment must be placed where it will use such structural strong points of the overturned vehicle as the firewall area, rocker panel areas, and base of the rear roof posts. Stabilization equipment should generally *not* be placed in contact with the front or rear bumpers of the accident vehicle because the bumper may fail when force is exerted on it. Arranging stabilization equipment to secure the vehicle effectively in its inverted position provides a safe working environment for medical and rescue personnel.

GLASS EVOLUTIONS

When a vehicle is involved in a collision and occupants are trapped in the wreckage, emergency service personnel must work both in and around the vehicle. One barrier to acceptable access to injured passengers is the safety glass in window and windshield openings. Safety glass may remain undamaged by the collision and have to be moved or removed by emergency personnel, it may crack and resemble a spider web, or it may completely disintegrate into small glass nuggets, injuring unprotected persons who come in contact with it.

When confronted with a vehicle that has been involved in a motor vehicle collision with occupants trapped inside the wreckage and using available basic vehicle glass-removal tools, the rescuer should be able to do the following:

- Correctly identify the various types of manufactured vehicle safety glass that may be present in window or windshield openings.
- Accurately describe and correctly identify the various glass-mounting procedures used by manufacturers to hold glass in the opening.
- Recognize that safety glass in selected locations can present an unsafe working environment in and around the vehicle and can pose potential safety hazards to operating personnel if left in place during disentanglement evolutions.
- Determine the specific pieces of safety glass in the vehicle that require removal.
- Determine the presence of problems or hazards that exist or may arise during the glass removal evolution.

- Determine the most appropriate glass removal tools, equipment, and techniques necessary for accomplishing the evolution.
- Work with one additional crew member to remove the laminated safety glass front windshield from a vehicle safely and efficiently and render the opening safe for access and egress as required in 2 minutes or less.
- Work with a minimum of two additional crew members to remove a patient impaled in the laminated glass windshield of the vehicle safely and efficiently without causing further injury to the patient or endangering operating personnel in 5 minutes or less.
- Safely and efficiently remove tempered safety glass from a vehicle and render the openings safe for access or egress as required in 60 seconds or less.

Most motor vehicles licensed and in use in the United States today are equipped with safety glass in their windshield, side window, and rear window openings. Exceptions to this rule include antique motor vehicles, buses, armored cars, and high-security vehicles used by corrections departments, governmental agencies or officials, and various corporate executives. These vehicles typically have special glass in the window and windshield openings. Certain commercial vehicles, such as city transit buses, may have thick plastic mounted in their large side window openings in lieu of safety glass.

Most vehicles encountered by emergency service personnel at a vehicle accident scene will have laminated safety glass in the front windshield opening and tempered safety glass in the remaining side and rear openings. Laminated windshields consist of multiple layers of glass and plastic sandwiched together to form the finished product. Standard laminations include an inner and outer layer of glass with a layer of plastic laminate material between the layers. The new technology windshield product, known by the trade name Securiflex, includes an additional layer of plastic bonded to the interior passenger compartment side of the windshield. The outer glass layer may actually be thinner than a standard windshield glass.

In a collision, laminated safety glass is designed to crack into large sections yet remain together in its sandwich design. Impacts to the laminated glass produce the familiar spider web glass fractures (Fig. 7-12).

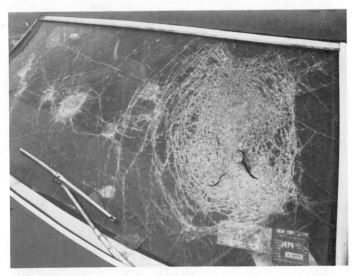

FIG. 7-12 Laminated windshield glass layers fracture in a circular pattern when impacted by heads or faces of unrestrained occupants or when struck by loose objects inside the vehicle. Glass breaks in a spider web impact pattern.

Tempered safety glass used for side and rear window openings is manufactured totally differently and therefore reacts differently when impacted. Molten glass is poured into a mold and rapidly chilled, causing it to develop a degree of tension across its outer surfaces. When hit hard enough to relieve this surface tension, the glass disintegrates into small pieces or nuggets, each approximately ¼ inch in diameter (Fig. 7-13). The glass nuggets expand outward in all directions parallel to the surface of the glass. If the window section is surrounded by a window frame and the glass is snug against the frame on all sides, the broken glass will generally remain in the window opening. If a window is rolled partially down or the window does not have a frame surrounding it, the outward expansion of glass at the moment it is broken creates a miniature explosion of flying nuggets of glass.

Tempered or laminated glass may have to be removed to allow access to a vehicle's interior, ventilate a passenger compartment area, or allow personnel to perform disentanglement and extrication evolutions safely. Some glass may break partially during the collision, while other panes of glass will require removal by emergency service personnel. Regardless of the circumstances, all glass-breaking and removal evolutions must safeguard the rescuer, assisting crew members, and the patient. Glass must be broken or cut as necessary, completely removed from all edges of the window opening, and disposed

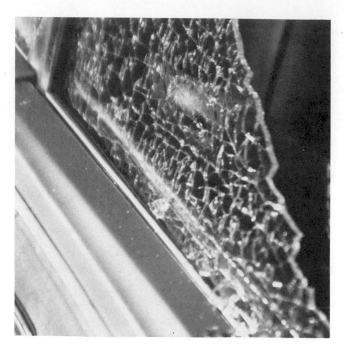

FIG. 7-13 When the surface tension of tempered safety glass is broken, the glass breaks into nuggets of approximately ¼ inch in size.

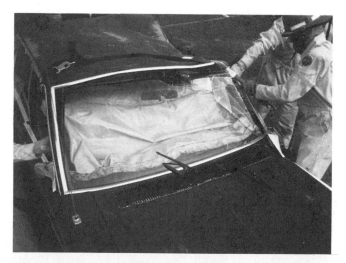

FIG. 7-14 Total windshield removal produces large quantities of broken laminated glass slivers known as *salt and pepper* glass. During evolution, protection for the patient and inside medic is provided by a Holmatro Windshield Blanket secured to the roof of the vehicle.

of efficiently in ways that minimize the potential for additional injuries. Any broken glass, particularly cracked sections of laminated safety glass, should generally be placed under the damaged vehicles.

If tempered glass nuggets penetrate an open wound, delicate removal on an almost piece-by-piece

basis at a medical facility is required. The salt-and-pepper glass residue produced by broken laminated glass, on the other hand, can penetrate so deeply into open wounds that it cannot be totally removed. This minute glass residue material can cause serious infections days after the original injury.

Protecting medical personnel and injured patients inside the vehicle during glass removal evolutions is typically accomplished by covering them with a protective blanket or tarp (Fig. 7-14). Safety conscious rescue teams now also position a wooden shortboard or longboard between those inside the vehicle, the glass pane to be broken, and the tool performing the evolution. The ¾-inch-thick board acts to insulate the people inside, protecting them from both the broken glass and the tools.

The most effective vehicle glass removal tools are basic hand tools. Laminated glass removal requires either cutting, sawing, or chopping tools such as the fire axe, hay hook, can opener style of metal-cutting tools, a specially designed windshield saw, reciprocating saw, air chisel, or air gun (Fig. 7-15). Air tools must be operated with flat chisel bits in place and the air operating pressure reduced to a flowing pressure of 50 psi or less.

Tempered glass can also be removed with basic hand tools. Removal requires the use of a sharply pointed tool to break the surface tension of the glass pane. The spring-loaded automatic center punch or the sharp point of a forcible entry tool are the hand tools most commonly used for this evolution (Fig. 7-16). It is not difficult to assemble a multitude of sharply pointed hand tools from those carried in a typical vehicle rescue tool inventory.

If the passenger side windshield wiper arm found on most automobiles has a protruding point to attach the wiper blade to the arm and is of one-piece construction without a swivel head, it can also be used successfully to break tempered safety glass. The small point of the wiper arm can be used to strike the glass and fracture it, as can the one-piece solid metal radio antenna rod. If smacked across the pane of tempered glass properly, this rod will fracture the glass.

An air chisel or air gun with its flat chisel bit placed in direct contact with the surface of the glass can also effectively break tempered glass. Placing the corner of the chisel bit in direct contact with the glass, restraining the chisel bit slightly with one gloved hand, and momentarily operating the air tool causes the tempered glass to shatter instantly.

Before personnel break any tempered glass, it may be desirable to apply adhesive material to the outside or inside surface of the window to minimize glass scattering and fallout. Rescue crews may apply either adhesive contact shelf paper, 2- or 3-inch-wide duct tape, or a glue adhesive in an aerosol spray to the surface of the glass. When applied properly, the adhesive agent restrains the glass when it disintegrates into small nuggets, binding them together into larger, more manageable sections of glass. It is important to remember that adhesive materials will not function when applied to wet, damp, excessively cold, or dirt-covered glass surfaces (Fig. 7-17). Applying the adhesive also takes time, and the results cannot be guaranteed. Adhesive application of shelving paper, tape, or aerosol spray should *not* be considered a routine or necessary action before breaking each and every piece of tempered glass.

If adhesive duct tape is used, it should be applied in a criss-cross pattern on the glass. Two or more vertical pieces of tape are first applied, with slack remaining in the center of the tape to form handles. Horizontal strips are then applied to complete the grid. It is important to apply all adhesive tape only to the glass and not to allow it to extend beyond the edge of the glass to contact any surrounding metal or window trim material. To remove the glass when the grid of duct tape is in place, one rescuer holds onto the tape handles while a second rescuer breaks the glass. The two crew members then work together to move the broken and taped glass out of the window opening and away from the interior of the vehicle (Fig. 7-18).

When rescue personnel are using the larger forcible entry hand tools such as the pick-headed axe or Halligan type of bars to break tempered glass, only the point of the tool should contact the glass surface. The tools perform best when the point contacts the surface of the glass pane at a 90-degree angle. This minimizes the chances of the point glancing off the surface of the glass. Rescue personnel must be sure that the momentum of the heavy forcible entry tool does not propel the tool into the interior areas of the vehicle. Glass can be safely and efficiently removed with these large hand tools if the rescuer designs the attack upon the glass with a shock-absorbing safety consideration in mind. The body of the striking tool must be positioned so that while the tool fractures the glass, solid portions of the vehicle contact solid portions of the tool, absorbing its momentum and stopping its forward motion (Fig. 7-19).

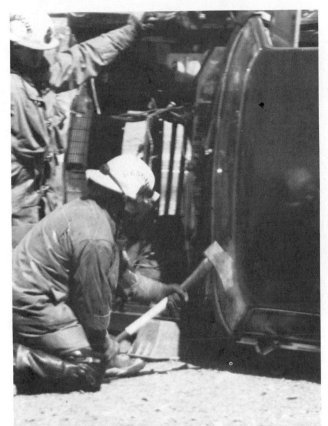

A

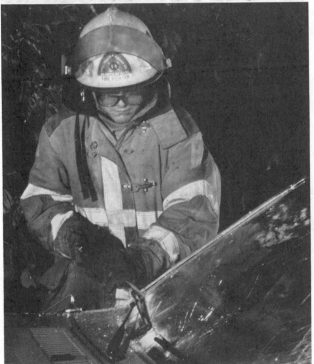

B

FIG. 7-15 A, To remove a windshield, rescuers chop along the two short sides and the one long side of the glass and pry it off the vehicle. **B,** Alternative windshield removal tool is a specially constructed windshield saw using a metal handle and frame fitted with an industrial 1-inch thick hacksaw blade with a coarse tooth design.

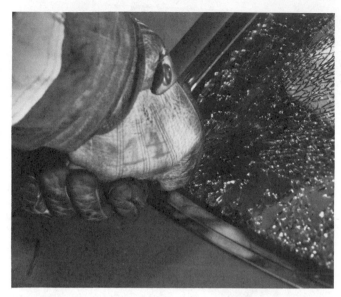

FIG. 7-16 Tempered glass removal is accomplished with a spring-loaded automatic center punch. Note the rescuer cups the hand together for support during the fracture.

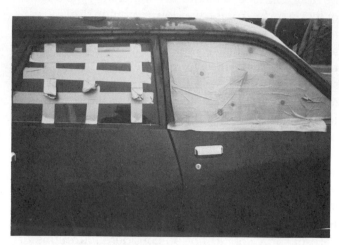

FIG. 7-17 Adhesive materials applied to tempered glass should bond nuggets together for a safer and more efficient removal from the window opening. Adhesive materials include 2- or 3-inch wide duct tape, contact shelving paper, or spray glue adhesives such as Rescue Web (a commercially available product).

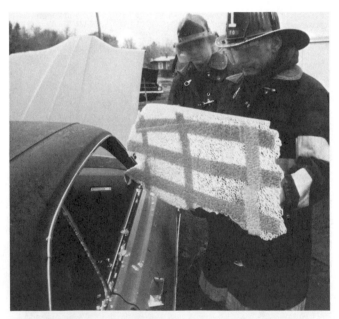

FIG. 7-18 Under ideal conditions, properly applied tape or spray adhesive permits most of the glass to be removed from the window opening in a large sheet. Rain, excessive moisture, or cold temperatures make the adhesive less likely to bond to the exterior of the glass.

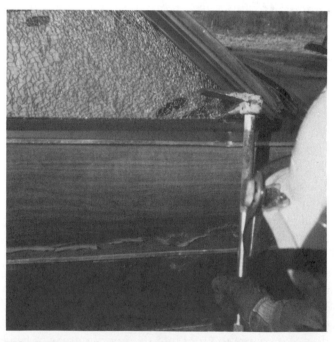

FIG. 7-19 Use of a heavy tool, such as a Halligan bar or pick-headed fire axe, requires a shock absorber to cushion the tool impact and prevent movement of the tool into the vehicle. Note how the shaft impacted the top edge of the door while the pointed end fractured the glass. A wooden shortboard held inside the window glass insulates the patient and inside medic from danger.

Laminated Windshield Glass Removal

Laminated glass can be secured in vehicles in several ways. Trucks, buses, vans, and some automobiles have a multipiece rubber gasket material bonding the glass into the windshield opening. Rescue personnel can readily remove the glass from this type of windshield mounting by first removing any decorative molding and then cutting and peeling away the rubber-mounting gasket. Once the gasket has been loosened or removed sufficiently, pushing, prying, or localized chopping with a forcible entry tool will dislodge the entire windshield from the vehicle.

The most common windshield glass-mounting systems for automobiles use adhesive materials to glue the glass into position. Adhesive butyl rubber mounting material, which resembles weatherstripping, or polyurethane spray foam are now widely used.

Total Windshield Removal

Rescue personnel have one of two strategic choices to make when considering windshield removal: total windshield removal or simultaneous removal with the roof. The most common strategy is to consider total windshield removal as a separate rescue evolution in which two rescue personnel remove the entire windshield glass in 2 minutes or less. When removing a windshield that is glued into place, rescue personnel should leave all decorative molding or trim material in place and attack the glass with cutting, sawing, or chopping tools. The attack is first made along the two short sides of the windshield and then across the long bottom edge just above the dashboard. The glass residue from the short-side cuts falls down the side of the door panel area, and the broken glass from the dashboard cut falls onto the dashboard and defroster area. There are two reasons for this long dashboard-side cut: The glass falls safely out of the way, and the aerodynamic contours of today's windshield make for easier and more efficient removal if the glass is flipped rearward over the roof of the vehicle (Fig. 7-20). Folding the windshield glass forward onto the hood of the vehicle (once common practice) can be thwarted by the aerodynamic curves of these newer windshields.

If a chopping tool such as a fire axe is used, the tool should be held so that one corner of the blade pierces all of the windshield's layers of glass and plastic. Sawing or chiseling tools must also penetrate all these layers. Once all three sides are completely cut through, two rescuers can lift the glass up from the bottom edge and flip it rearward onto the roof. They can

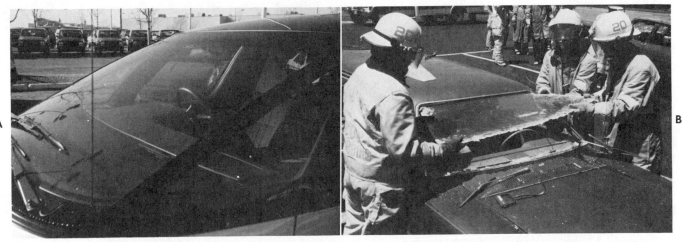

FIG. 7-20 A, The all-plastic Trans Sport, Lumina, and Silhouette vans from GM have an unusually large front windshield with separate laminated glass panels at each side. A solar-reflective layer of clothlike material is also bonded into the windshield.
B, Total windshield removal can be accomplished as a separate evolution or be completed in conjunction with roof removal. Note that the windshield is removed by being flipped rearward.

generally pull the windshield off its top edge mounting and slide the glass across the roof and down over the rear trunk or hatchback area. The broken windshield glass should then be placed safely underneath the rear of the damaged vehicle.

High-pressure air bags *should not* be used for total windshield removal, despite the recommendations of some manufacturers' representatives during sales promotions for these tools. The sales representative typically places one or two air bags along the dashboard at the point where the dashboard meets the windshield. When inflated, the expanding bag is supposed to push the windshield outward, removing it from its mounting. This evolution is unrealistic and can be unsafe. In real-world crash situations, rescue personnel would face several serious obstacles in such an attempt. A collision usually shatters a dashboard constructed of lightweight plastic in many places. A broken dashboard offers no firm base of support while the bags expand and is only crushed further into or onto trapped patients in the front seat area. The high-pressure bags, along with their air supply hoses, become cumbersome to work with in the limited space along the top of the dashboard, and their setup is more time consuming than recommended standard windshield-removal techniques with simple hand tools. The tool's action during inflation is also unpredictable; it may fly off the dashboard without warning, endangering nearby patients and emergency service personnel.

Simultaneous Windshield Removal

Simultaneous windshield removal presents both advantages and important disadvantages. In this second strategy, windshield removal is not a single or separate evolution but rather one that incorporates partial or total vehicle roof removal. In simultaneous removal, the glass is cut or chopped through only along the bottom edge at the dashboard. The remaining two short sides and the top edge are left intact in their mounting. When the front roof posts are cut and the roof either flipped rearward or totally removed, the windshield glass moves away with the roof section (Fig. 7-21).

The advantage of this evolution is that it can save time. The major disadvantage is that the windshield is removed over the passenger compartment area, which means that loose sections of glass could fall onto patients or personnel below or that the entire sheet of glass could suddenly become dislodged when the roof

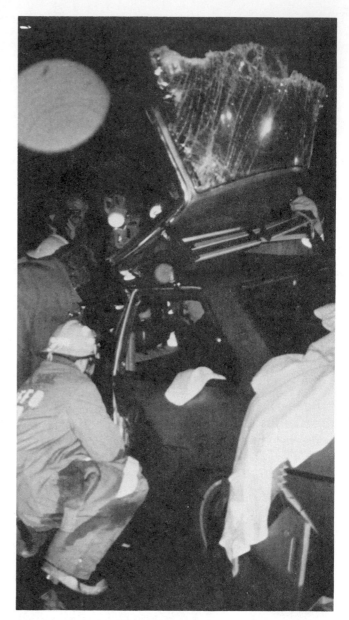

FIG. 7-21 Personnel should tarp and secure the flipped roof and windshield assembly. A sudden gust of wind may move the glass and roof back onto rescuers and patients.

is moved above the patient area. If the roof is to be totally removed, these hazards may be justified, but if a section of the roof is only to be flipped and not removed from the vehicle, the hazards may not be worth any savings in time.

Regardless of the method used, the windshield glass should be totally removed from the vehicle and precautions taken to insulate those inside the vehicle by covering them with a blanket or tarp and placing a wooden longboard or shortboard between them and the work area. Holmatro, Inc. has introduced a new

Windshield Blanket, which is designed to minimize windshield glass scattering and reduce the likelihood of injury from windshield glass fragments. The orange device has a small plastic cover with a strap along one end and a weighted edge at the other. It is positioned between the passenger compartment area and the windshield. While the windshield glass is being removed, it falls onto the blanket where it can readily be bundled up and moved away from those inside the vehicle.

Victim Impaled in Windshield Evolution

On fortunately rare occasions, first-arriving emergency service personnel find that a vehicle occupant who was unrestrained at the time of the collision has been impaled in the windshield glass. The victim's head has passed completely through the layers of the glass and is protruding from a hole in the windshield. The force of the collision with the windshield caused the laminated glass to fracture and tear open while the occupant's head squeezed through the opening (Fig. 7-22). The process has been likened to ramming the occupant's head into a brick wall while the individual was putting on a turtleneck sweater made of razor blades. The grotesque physical injuries that result can include skull and facial fractures, extensive bleeding, and debridement of face and ears.

This rescue problem demands rapid and systematic action to minimize further injury to both patient and rescue personnel. Initial steps must be taken to stabilize the vehicle, with the understanding that personnel must eventually climb into the vehicle during the rescue process. When the vehicle is stable, a crew member who has been assigned EMS responsibilities moves into position to apply manual support to the patient's head, neck, and spine. Another crew member then moves to stabilize the patient to the greatest extent possible.

With the patient secure and protected from exposure to broken glass or rescue equipment to be used, additional crew members begin to free the patient from the hole in the glass. This can be accomplished by manually peeling the shattered laminated glass away from the patient, using basic hand tools to assist in this effort. One very effective hand tool for this task is a large pair of tin snips or shears. This tool severs the glass and the laminated plastic layers without causing further injury to the patient. While the opening gradually enlarges, a makeshift immobilization collar, then

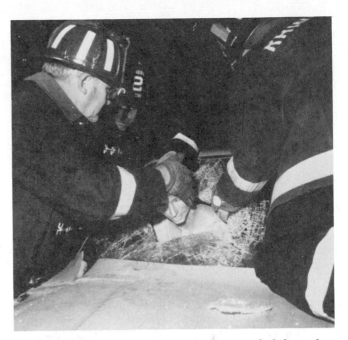

FIG. 7-22 A simulation of an occupant impaled through laminated glass. This process requires initial vehicle stabilization, stabilization of the patient, and subsequent glass removal to permit patient to be lowered back into the vehicle for extrication from within.

a rigid immobilization collar, and eventually a shortboard immobilization device can be positioned on the patient as appropriate. When the disentanglement work has been completed, rescuers pass the patient back inside the vehicle to be extricated from the front seat.

This evolution is a delicate and highly coordinated operation, requiring effective supervision and dedicated teamwork from a minimum of four working emergency service personnel and a supervising individual.

VEHICLE DOOR EVOLUTIONS

One of the most frequent vehicle rescue evolutions to be performed at a vehicle accident is work with the vehicle's doors. As the structural components of automobiles become lighter and less substantial, collision impact can easily render one if not all of the vehicle's doors inoperative. Experience has shown that a vehicle's most likely position after a collision is with its tires or wheels on the ground. In this position the vehicle's doors and door openings are most often used for access to and egress from the interior passenger compartment.

When access to the interior of a vehicle involved in an accident must be gained and using one assistant and available vehicle rescue equipment, the rescuer should be able to do the following:

- Determine that a door of a damaged vehicle interferes with safe and efficient disentanglement and extrication.
- Determine that a closed door presents a hazard to operating personnel if left in the closed position.
- Recognize and determine the need for opening a particular vehicle door found closed on arrival at an accident scene.
- Determine why a given vehicle door is inoperable.
- Determine the extent to which a given door is or is not operable by normal means.
- Determine the most appropriate rescue tools and equipment necessary for accomplishing the desired door-opening evolution.
- Determine the safest and most efficient series of vehicle rescue door evolutions that will yield the greatest benefits to the overall rescue and extrication process.
- Safely and efficiently perform any desired door evolution within 2 minutes or less.

Vehicle rescue evolutions involving doors range from the simple to the complex. In all cases, however, common sense, the ability to look beyond the physical damage of the particular door, and a systematic analysis of the specific rescue problem must prevail. Rescuers must understand that the appearance of a damaged vehicle door is *not* a true and reliable indicator of its status. Particularly during the early moments of an incident, a mutilated door that nearly everyone assumes to be jammed may open or unlatch when a rescuer simply reaches inside and operates the interior door handle mechanism. Remember, the door may simply be locked. All emergency service personnel, particularly those with command responsibility, must develop the ability to read a door. A trained and experienced rescue officer will not be fooled into basing decisions about the operation of a door on its external appearance alone.

Reading a damaged door means systematically exploring all aspects of the door to fully understand any rescue problems that it may present. There is a recommended three-step process for surveying a damaged door. Personnel first must *size up*, then *set up*, and finally *open up* the door (Fig. 7-23). All three steps are necessary, even when the door appears only slightly damaged. Door size-up activities include all survey and inspection work done before applying any

tools or equipment to the door. Setup work includes activities performed to prepare the door to be worked on by additional rescue equipment, for example, when a rescuer uses a Halligan type of forcible entry bar to pry the edge lip of door metal outward so that the spreader tool of a power rescue system can be positioned properly. The act of actually opening a jammed door by any of several methods is the open-up step in the jammed door evolution process.

Door size-up work is crucial to a safe, efficient rescue evolution. A trained emergency service person aggressively works to determine whether the door is inoperable and, if so, to what extent and searches for the most likely reason for the door being jammed. For example, it may be held shut simply because it is locked or because substantial body damage is causing pressure against the door. In a rollover collision, for example, the window frame can become wedged into the roofline area above a door, jamming the door closed.

Door size-up work also considers the location, function, and condition of the door's many components, which generally number fifteen or more. Any individual component that no longer functions as designed may make the door inoperable. By the same token, a small component may be the very item that keeps the door operable.

A door's components consist of the body of the door, the window, and the necessary window controls. Visible from the outside are the handle and key-lock cylinder, which usually has a cam arm located inside the door's outer panel. On the inside panel are an inside door handle and an interior door lock button or lever. Between the inner and outer door panels are the important safety lock-and-latch mechanism and various linkage rods and connectors that enable the handles and lock devices to function. This assembly resembles a plastic or metal box about the size of several packs of cigarettes (Fig. 7-24). Inside this box are the safety latch and lock cogs, which consist of small metal disks that operate to grab, hold, or release the companion safety bolt mounted to the body of the vehicle. The grabbing power of the cogs inside the typical safety latch-and-lock assembly ranges from 2500 to 4000 lb of force, with the latest designed Nader latch assemblies rated up to 6000 lb.

The door opens, closes, or slides by the actions of its hinges, which are generally cast-white metal or pressed metal construction and bolted or spot welded to the door and the body of the vehicle. The front and rear passenger doors of four-door vehicles have many

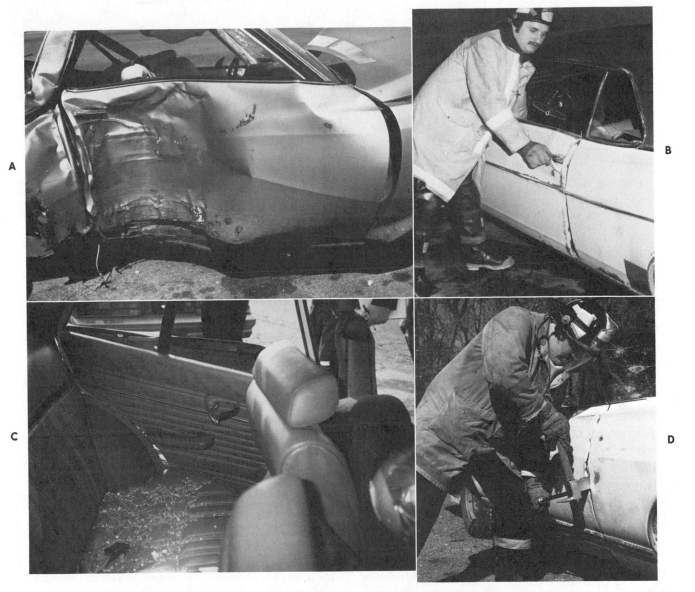

FIG. 7-23 A, Procedure for working with any vehicle door suspected of being jammed is to size it up, set it up, and open it up. **B,** Door size-up work involves looking at the door's physical condition, determining if it is unlocked, then trying outside as well as inside door release mechanisms. **C,** Wisconsin firefighters developed a small piece of steel angle iron to use during door size-up work. The rescuer assigned to open the door inserts a metal bar under the inside door-release mechanism to hold it in an open position. While firefighters work on the outside to force open the jammed door, internal mechanisms have already been positioned to release from the Nader pin. **D,** Setup work for a jammed door involves creating a purchase point for the spreading operations. Work at the hinge or latch side depends on how the attack will be conducted.

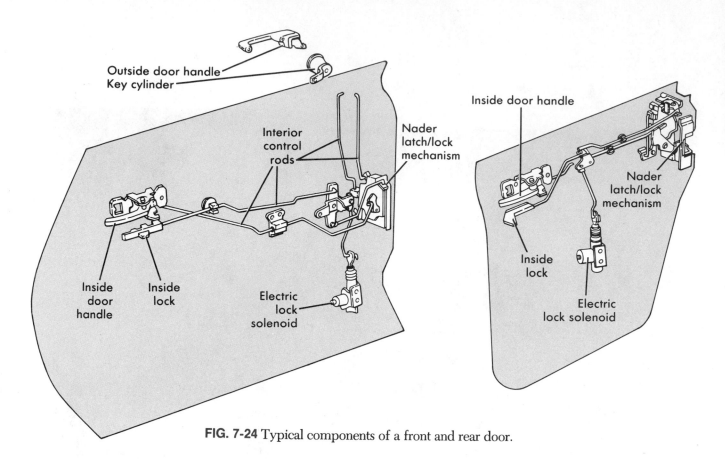

FIG. 7-24 Typical components of a front and rear door.

of the same features except that rear doors require different locations for their components because of differences in size and shape. Sliding doors, popular on mini vans, contain additional components related to their operation, with door locks, windows, or mirrors that are electrically controlled. The switch mechanisms, solenoids, and levers are also found inside the door.

The most important thing to remember about the components of a typical door is that the separate outside and inside door latch-and-lock controls go to a common latch-and-lock box assembly. The outside handle and its linkages may be damaged during a collision, yet the interior control linkages and handles on the same door may function normally. It is therefore crucial to remember that although exterior damage may be extensive, suggesting a jammed situation, it is important to try before you pry because there is a possibility that the door is only locked or that the interior mechanism is still intact and operable. Locking a door simply disconnects the inside and outside door handle linkage mechanisms from the lock assembly inside the door, making them unable to release the door latch mechanism. The rear door childproof lock works on this same principle.

Opening a Locked Vehicle Door

Emergency service personnel are often asked to open a locked vehicle door without damaging the vehicle, generally because an owner has locked the keys inside. When handling such a request, the command person must first determine whether a life-threatening situation exists (Fig. 7-25). Is there a passenger inside who appears to be in immediate need of medical attention? Is there a potential for a hazardous condition to develop? If the answer is "yes", the justifiable emergency action is to employ force to gain quick access to the interior of the vehicle. This is most efficiently accomplished by breaking out tempered glass.

If no immediate life-threatening situation exists, such as with the typical vehicle lockout service call, the command officer must consider the relevance of a number of other important factors. Initially, proper verification of vehicle ownership should be obtained from the individual claiming to have keys inside. If the automobile engine is running, the vehicle could move under its own power, in which case vehicle stabilization should include chocking or blocking the wheels. When there is an outside hood release, crew members working from the side may be able to raise the hood,

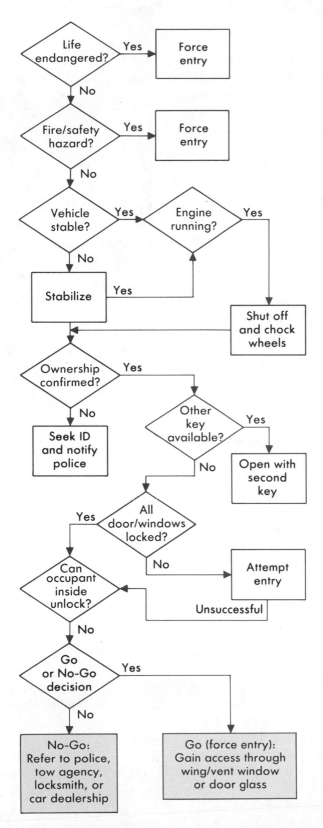

FIG. 7-25 Decision tree. (Courtesy Fire Engineering, New York, NY.)

stall out the engine, and disconnect the electrical power. When access to the engine is denied because the hood releases from inside, crew members may consider quickly jacking the vehicle's drive wheels off the ground. If a child is locked inside a vehicle with the engine running, the child should be distracted away from the driver's seat. Remember — if a child is playing with the gear selector lever, after "P" for park comes "R" for reverse.

At vehicle lockout incidents, the emergency crew should determine for themselves whether all doors are locked. Asking the owner about a second set of keys may jog the person's memory about a forgotten spare key set. Small children locked inside a vehicle may be able to be directed to unlock the door or roll down a window for quick access to the interior by emergency crews. Once all possible alternatives have been explored, the officer and emergency crew must make a *go* or *no-go* decision. In the no-go entry decision, the owner is advised to summon assistance from a police agency having jurisdiction, a locksmith, a car dealership, or a tow truck agency. A decision to go with the entry evolution requires forced entry by working with the window glass.

In recent years, both foreign and domestic automobile manufacturers, have increased the theft resistance of their vehicles. Mushroom-shaped door lock buttons have been replaced with slender antitheft styles mounted flush with the top of the door panel. Door lock mechanisms are increasingly being hidden inside or under door armrests, making access to them difficult. In addition, metal plates are being installed inside doors above the internal lock mechanisms. These plates serve to limit the effectiveness of door-unlocking tools sold under such tradenames as Lock Jok, or Slim Jim (Fig. 7-26). New plastic latch-and-lock components inside vehicle doors are designed to fall apart inside the auto door if contacted by these door unlocking tools.

The safest policy in terms of avoiding future legal complications is to act only if a verifiable, life-threatening situation exists. Because many vehicle owners have full glass coverage automobile insurance, the only action recommended is forcible glass-removal work. Other agencies that are willing to accept the responsibility and the liability should be left to handle the routine vehicle lockout service calls. If they choose to work with the door-unlocking bars, that is their prerogative. We know the potential for problems that can develop.

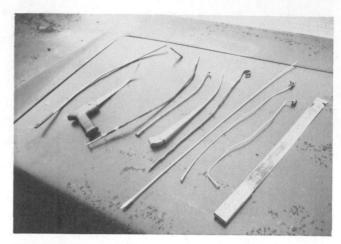

FIG. 7-26 Door-unlocking tools used by fire departments for lockout incidents have limited effectiveness because of theft-resistant door lock features on late model automobiles.

Opening a Jammed Door

When a collision has physically damaged either the door or the structure of the vehicle in close proximity to it, the door may be jammed and inoperable. Getting the door to open, regardless of the specific tactics used, always requires the basic three-step process of size up, setup, and open up.

Size up begins with a physical survey of the exterior and interior components of the door itself, taking into consideration the type of collision that the vehicle has undergone and the location of the major impact in relation to the damaged door. A door may be inoperable because it is locked, compressed shut during a head-on or rear-end collision, crushed downward during a rollover accident, or bowed inward or outward as a result of side impact (Fig. 7-27). The crew member conducting the size up must test both the outside and the inside door handle controls and the manual door lock/unlock mechanism while they physically survey the door and surrounding areas of the vehicle. The three-part goal of door size up is to confirm that the door is actually inoperable, assess what has happened to cause it to be inoperable, and plan the strategy and tactics necessary to get it open.

Once the door has been confirmed inoperable, rescue personnel move to the setup activities. Jammed door setup work includes removing tempered glass from the door and nearby vehicle openings, fulfilling patient and inside medical personnel safety precautions, and accomplishing necessary door preparation work. If tempered glass is rolled down inside the jammed door, the top edge of the glass should be covered and intentionally broken inside the door to prevent the glass from exploding unexpectedly under stress generated by the door-opening evolution. Other necessary door preparation work depends on the specific tactics used to open the door.

Jammed doors can be opened by two methods, forcible entry or safety lock deactivation. Forcing a jammed door open can be accomplished by attacking the door with spreading rescue equipment at one or more of three attack points: the safety lock-and-latch mechanism, the top and bottom hinges, and the structure of the door itself by using the vertical-crush attack.

Deactivation of the safety lock-and-latch mechanism is a simple but effective technique for opening jammed doors. This evolution can be considered an alternative, backup technique to forcing a door with power rescue tools, or it can become the primary attack evolution when power rescue equipment is not available. To set up for the lock-and-latch deactivation evolution, personnel use either air-powered or manual metal-cutting equipment to make a large opening in the outer skin of the damaged door. The opening should begin above the door handle, proceed across the top portion of the door for a distance equal to one half of the length of the door, continue vertically for one half the distance down the door, and return to the latch edge (Fig. 7-28). This three-sided cut allows the skin to be folded outward and rearward. The desired opening in the door should cover at least a 16 in x 16 in area.

The final opening-up phase of the lock-and-latch deactivation evolution involves using rescue tools to destroy the integrity of the internal door latch-and-lock mechanism (Fig. 7-29). This is best accomplished with an air chisel or air gun tool equipped with a

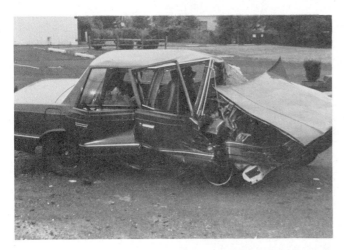

FIG. 7-27 Doors can jam because of crushing or compression actions that occur during the dynamics of a collision.

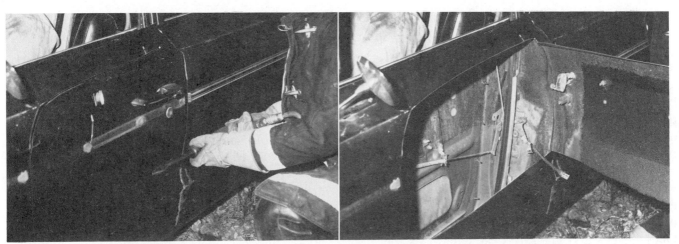

FIG. 7-28 A, Initial stages of lock deactivation evolution require that outer door panel be removed. Air chisel with panel cutter bit is shown making large, three-sided, horseshoe-shaped opening around the door handle. **B,** Opening should be made from above the door handle and proceed at least half the distance across and half the distance down the door. Remember, this access opening can never be too big for what you need.

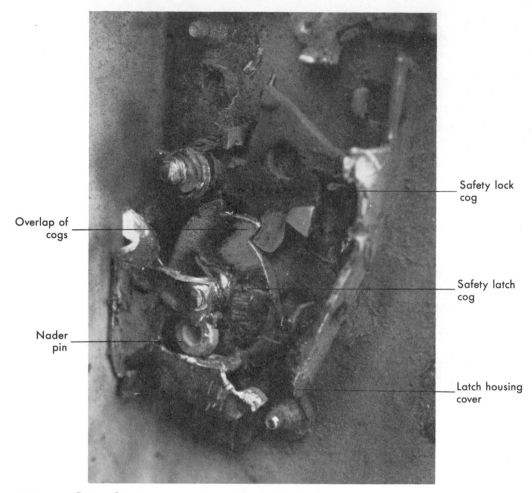

Overlap of
cogs

Nader
pin

Safety lock
cog

Safety latch
cog

Latch housing
cover

FIG. 7-29 Internal components of a typical safety latch assembly include the safety latch cog, the Nader pin or bolt, and the latch housing. Overlap of latch-and-lock cogs holds entire Nader assembly in the closed (latched) position.

long-shanked flat chisel bit. Manual equipment, such as a Halligan forcible entry bar or carpenter's crow bar, can also function well for this task. The deactivation work involves splitting the casing of the latch mechanism apart and moving or removing the two or three metal latch cogs holding the door mechanism to the safety bolt mounted into the structure of the vehicle at the "B" post (Fig. 7-30). When these components are freed, the door can be easily pried open at any point if it is still bound shut (Fig. 7-31). Once deactivated, the safety latch-and-lock mechanism no longer functions to hold the door shut. If done by a trained crew of two persons, the total door deactivation evolution can be accomplished in 90 seconds or less.

Opening a jammed door by using spreading equipment to force the safety latch mechanism away from

the safety bolt mounted into the body of the vehicle is the oldest and most commonly performed jammed-door evolution. This evolution's setup work depends on the method of door attack, which is determined by information gained from the door size-up work. Safety work for forcing a door open includes insulation of the patient, glass removal from the door and its immediate vicinity, and the application of a safety strap to the structure of the door (Fig. 7-32). Placing a rescuer's body against the door to attempt to butt the door while it is being forced open is no longer accepted as an appropriate technique by progressive rescue personnel. A safety rope or strap is used to *safety* the door by remote control, allowing the rescuer to remain at a safe distance.

If the jammed door attack is to be directed at separating the Nader safety latch mechanism from

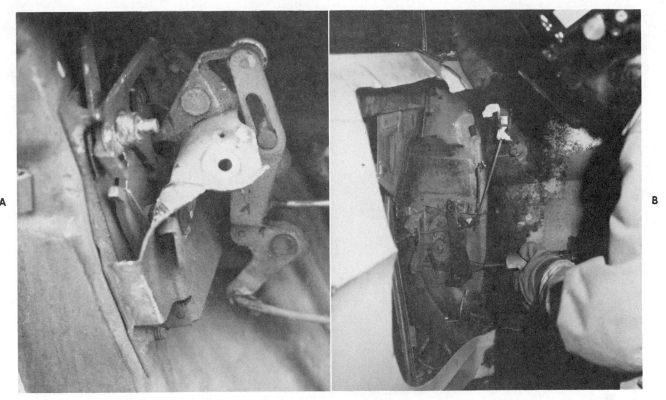

FIG. 7-30 A, The latch housing or cover plate should be cut off or pried off for access to the overlapped Nader latch-and-lock cogs. Do not attempt to remove the entire housing from the end of the door. Deactivation means to take the latch-and-lock housing apart only. **B,** Once access has been gained to the cogs, the entire assembly can be deactivated. Use of a flat chisel bit on an air chisel or air gun is the most effective deactivation tool and technique.

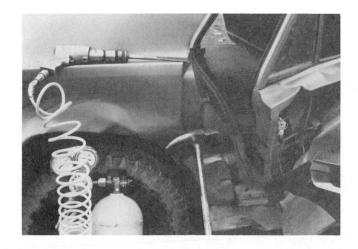

FIG. 7-31 Once the Nader assembly has been deactivated, a door can be pried open easily with hand tools such as the Halligan bar shown.

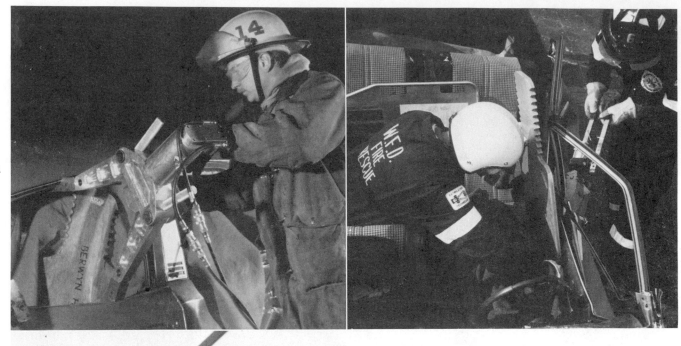

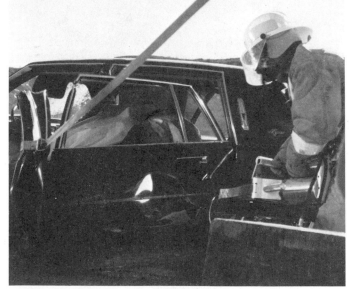

FIG. 7-32 Opening jammed doors with spreader tools requires proper tool positioning and special precautions to protect the patient and inside medic during the evolution. **A,** The shortboard protects the patient during a vertical crush evolution and **B,** during use of a manual spreader to open the front door. **C,** Door removal is underway as shortboard insulates the inside occupants and long strap serves as a safety tag line to hold the door and "B" post during the door release.

the safety bolt, the setup work involves flaring the rearmost lip of the door outward. Providing a purchase point for the tips of the spreading equipment allows for proper placement of the equipment and makes the task safer and more efficient. To obtain a purchase point, rescue personnel insert the bladed end of a Halligan bar into the door jamb area and move the shaft of the bar up and down. This action bends the metal lip outward, making an acceptable starting point for the tips of the power spreader tool. If a power spreader has the capability to close under pressure, one of its tips can be inserted into the door jamb area and the arms closed tightly. This squeezes the lip of sheet metal, allowing the entire tool to be moved toward the front of the vehicle, flaring the door lip outward. Amkus, Inc. advocates a door setup technique with their equipment that involves opening the arms of the power spreader, placing it vertically down over the top of the door itself, and then closing the arms to squeeze near the latch end of the door. Like squeezing a tube of toothpaste, this action causes the end lip of metal on the door to flare outward as desired.

Once the lip has been set up, the open-up procedures begin. Spreading forces must be directed initially above or below the lock-and-latch mechanism

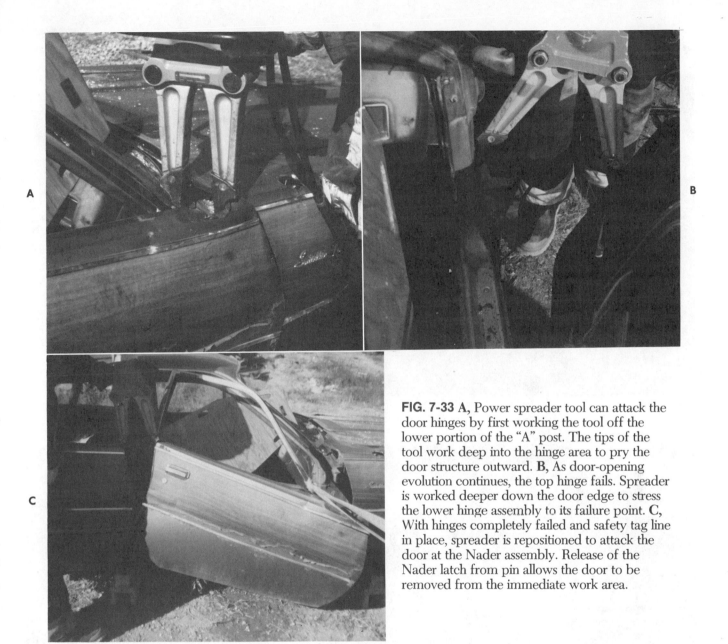

FIG. 7-33 A, Power spreader tool can attack the door hinges by first working the tool off the lower portion of the "A" post. The tips of the tool work deep into the hinge area to pry the door structure outward. **B,** As door-opening evolution continues, the top hinge fails. Spreader is worked deeper down the door edge to stress the lower hinge assembly to its failure point. **C,** With hinges completely failed and safety tag line in place, spreader is repositioned to attack the door at the Nader assembly. Release of the Nader latch from pin allows the door to be removed from the immediate work area.

and the safety bolt. As the structure of the door spreads away, giving more access to the latch and bolt, the spreading forces are concentrated deeper inside the door, closer to these mechanisms. Spreading too far too fast causes the outer sheet metal skin of the door to rip or peel apart, splitting the door structure and tripling the time necessary to force the door open.

Setup work for a jammed door attack at the hinges can include flaring the metal lip along the forward edge of the door and fender panels to expose the hinges. This provides access for the tips of the spreading tool either above, below, or into the hinge assembly. The attack can also be made by working

off the lower portion of the "A" post to stress the hinges (Fig. 7-33). While the evolution progresses, the spreader tool can be positioned to take deeper bites into the door or hinge structure until the hinges fail. If the door is still latched after both hinges and any wires are completely severed, the latch mechanism may still have to be forced off the safety bolt to completely remove the door.

The third attack method, the vertical-crush evolution, is particularly effective in side impact collisions where the door has bowed onto those trapped inside (Fig. 7-34). In these cases, hinge or latch attacks can actually force the door or the interior collision beam

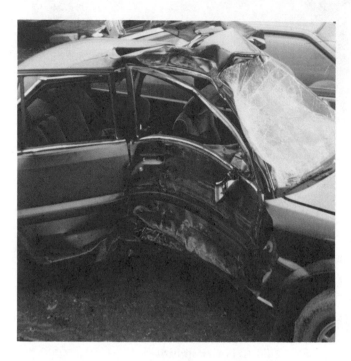

FIG. 7-34 A horizontal attack at the door hinge or latch area is complicated on a door that has crushed inward. If the roof structure is intact, a vertical-crush door evolution may be the most effective.

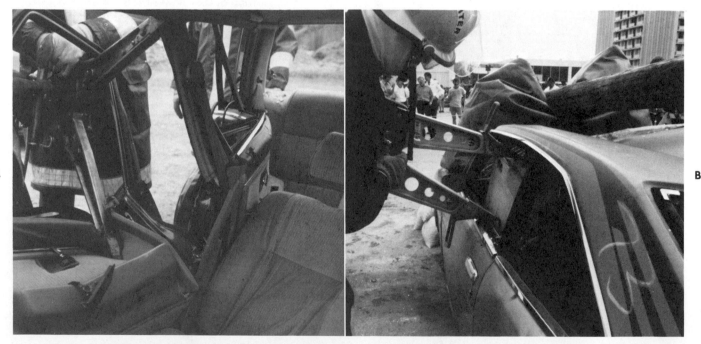

FIG. 7-35 Placement of the spreader tips is important during a vertical-crush evolution. **A,** The upper tip is into the roofline while the bottom tip is on top inside edge of the door. As the arms open in an arc, the door is crushed down and out, moving it away from the patient inside. **B,** Rockville, Maryland extrication team modified the tips of a power spreader with restraint loops to minimize the possibility of the tool slipping in through the window opening during the evolution.

inward toward the occupants. The vertical crush method is intended specifically to move the top of the door and then the interior panel of the door down and out in a smooth, rolling action.

When using this technique, rescue personnel place the tip of the top arm of a power spreader in the window opening of the door, centered along the roof-line area above the door. The tip of the bottom arm of the spreader tool is then positioned at the top of the inside door panel, again near the center of the door (Fig. 7-35). While the arms of the spreader tool are opened, the tool control operator must anticipate possible movement or slippage of the tool inward toward the occupant area. Tool operators must be careful to keep proper body posture and maintain good balance while using the spreader in this mode.

The vertical crush will expose a V-shaped opening at both the top door hinge area and the area above the safety latch and bolt at the rear edge of the door. With a large size power rescue spreader, the vertical-crush evolution may open the door in one action, particularly if the spreader tool can attain an opening distance of 30 inches or more measured tip to tip. The vertical crush, however, is most frequently used simply as a preliminary step to a standard door hinge or latch attack, making this work easier to accomplish.

In a rare circumstance, access may be necessary through the very structure of a closed and latched door, for example, when size-up work indicates that there is no access to the hinge or latch mechanism and no space immediately available outside the door to force it open. This can occur when a vehicle is wedged between large stationary objects and only a portion of the door is exposed.

Setup work is minimal in this case because the evolution consists primarily of cutting through the door. The door is dissected as the outer skin, inner structure, and innermost panels are removed, providing access to the interior through the door itself. This is a good training evolution for learning to work with assorted metal-cutting rescue equipment.

Widening a Door

When rescue and medical personnel decide to use a door opening as a pathway to extricate a patient, the pathway must be made wide enough to extricate the patient safely on a longboard. Even though a door may already be open, it can still restrict the available working space for medical and rescue personnel, making patient handling procedures difficult or unsafe. The position of the open door or the size of the opening may also interfere with access to areas of the passenger compartment when additional rescue work must be accomplished (Fig. 7-36). Improving longboard patient extrication involves widening the door beyond its normal range of opening, completely removing it, or physically widening the opening itself. The door widening evolution size up must determine to what degree the actual opening needs to be increased. When only a slightly larger opening is needed, rescue personnel can widen the door by

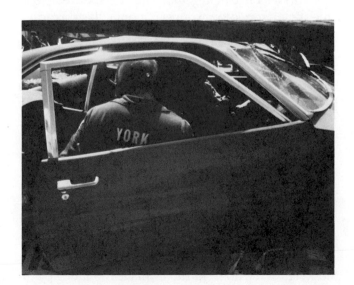

FIG. 7-36 Rescue personnel must be alert to the presence of a restricted door opening. Widening or removing a door can enhance care provided to the patient and make extrication safer and more efficient.

moving it past its normal opening range. If a larger access area is needed, widening plus total door removal may be required.

Rescue personnel have several specific methods to choose from when required to widen or remove a door or increase the door-opening area. Quick and simple evolutions can be tried first. If these are unsuccessful, personnel can logically proceed to the next method. One method can build on and complement another.

Setup for widening the door involves removing door window glass, protecting against any sharp metal areas of the damaged door, and insulating the patient from the work area with wooden shortboard devices.

The simplest door evolution is to widen the door by a controlled brute force effort applied against it. This requires several rescue personnel working together in a steady push or pull to move the door past its normal opening range. The door must then be secured in the open position. If this steady, direct push on the door is unsuccessful, a 12- to 15-foot length of rescue chain can be wrapped first vertically around the structure of the door and then brought horizontally around the end of the door from the inside. Rescue personnel can still apply direct force to the door to widen it while additional personnel are employed on the chain in a tug-of-war to widen the door in a smooth arc.

The door chain wrap is specifically designed to serve five important functions:

- It gives an increased mechanical advantage.
- It works with the strength of the internal door collision beam.
- It will not slip off the damaged door during the widening.
- It can secure the door in its open position.
- It can be easily used with pulling equipment if necessary.

Applying brute force against the door or wrapping a chain around it are generally successful. If more space is needed, pushing or pulling equipment can be quickly and easily positioned to complete the evolution. To pull, rescuers must secure an additional anchor chain to a structural point under the front end of the vehicle, position adequate rescue blocking across its front grille area, and connect a pulling tool such as the come-along to the two chain lengths (Fig. 7-37). Even though the doors are opened fully or even removed, a complete dashboard movement evolu-

tion may still be necessary or desirable at this point in a real-world incident. This evolution, which effectively disentangles the patient from the steering wheel, column, dashboard, and pedals and clears the patient's extrication path, is discussed later in this chapter.

Door Removal Evolution

To justify complete door removal, the door size up must reveal that even with the damaged door widened fully, the opening is not large enough for adequate access to the interior or for patient extrication. Door removal evolution setup involves securing a safety strap to the door, covering sharp metal, removing door window glass, and insulating those inside from the rescue procedures. One method of door removal employs power-spreading equipment to break the weakest point of each hinge assembly. When force is applied against the bolts or welds holding the hinge to the vehicle or against the hinge itself, a failure will occur that releases the door from the vehicle (Fig. 7-38).

The recommended tactic for door removal with power-spreading equipment is to attack the top of the top hinge until that hinge fails (Fig. 7-39). The spreader is then positioned at or near the bottom of the bottom hinge. Spreading at this location generally moves the door into a horizontal position; when the final hinge breaks, the door moves smoothly off the vehicle. Spreading too far at the top of the door may actually drive the lower corner of the door into the ground, which can lift that side of the vehicle if emergency service personnel continue this spreading operation.

Special safety precautions must be taken by rescuers during this door removal evolution. All personnel must remain away from the path that the door is likely to take as it is pried off the vehicle. When the door disconnects from the vehicle, all feet, hoses, cords, and other equipment must remain clear of the area directly under the door itself. The safety strap that was applied to the door must be held firmly by a rescuer to aid in restraining the door as the final hinge is broken.

Other door removal equipment includes hand tools to unbolt the hinges and sawing, chiseling, or power-cutting equipment that can sever the door hinges or the layers of the door skin at the hinge mounting plates (Fig. 7-40).

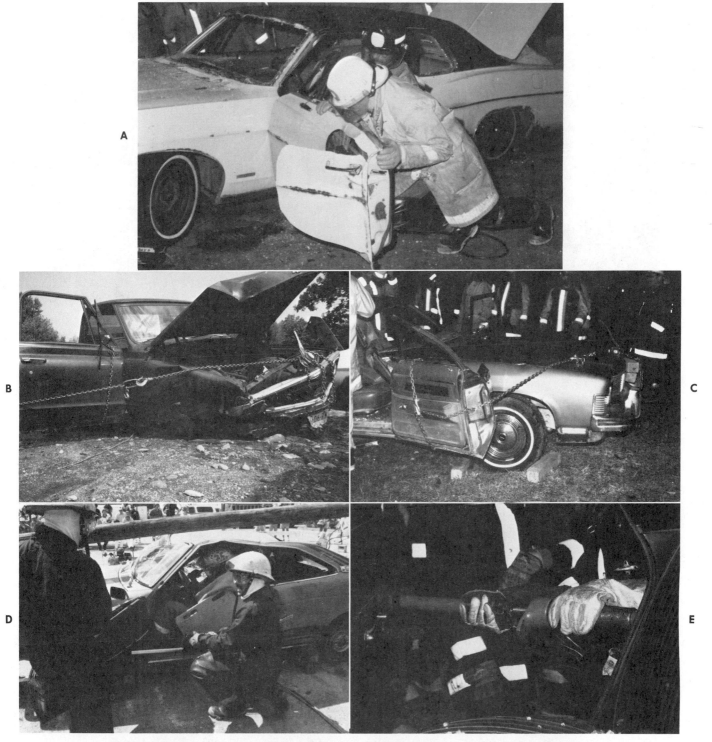

FIG. 7-37 A, Brute force used to widen a door bends the hinges and increases the working room near occupants. **B,** Chain come-along with two rescue chains is used to widen the front door of a truck. Observe the vertical chain wrap on the door and the horizontal chain positioned around the end of the door to increase pulling leverage of the rescue equipment. **C,** Chain wrap shows the effectiveness of chain's vertical and horizontal positioning. Collision beam inside the door actually acts to stiffen the door, allowing it to be widened more effectively. **D,** Widening of a door is accomplished with a power ram pushing from the bottom area of the "B" post onto a strong point of the door. **E,** Widening of rear door is demonstrated by applying porto-power ram, extension tubing, base plate, and rubber flex head. Action is slower than with power rams, but the end result can be the same.

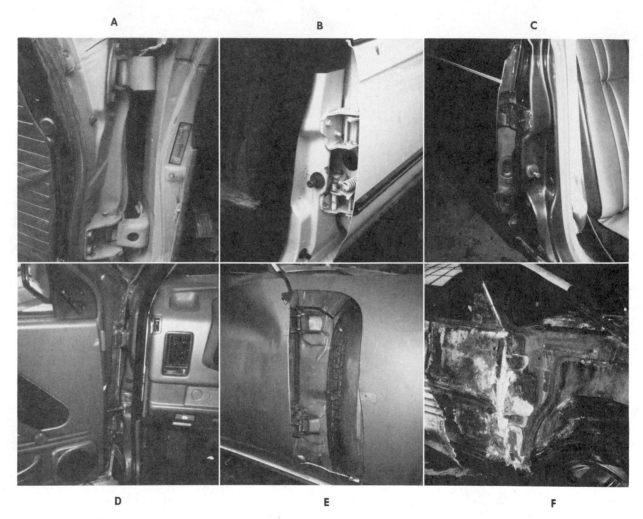

FIG. 7-38 A, Hinges are constructed of various materials. In this instance, the top door hinge is solid cast metal while the bottom hinge is stamped or pressed metal. **B,** Hinges are commonly secured to vehicle with steel bolts. Note that the top hinge has the head of one bolt inserted from outside while the second bolt is placed into the hinge from inside the vehicle's "B" post. This manufacturing method is used to deter auto thieves stripping a vehicle for parts. **C,** Door hinges are secured to the "B" post by welds applied during manufacture. Compared to the ease of unbolting a standard door hinge, this attachment method makes door removal with hand tools more difficult. **D,** Note small linkage found just above the bottom door hinge. This pin and metal bar function to limit the degree that a door opens. Removal of this linkage allows the door to be widened efficiently. **E,** Access to the front door hinges has been gained by removing the sheet metal fender. **F,** Close-up view of a fire-damaged Pontiac Trans Sport van reveals steel hinges and hinge-mounting plates. The door structure consists of combination plastic and fiberglass materials.

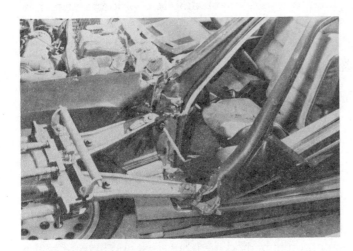

FIG. 7-39 When accomplishing door removal with a power spreader, rescuers should break the top of the top hinge and then the bottom of the bottom hinge.

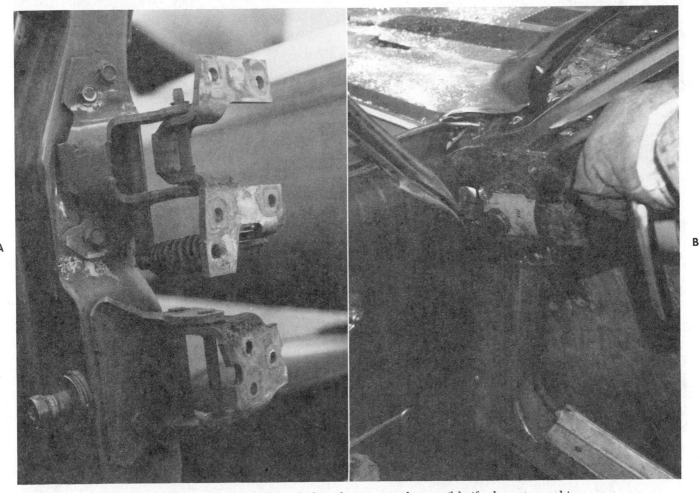

A

B

FIG. 7-40 A, Door removal by unbolting hinges may be possible if adequate working room exists and rescuers have the proper size and type of hand tools. **B,** A hand hacksaw or reciprocating saw can cut hinges. Power cutters should only be used if rated and approved for this application. Be cautious when attempting to cut solid cast-metal hinges.

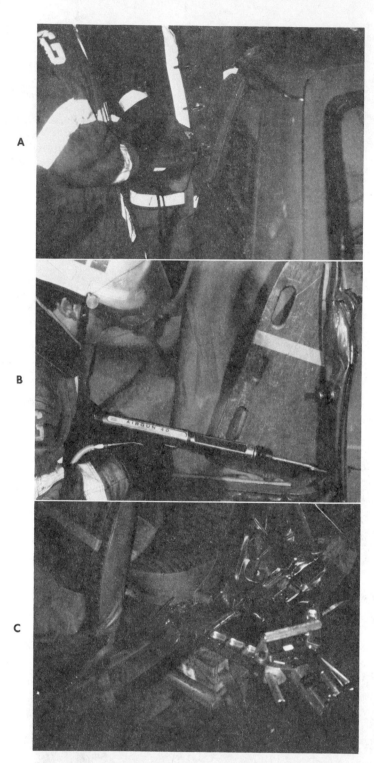

FIG. 7-41 Making a three-door evolution requires that the "B" post be cut at both top and bottom. **A,** Upper cut is being made with an electric reciprocating saw while soapy water is sprayed onto the blade. **B,** A lower relief cut is made in the "B" post with an Airgun 40 tool and a flat chisel bit. **C,** A power spreader breaks the three-door panel down and away from the patients inside the vehicle.

Three-Door Evolution

With a two-door automobile, collision damage may so severely deform the body of the vehicle that access to or egress from the rear seat area is greatly hindered. Even though both front doors have been opened, widened, or even removed, patients in the rear seat area may be difficult to access or extricate on a longboard. Effective rear seat access and patient extrication in such situations can be accomplished by using the *three-door* evolution.

The size-up portion of the three-door evolution confirms that body damage to the vehicle is restricting access to those in the rear seat passenger area. The size up also must verify that removal of one or both side body panels — the area of the side of the two-door automobile behind the front door and in front of the rear wheels — would provide the necessary patient working room and result in a large enough extrication pathway. Setup for the three-door evolution includes insulating those inside the vehicle from the work that is to be initiated, removing tempered glass in the immediate vicinity of the work area, and opening the front door on each side where the three-door evolution is to be accomplished.

The open-up phase of the evolution can be accomplished in several ways. The body panel that is to become the third door can be cut open one layer of metal at a time until it is completely removed. The panel can also be cut at selected reinforcement points and pried downward or pried out and rearward similar to a rear door on a limousine. The strategic relief cuts must be made at the bottom of the "B" post at its junction with the side rocker panel and at the top of the "B" post if the vehicle has a full-height post. An additional relief cut should be made by EMS personnel at the top rear portion of the body panel where it begins to form the contours of the "C" post. When these necessary cuts are completed, the third door body panel can be pried outward by pushing off the seatbelt recoiler unit, rocker panel, or floor-mounted track of the front seat (Fig. 7-41). The body panel can also be pried downward in a vertical crush type of evolution by rescuers pushing off the "C" post itself or the roof if it is still intact. The evolution is completed when the body panel is at or below the level of the seat cushion of the rear seat or is completely removed. Final safety work necessitates that EMS personnel tape or tarp the sharp, exposed sheet metal to minimize any injury potential to themselves and the occupants.

Widen or Remove the "B" Post Evolution

If a four-door automobile is involved in a collision, occupants can be trapped by the full-height "B" post. This is particularly true in the case of a side collision. The full-length "B" post, even when undamaged, can seriously interfere with patient extrication. Rescue personnel can provide access to the crushed passenger area and allow for the safest and most efficient patient extrication by either widening the "B" post or opting for its removal. This evolution series is referred to as making a four-door automobile into a *wide body*.

Justification for widening or removing a "B" post comes from a size up indicating that the post obstructs patient removal in its current position. This obstruction may be due to the normal post location, the location of the injured patient, or a result of accident crush damage that has moved the post into or onto an occupant seated in the outboard front or rear seat area. Wide body evolution setup work includes standard safety concerns for those inside the vehicle during the evolution. The rear door where the work is being done must be opened before completing either of these "B" post evolutions. The rear door can be left attached to the "B" post without interfering with the evolution. The front door must be either opened or removed from the "A" post at the door hinges. It is also important to accomplish effective vehicle stabilization before working with the vehicle. The task of cutting, prying, and bending the post could radically move an unstabilized vehicle. Once the doors are opened as necessary, several strategic relief cuts in the strongest structural areas of the post must be made. The "B" post must be completely cut through at its highest point. Low relief cuts must also be made at the base area of the post where it joins with the rocker panel. These cuts are strategically designed to influence the direction in which the "B" post can be moved, much as a woodsman uses a wedge-shaped notch cut in the trunk of a tree to determine the direction in which a tree will fall.

The open-up phase of the evolution, designed to move or remove the "B" post to widen access to the passenger area of the vehicle, can be started after the relief cuts have been made. Force is applied with manual or power tools against the post, forcing it to fall out toward the ground and widening the body of the vehicle like wings on an airplane (Fig. 7-42). If total "B" post removal is needed to solve the disentanglement or extrication problem, the bottom cuts near the rocker panel must completely free the post

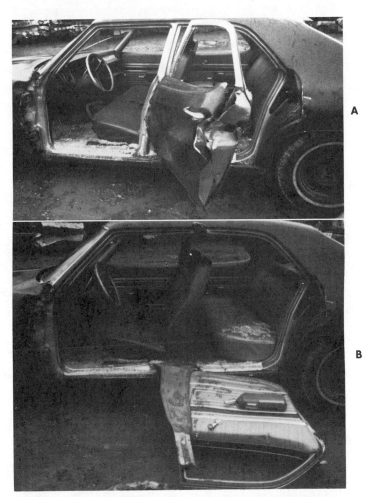

FIG. 7-42 **A,** A "B" post obstruction on a four-door automobile can be eliminated with proper vehicle stabilization and the wide body evolution. **B,** The rear door and "B" post have been moved from the occupant area of the vehicle. Rescue personnel would follow with total removal of the door and post to create a safer work area during patient extrication.

from the rocker panel area. Finishing safety work requires taping or tarping of the sharp metal exposed during the evolution.

With the increased popularity of mini vans, EMS personnel are frequently confronted with incidents involving vans or station wagons equipped with sliding side doors. Two concerns with the sliding door design include its potential for an invisible "B" post (Fig. 7-43) and its tendency to jam. To open a jammed sliding door, rescuers may consider a total roof removal evolution, or they may use the *fourth-door* evolution. This involves opening the sheet metal or plastic skin segment of the vehicle opposite the sliding door (Fig. 7-44).

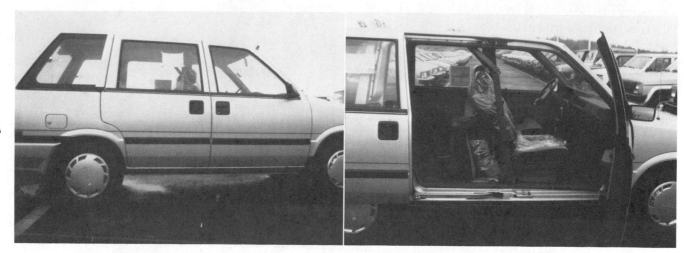

FIG. 7-43 A, Nissan Sentra four-door vehicle with both door handles close to each other indicates that an invisible "B" post is present on both sides of the vehicle. **B,** With either of the rear sliding doors and the adjoining front door open, rescuers can quickly see that only a seat belt remains where one would expect the "B" post to be. Note that both doors have safety latch-and-lock mechanisms at the top and bottom edges and not at the ends as is typically found.

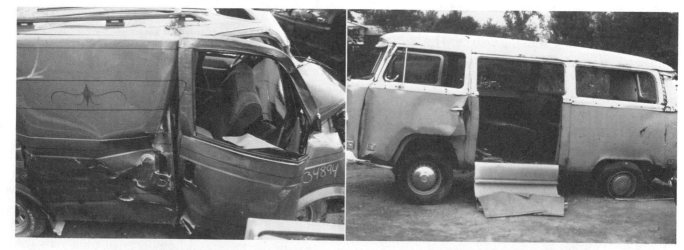

FIG. 7-44 A, Opening a jammed sliding door of a van may be a complicated evolution due to possible multiple latch assemblies, sliding track mechanisms, and large cast-metal hinges. Confronted with this situation, rescue personnel may opt for total roof removal as a means of rapid patient extrication. **B,** The fourth-door evolution, an alternative for opening a severely jammed sliding door, involves cutting the sheet metal or plastic skin of the vehicle opposite the sliding door. It is important to note that Ford Aerostar vans have fiberglass rear hatch doors, and the GM Lumina, Trans Sport, and Silhouette have all-plastic body materials.

Five-Door Evolution

In the five-door evolution, a front door, its hinges, and the side body area near the door hinges are moved or removed to aid in front seat patient access or extrication. The evolution size-up work associated with this assignment indicates that a front seat occupant is trapped by the side body area of the vehicle or that safe and efficient extrication would be compromised unless increased access to the patient's lower extremities is provided. The five-door evolution concentrates on the bottom of the "A" post and the side body of the vehicle located in front of the door hinge area and behind the front wheelwell. This area is near the front seat occupant's legs and feet and is generally where the fresh air vents are located on a vehicle not equipped with air conditioning. This portion of the vehicle can be quite a substantial structural area; the thick firewall of the vehicle begins here, and the front door is hinged to the vehicle at this point.

The five-door evolution setup work requires patient and inside personnel protection, opening the front door of the vehicle, and complete door removal. Again, effective vehicle stabilization must be in place before starting this evolution.

The open-up phase of the evolution is much the same as the three-door evolution except that a different area is being moved or removed. Relief cuts are made in the vehicle's structural areas by cutting completely through the front "A" post at or above the dashboard. Cuts are also made at the bottom of the same post below the bottom door hinge and hinge mounting plate at the point where the "A" post joins with the side rocker panel. Equipment is then used to pry this five-door panel outward and away from the patient area, rolling it toward the front of the vehicle (Fig. 7-45). Spreading or pushing equipment must be positioned properly at a point along the rocker panel area to exert an outward pushing or prying force against the panel. When the proper angle is achieved, the panel bends outward and forward as if it were a small door hinged to the vehicle at the pivot point. When this area opens up, the floorboard area becomes readily accessible. This evolution increases the efficiency of front seat patient extrication and provides good access to the dash, floorboard, and pedal areas on the driver's side.

The five-door side panel can also be lifted upward by applying a spreading tool into the lower cut of the "A" post. While the spreader opens into the cut, the major portion of the five-door panel, the "A" post, and portions of the dash are lifted up and away from the passenger area.

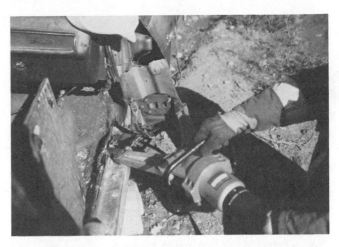

FIG. 7-45 The five-door evolution involves cutting away and bending lower portions of the "A" post forward as if it were a miniature door. This evolution provides increased access to the patient's legs and feet.

STEERING WHEEL AND COLUMN EVOLUTIONS

When confronted with a vehicle that has been involved in a collision and using vehicle rescue tools and equipment as necessary, the rescuer, as part of a four-person team, should be able to do the following:

- Recognize that the steering wheel or column of a damaged vehicle presents treatment and extrication problems for both the trapped patient and the attending emergency service personnel.
- Determine to what degree the steering wheel and/or steering column must be moved or removed to treat, disentangle, and extricate the trapped patient properly.
- Determine the presence of any safety problems or hazards that exist or may arise during the fulfillment of the steering wheel and column evolutions.
- Determine the most appropriate rescue tools, equipment, and techniques necessary to accomplish the necessary wheel and column evolutions.
- Safely and efficiently move or remove the steering wheel or portions of it in 30 seconds or less.
- Safely and efficiently move the steering wheel and steering column away from the trapped front seat occupant in 3 minutes or less, or safely and efficiently remove the steering column from the vehicle in 5 minutes or less.

Steering Wheel Evolutions

When rescue personnel believe that the driver of a damaged vehicle may be trapped by the wheel and column, a rescue evolution size up is initiated. This requires running through a mental checklist beginning with a close look at the actual situation. Rescue personnel must confirm that the patient is truly trapped. Some situations appear to indicate entrapment when in fact the steering wheel or column is not even touching the patient. There is no extra credit given for doing something that does not need to be done! Evolution size-up work must also determine whether the patient is physically pinned not only by the wheel or column but also by the dashboard or protruding metal such as gear shift levers, hand brake controls, and floor pedals. If a trapped occupant is actually contacting the steering wheel, it must be determined to what degree. The stomach of an obese person may normally extend over, under, or around the steering wheel yet not be trapped by it. Rescue personnel must examine — by sight and by feel — the path that the steering wheel ring takes as it goes around its circle. Collision damage to the front of the vehicle, combined with serious deformation of the wheel and obvious contact between the wheel and the patient, strongly suggest an actual entrapment situation (Fig. 7-46).

It may seem at first to be the lazy way out, but if there is anything rescue personnel can do to avoid having to move the column, they should consider doing it. For example, simply operating a tilt-steering column control lever may permit a fast and effective raising of the upper steering column at the tilt joint, giving rescue personnel enough working room to extricate the patient.

When occupants slide forward during a head-on collision, vehicle components in the passenger compartment are also likely to do so. In a head-on collision, the forward movement of the driver's seat may in and of itself be the reason that the driver is trapped. Rescue personnel must check out the possibility of using still-functional manual or electric controls to move the driver's seat rearward. Remember to try the simple, obvious methods. They can make a potentially difficult and time-consuming task relatively easy.

Once all of the simple solutions have been tried and it is clear that the patient is trapped, the second step of the process, the setup work, begins. The second step is to move or remove the lower portion of the steering wheel ring and any supporting steering wheel spokes that are near or in contact with the trapped patient. This cutting action should be performed whenever the column is to be moved because movement of the column during a rescue evolution causes the lower portion of the steering wheel to swing in an arc, moving closer to the trapped driver before moving clear. If rescue personnel were to move the column without first removing this part of the steering wheel, a pinned driver could be further injured by the lower portion of the wheel being forced into or onto the occupant during the evolution.

Typical steering wheel rings for automobiles are constructed of a ⅜-inch round core of cold-rolled steel. The metal is *not* spring loaded as many rescue personnel are led to believe. This metal core is generally

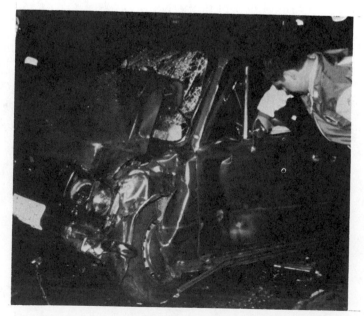

FIG. 7-46 Collision dynamics involved in a head-on accident compress the vehicle into the occupants' survivable space. Medic is assessing the adult driver; three other adults also were trapped inside.

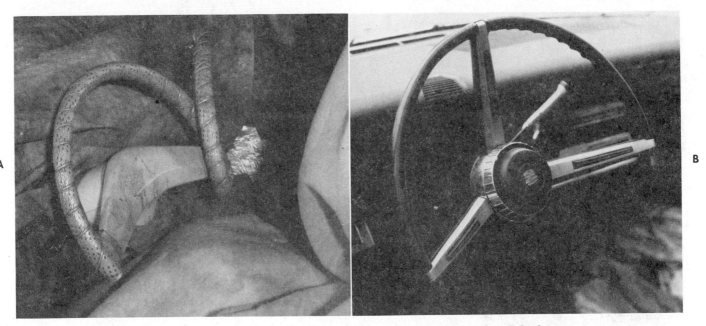

FIG. 7-47 A, One cut of a steering wheel ring may allow rescuers to bend the lower portion of the wheel away from the patient. **B,** Cutting the ring at the nine o'clock and three o'clock positions allows for total removal of the lower portion of the ring.

covered with vinyl or a similar material. The overall thickness of the ring is about 1 inch in diameter. Although larger vehicles may have larger diameter steering wheel rings, they are constructed of the same cold-rolled steel. Work with the ring involves a complete cut of the ring at the nine o'clock position when seen from the driver's vantage point. Once cut through, the lower portion of the ring can then be manually bent up and away from the driver toward the driver's right. This causes the ring to pivot and bend at the three o'clock position. Once the ring is bent far enough to clear the trapped patient, the initial task is completed. This relatively simple yet delicate procedure should immediately provide an additional clearance of 6 to 12 inches between the driver and the center portion of the steering wheel.

A more common method of providing this clearance is to cut away all or a portion of the wheel. Cuts can be made at both the three o'clock and the nine o'clock positions to remove approximately 50% of the ring (Fig. 7-47). Use caution if cutting away a steering wheel ring with a power cutter unit. The portion of the wheel being cut must be held firmly to restrain it as the cut is accomplished. All of the steering wheel spokes attached at the horn button area of the column can also be cut through. Two or three cuts of the

spokes at the steering wheel hub permit complete removal of the wheel and spokes in one action. Although this is effective, the cutting process can be difficult due to the positioning of the trapped patient near the wheel. There may also be very little working room inside the automobile, making any cuts difficult to accomplish in some rescue situations.

Tools for cutting away the steering wheel ring or spokes include hand tools such as a hacksaw (with lubricating fluid), a 36-inch size or larger bolt cutters, or a ratchet type of bolt cutter (Fig. 7-48). If the steering wheel spokes are wide or extra thick, the bolt cutters or ratchet cutter may not be usable. An electric reciprocating saw with adequate lubricating fluid can also be used for this assignment, as can hydraulic cutting units of power rescue systems.

When selecting primary and backup tools for cutting, rescuers should consider the amount of working room between the steering wheel and the trapped driver and the amount of time needed to get the tools in service. Although a hacksaw may be a slow tool, it may accomplish the job long before bigger, more sophisticated tools can be readied. Remember, it does not take a shotgun to shoot a mosquito.

Once the necessary portion of the steering wheel has been cut and bent or cut and removed, it may be

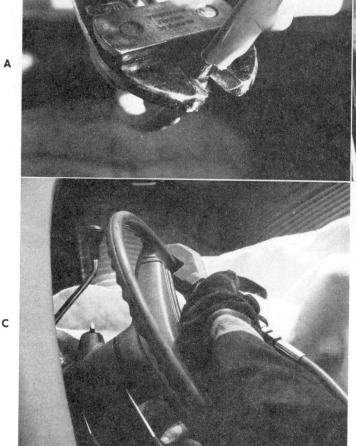

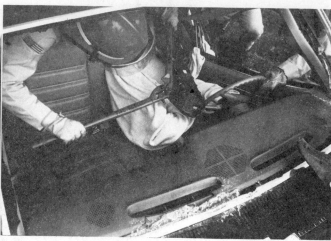

FIG. 7-48 A, Severing of cold-rolled steel steering wheel ring is possible with a hacksaw, reciprocating saw, or bolt cutter *(shown)*. **B,** Patient positioning or vehicle damage may make using bolt cutters cumbersome. **C,** Separate hydraulic cutter unit from the Lukas Co. can safely cut the steering wheel ring and requires very little room to operate.

possible to extricate the driver. Further analysis at this point is required to determine if moving the column is still necessary. More than likely, moving or removing the wheel has provided sufficient clearance to remove the driver safely and efficiently.

Steering Column Movement Evolution

If the driver is still obstructed by the column, a number of factors enter into the decision on the next necessary action to free the driver. Rescue personnel must consider all accident scene information including the type of vehicle involved, its condition and location, the extent of damage, and patient positioning within the wreckage. EMS work already done or still to be accomplished influences the specific column movement evolution to be chosen, as do the rescue tools, both primary and backup, available for the task. Complicating the decision-making process are the

rescue evolutions that may have already been accomplished or those that remain to be done. Completed rescue evolutions can greatly affect decisions on how to free the occupant safely and efficiently.

Specific column techniques are categorized by the area of the vehicle in which the column work is to take place. All column evolutions fit into one of the following four categories:
- Movement across the front
- Movement across the windshield
- Movement from inside the vehicle
- Steering column removal

A basic method of moving the column is to place rescue equipment across the front hood. This grandfather of column movement techniques is also considered by some rescue instructors to be something of a dinosaur. Unfortunately, many rescue teams are locked into this technique as their one and only method of moving a steering column.

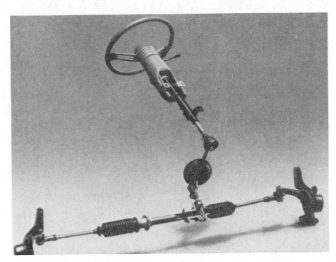

FIG. 7-49 Rack-and-pinion steering systems, which dominate today's vehicles, are referred to as split steering columns by rescue personnel because of their multipiece assembly.

The once smooth and horizontal hood and fender area can be so crumpled by the impact of a collision that there may no longer be a surface for rescuers to use as a platform for their equipment. This problem, combined with the danger of the potential seesaw action of the rack-and-pinion split steering column, makes it clear that this method can no longer be relied on as a primary method (Fig. 7-49).

The across-the-front method involves pulling or lifting a length of chain or strap that is placed across the front. Regardless of the equipment used, certain support activities must take place. Initially, the vehicle's front area must be surveyed in terms of desired equipment position, status of the shock-absorbing bumper, possible chain anchor points, and the general strength of the area. The frameless, new technology vehicles that have plastic bodies, lightweight space-frame metal underbodies, and crushable front end areas are becoming increasingly common and can make column pulling a difficult and time-consuming evolution.

If equipment or personnel are to work across the front of the damaged auto, the bumper must be reported safe and the front of the vehicle determined to be capable of supporting the pull required. A secure anchor point, such as the front axle, torsion bar, or tie rod, must be found under the front of the vehicle to serve as the basis of the column-pulling setup. Once the anchor point is secure, rescue chain or strapping can be secured to it. The use of rescue strapping for this evolution as required with power rescue systems, such as Phoenix or Holmatro, rather than the appro-

priate capacity chain requires extra safety precautions. The nylon strapping is more vulnerable to injury than the chain. Sharp glass and metal may cut the straps, particularly when drawn tight during a pull, and contaminating fluids from the car (oils, battery acid, gasoline, or diesel fuels) may cause permanent damage. When strapping is used, sources of physical damage or contamination should be removed, taped over, or covered with a safety tarp. The strapping material also tends to stretch under load applications. In hot weather, the strap can elongate so far that the rescue equipment actually runs out of travel before the column has been moved.

All vehicle rescue evolutions that can be carried out with the nylon strap and ratchet provided with some rescue equipment can be done just as efficiently with appropriate rescue chain. The chain is not as susceptible to physical damage and does not stretch under load conditions like the strap.

By this stage of the rescue the windshield glass should have been completely removed, and the doors opened and widened. The roof may also be flipped or removed completely at this point. For personnel and patient safety, glass shards and exposed sharp metal must be taped and tarped. Strengthening of the front grille area should be undertaken next. Blocking is placed parallel to the front bumper, reinforcing this area for the upcoming pull. It is generally not effective to place blocking material on top of the damaged hood area of the vehicle or under the rescue equipment. Blocking placed in these areas may look good but does not strengthen the front end and may actually interfere with the movement of the steering wheel and column. Blocking should only be placed over the grille and bumper area of the vehicle and on top of the firewall near the dashboard.

Two very effective methods exist for strengthening the critical front end area of the damaged vehicle. One method uses four footers, 4-foot long, 4 in x 4 in hardwood blocks. Two or three of these blocks are placed parallel to the front bumper area, resting either on the bumper or just above or below it. A second and newer technique that is also very effective uses the flexible ladder-cribbing assembly (Fig. 7-50). With this cribbing setup, a rescuer holds a rope handle and drapes the cribbing blocks over the front area of the vehicle. Using a bungee stretch strap, rescuers attach the rope handle of the ladder crib to a point near the windshield area of the car (wiper arm, hood lip, or louvered vent area). The ladder cribbing is thus temporarily secured in position, freeing rescue personnel for other work.

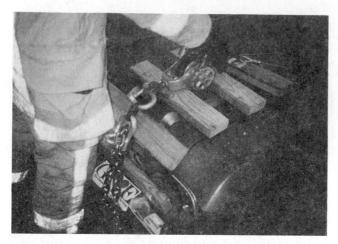

FIG. 7-50 Ladder cribbing in position over the front end with come-along in position for pulling evolution.

Once the front has been adequately blocked and secured, the anchor chain or strapping is brought around the front end, passing over the cribbing. Using another bungee stretch strap, rescue personnel can secure the anchor chain or strap in this position.

While this preparation work is done, other personnel work to secure the rescue chain or strap around the steering column and wheel assembly, bearing in mind the two major concerns that relate to column hookup work: the column may either seesaw or fail completely during the pull, endangering everyone in the immediate area. Because failure of a steering column evolution usually results from improper rescue equipment setup, the problem can be prevented by doing the work correctly in the first place.

One column-pulling strategy is to concentrate the pulling forces as low as possible on the column itself. A low pull minimizes stress on a tilt column knuckle joint and reduces the potential seesaw action of a split column. Accessing a low pulling point on the column is made easier by removing the plastic top portion of the dash and instrument panel, which can easily be done in a few extra seconds. A second strategy recently introduced involves intentionally wrapping a tilt-steering column at a point as high as possible. The intent is to fracture the tilt knuckle joint, allowing removal of the upper portion of the column and wheel.

The equipment used to wrap the column depends on the devices doing the actual pull. With power rescue tool systems, rescuers must use chain or strap provided by the manufacturer of the system. Substitute chain or strap can be used only if it meets or exceeds the specifications of the original equipment.

Many rescue teams that use ½-inch alloy chain with their power rescue tool systems have purchased equivalent quality 10- or 12-foot lengths from local supply sources in their community. Those who use nylon strap material for column wrapping must remember to deploy safety tape or tarps to protect the strap against sharp glass and metal that may exist along the dashboard, defroster, and windshield area.

Crew members have several options when ready to begin the actual securing of the chain or strap around the column. Precision is critical in this procedure. Those who are to do the work should put themselves in the victim's place — imagine that *they* are the ones who have to rely on the ability of those wrapping the column. This particular task leaves no room for error. With the relatively large and bulky chain required with some rescue systems, rescuers make one or two wraps with the slip hook end of the chain low around the column and ensure that when the chain pulls, it pulls into the rounded backside, the *heel* of the slip hook. The load of the pull should not stress the open end portion, the *toe* of the slip hook. Proper positioning of the hook is important.

If rescue equipment, such as a chain or cable come-along tool, is used for the pull instead of power rescue tool systems, smaller, more easily maneuvered chain or strap is generally secured to the column (Fig. 7-51). Column pulling across the hood of a typical automobile can be accomplished with about 4000 lb of pulling power. This means that the strap or chain should exceed this load requirement by a suitable safety margin to be considered for this application.

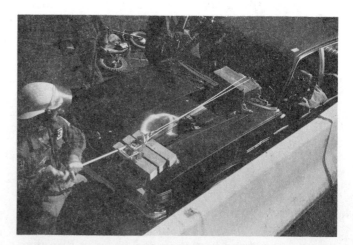

FIG. 7-51 Chains, come-along, and ladder cribbing employed to move a column while a rescuer holds the shortboard to protect the patient.

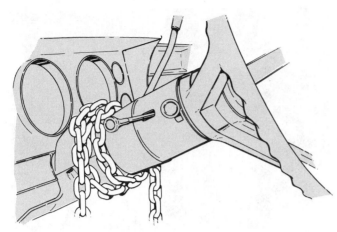

FIG. 7-52 Initial application of the chain for a column cradle wrap requires the center of the chain to be positioned over the column. One end is wrapped around the column to form a low anchor point.

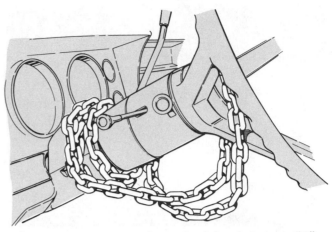

FIG. 7-53 Rescuers cross the ends of the chain in an "X" under the center length of the column. This cradle wrap also provides support to the knuckle joints of the tilt-steering column assemblies.

A very successful column-wrapping method is the *cradle wrap*. It is intended to secure the chain or strap to the column safely, support the vulnerable middle section of the column, and use the mechanical advantage of leverage to maximize the effort of the pulling equipment. The cradle wrap works well with chain up to ⅜-inch diameter or strapping up to 1-inch wide. The recommended minimum length required would be 10 feet. The ½-inch rescue chain of some power rescue tool systems is too large and bulky for this particular wrap.

The cradle wrap begins by placing the center of the length of chain over the top of the steering column and sliding it down as low as possible into the dashboard and instrument panel area. One of the two ends is then placed under and around the column completing one full wrap, leaving two free ends hanging on opposite sides of the column (Fig. 7-52). Next, as seen from the driver's vantage point, the chain end on the left crosses under the column to the right side, passing under and then over the right side steering wheel horn button and spoke area. The end on the right side of the column is crossed under and around the column, wrapping under and over the left side steering wheel horn button and spoke (Fig. 7-53).

Positioned close to the column, each end passes under the top portion of the steering wheel ring and out onto the dashboard area (Fig. 7-54). The chain ends are then available to be joined together to form a loop or used as separate pieces when two separate lines of chain are desired. The safety advantage of the cradle wrap is that the chain or strap is secured low on

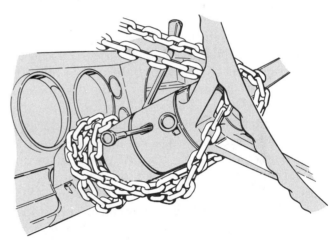

FIG. 7-54 Increased leverage of a light-duty pulling tool, such as come-along, is achieved by positioning the chain around the supports of the steering wheel and passing them over the dashboard and out towards the pulling tool.

the column, below any failure areas. The crossing of the chain or strap underneath the center section of the column, the actual cradling of the column, supports the upper column section and minimizes the seesaw action of the column during pulls. Placing the chain or strap over the free end of the steering column increases the mechanical advantage of the pull.

In addition, if the column slips or fractures during the pull (for example, when a tilt-steering column breaks), the cradle wrap continues to act as a restraint for the upper end of the column, moving it away from the trapped driver.

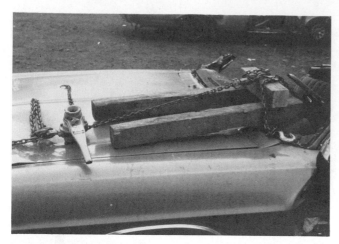

FIG. 7-55 Sliding box crib is constructed using two parallel wood blocks and a third block as a slider. The assembly should be centered above the point where the dashboard meets the front hood.

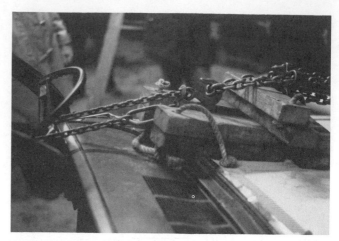

FIG. 7-56 With a properly positioned crib assembly, the top block slides as the column moves away from the trapped occupant. Note that the lift or pull generated by a porto-power and chain head attachment was directed over and above the dashboard by the sliding box crib.

If a 20-foot length of nylon strapping is used for the cradle wrap technique, the only difference is in the initial placement of the strap. Instead of locating the center of the strap over the top of the column (as is done with the 10- or 12-foot chain) a point of the strap approximately 6 to 8 feet from the ratchet device is placed over the column. The ratchet end of the strap and the other long strap section are passed under and around the column just as with the end of chain. If positioned properly, the ratchet will end outside the car on the front hood area and usually near the top of the firewall, where it is readily accessible to rescue personnel.

Regardless of the tool chosen for the pull, the addition of wood blocking at the dashboard and top of the firewall area is recommended. In the simplest and easiest procedure, several 4 in x 4 in hardwood blocks are placed parallel to the dashboard to provide lift for the chain or strap that will move the column. A more effective form of blocking is the *sliding box crib*, a moving and self-adjusting system that gives the column the necessary lift and makes maximum use of the rescue equipment pulling power.

Composed of three blocks of hardwood, the sliding crib is best constructed with three 4-foot long 4 in x 4 in blocks. Two of the three blocks act as rails. These blocks are placed in line with the column pull, parallel to the side of the vehicle, and spaced 12 inches apart. They resemble the rails of a railroad track. The remaining block of wood, which becomes the slider, is placed over the rails at a 90-degree angle to them (Fig.

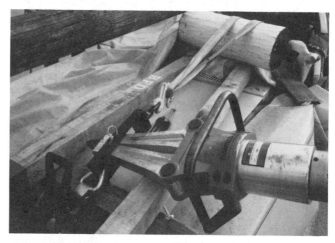

FIG. 7-57 A lifting action with a sliding box crib can also be accomplished by positioning a log roll at the front edge of the dashboard. Note that the power rescue tool strapping rolls over the short length of the telephone pole as the column moves.

7-55). Starting at the end of the rail blocks nearest the column, the block slides toward the front of the auto during the column movement (Fig. 7-56). This sliding action automatically adjusts the cribbing as the column moves, yielding safe and effective results. An alternative arrangement uses a 16-inch section of a power company pole (Fig. 7-57) or one half of a vehicle wheel rim (Fig. 7-58) placed at the top of the firewall area and parallel to the dash to perform a similar function as the column is moved forward.

Patient safety considerations during the column-

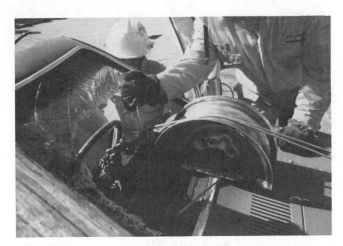

FIG. 7-58 Come-along and chains pull a column while the lifting effect is created by using a half rim. The rescuer is steadying the cable come-along's pulley to prevent jamming it inside the grooves at the center of the wheel.

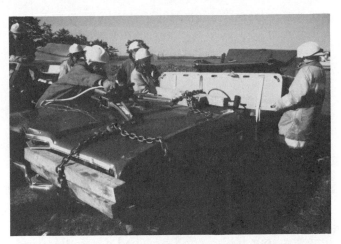

FIG. 7-59 Safety activities include the longboard on edge for patient safety and the positioning of the rescue tool and operator on the passenger side for increased rescuer safety.

pulling evolution include proper tool and equipment hookups, adequate covering for those inside the vehicle, and the companionship of at least one rescue person, preferably a medical person, for the trapped patient as the pull is accomplished.

An additional measure of patient safety involves the use of the ¾-inch-thick medical longboard or shortboard.* Once considered strictly medical tools, these wooden boards have proven themselves to be valuable patient safety tools. In the case of column movement evolutions, for example, persons inside the vehicle are typically covered with a blanket or tarp during the column pull. In the event of failure of a component of the steering wheel, column, dashboard, or the working rescue tool itself, a simple cover or blanket would probably not deflect the flying object enough to prevent injury. More than likely, the blanket would be penetrated and those underneath it struck by the object.

When a wooden longboard or shortboard is positioned on its edge inside the vehicle, an added measure of safety is provided for those inside the vehicle (Fig. 7-59). Two rescuers, one at each end of a longboard, can hold it across the inside of the vehicle, placing it between the trapped persons and the column to be moved to deflect any broken glass, plastic, or metal that might fly off unexpectedly during the

*The patient safety items discussed here are the standard plywood construction shortboard or longboard, not the popular K.E.D. type of immobilization devices.

pull. If access is inadequate for a longboard, a shortboard can be positioned as a chest protector. The shortboard serves to insulate the person directly behind the column from potential injury.

Next the rescue equipment that will be used to accomplish the actual pulling of the column is placed in position. If power rescue tools are to be used, the pulling tool itself, the power plant, hydraulic hoses, and the tool operator should be positioned on the *passenger* side of the vehicle if possible. This clears the driver's front fender area of obstructions for assisting crew members hooking up the equipment and places the tool operator in a safer position during the pull. The operator is an arm's length plus the length of the tool away from the pulling tool's line of fire.

If a come-along pulling tool is used, the body of the tool should be placed near the front end of the accident vehicle with the working end slip hook secured to the chain at the steering column. This positioning allows for the safest use of the come-along and maximizes the tool's pulling power. If a rescue vehicle winch line or cable from a tow truck are used for the column-pulling evolution, the slip hook again must be properly attached to the chain secured around the column itself. Any pulling work using tow truck or rescue vehicle winch cable means paying additional attention to securing the vehicle in place to prevent movement during the pulling evolution.

With blocking and chain secure at the anchor point and column, inside personnel protected, longboard in place, and all personnel ready, the pulling equipment is cautiously operated. While the pull takes place, column action and reaction are closely monitored. The tools are stopped when either the desired result is achieved, a problem is detected, or the tool runs out of travel. If the operation is successful, the tool may be left in place to hold the column in its "up" position.

If the equipment has to be reset and releasing pressure from the pulling tool would lower the column back on the trapped person, a method of securing the column in the "up" position must be devised. A simple technique is to take a chain or strap and secure it around the column, attaching the other end to a stationary point somewhere on the vehicle. If the roof is intact, a four footer can be placed across the windshield area above the column. A chain or strap is looped over the block and then placed around and under the bottom of the column. Once drawn tight, the loop holds the column up as the primary rescue equipment is released.

LIFTING A LENGTH OF CHAIN EVOLUTION

The second basic column movement technique, *lifting a length of chain,* also uses the front area of the automobile. With this method, a length (or lengths) of chain or strap is anchored at the front of the vehicle, run across the front hood area, and secured to the column as before. The difference with this method is that instead of being used to pull horizontally, the rescue equipment is used on top of the firewall area of the vehicle to lift the chain or strap vertically (Fig. 7-60).

To prepare for the lift, rescuers place either the four footers or the ladder crib blocking at the front of the

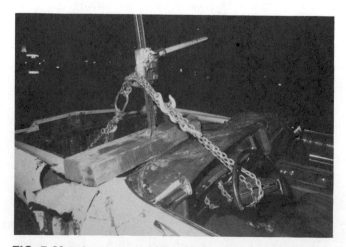

FIG. 7-60 Lifting action of a 7000-lb capacity mechanical jack along with rescue chain and blocking can be used to move a steering column by lifting a length of chain.

vehicle. At least one block is needed as a baseplate at the dashboard and firewall area, placed parallel to the windshield, where a lifting tool is then positioned on the wood. The chain or strap is placed from the front anchor point to the movable column so that it is relatively tight on the lifting tool. When all appropriate safety measures have been taken, the length of chain or strap is literally lifted at a point directly over the top of the firewall.

Power rescue tool spreader units can move columns more quickly in this manner and are less labor intensive than when they are set to pull horizontally across the hood. The spreader is positioned with its lower arm on the wood base plate. The tip of the upper arm is located under the rescue chain or strap. While the arms of the spreader are opened slowly, the upper tip lifts the chain. Rescuers should be alert to the possibility that when the spreader arms open more than 12 inches, the chain may slip off the tip of the upper arm or the spreader unit may torque to one side and slip out of position.

Spreader units that have a chain grab hook and shackle accessory can be used in a modified lifting technique. This requires the spreader to work much like a crane as it lifts the length of chain. An advantage of the modified lifting technique is that it reduces possible tool slippage. In setting up for this evolution, rescuers first open the spreader unit arms approximately 14 inches. A single grab hook and shackle unit is then placed on the upper arm but, unlike its conventional use, is positioned to hang down from the underside of the upper arm. The spreader is then put in position on the baseplate with the standard automotive tip on the bottom arm contacting the plate. The chain length running from the column is attached to the dangling grab hook at the appropriate point and the chain is lifted when the arms of the spreader are opened. Lifting the chain attached to the grab hook reduces the likelihood that the spreader unit will slip off the chain.

Many lifting tools can accomplish the task of lifting a length of chain, including tools such as the 7000-lb capacity mechanical jack, the standard hydraulic jack, the porto-power ram, air bags, or air cushions.

If a standard hydraulic jack is used, keeping the chain on the top serrated head of the jack unit can become a problem. A possible solution is to place a porto-power vee head loosely over the serrated head of the jack. The chain is run over the vee head and is lifted as the jack operates, pressing the vee head on the unit.

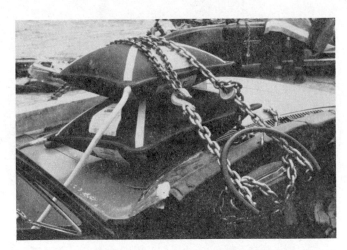

FIG. 7-61 Stacked high-pressure air bags, blocking, and rescue chain or straps can move a steering column. Observe the chain cradle wrap on the wheel and column.

If air-powered lifting tools are used, the largest capacity bags or cushions should be deployed. Because it takes only a few tons of power to lift the steering column, the large-capacity air equipment is used for its lifting height rather than for its strength. The larger capacity air bags or cushions offer rescue personnel the greatest lifting height for this evolution.

A maximum of two air bags can be used and are placed one on top of the other. Beginning with the bottom bag initially, both are partially inflated with the controlling operator alternating the inflation. The stacked bags are most effective if positioned directly over the top of the firewall area, near the column assembly itself (Fig. 7-61). This makes for more efficient movement of the column and uses the strength of the firewall for stability.

This rescue application of air bags or air cushions has specific safety concerns. First, in the initial setup the chain or strap that is to be used over the air bags must be placed in parallel lines. Parallel lines minimize the possibility of the bags shifting during inflation and slipping out accidentally. The two paths of chain or strap coming from the steering column toward the front of the vehicle in the cradle wrap column technique can simply be extended over the bags to make the necessary parallel lines required here.

Another safety concern mandates that the air bags not be fully inflated. A maximum of 70% to 80% of the peak inflation *height* of each bag should be the rule. The safety logic behind this inflation limitation is two-fold. Maintaining the bottom bag of a two-bag stack somewhat underinflated serves to maximize the gripping power of the two bags. If each bag were to

be fully inflated, it would be like trying to balance two basketballs on top of each other. Keeping the upper bag somewhat underinflated also serves to trench the chain or strap into the bag's surface. This long depression area, the trench, allows the strap or chain to nestle into the bag, maximizing the bag's gripping power and keeping the chain or strap from rolling off during the lift.

The limits of the air bags for this modified lifting task are reached when either the desired results are obtained, each of the air bags is inflated to its approximately 80% peak height, the stacked air bags shift off center and become potentially unstable, or some problem with the action or the reaction of the column develops.

In review, two of the five basic methods of disentangling a trapped occupant from the wheel and column both involve working rescue equipment across the front of the auto. Pulling a length of chain horizontally or lifting a length of chain vertically are options available to rescue personnel at an actual incident. Many tools can be used in either of these two basic methods.

ACROSS THE WINDSHIELD COLUMN MOVEMENT EVOLUTION

The third basic method of column movement uses a 4-foot-long block of wood placed over the windshield opening, parallel to and above the steering column. This method has both advantages and disadvantages over the methods just discussed. The disadvantages are that this method requires the roofline of the vehicle to be fairly intact and that the vehicle not be on its roof. If the roof has been removed in a previous rescue evolution or if the roof structure is severely damaged, this method may not be workable.

The advantages of this method are that it can be accomplished with very simple tools, can be done completely by one rescuer, and is very fast (the effort of the rescue equipment goes directly into moving the column). The most important advantage of this method is that it does not rely on the front end of the vehicle (Fig. 7-62). Considering the tremendous crush damage that automobiles can undergo in head-on collisions, a once long-nosed vehicle can be turned into a flat-nosed crunchie by the impact. Even if the vehicle is designed as a flat-nosed truck, school or city bus vehicle, full-size van, or mini van, working across the windshield area is effective for column movement.

The preliminary work for this rescue evolution includes evolution size up, moving or removing the

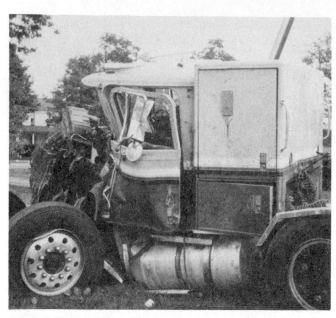

FIG. 7-62 Head-on collision between two fully loaded tractor trailer trucks resulted in the crushing of this vehicle's front end. Column movement by placing tools across the windshield would sufficiently move the column; standard across-the-front pulling efforts may be unsuccessful.

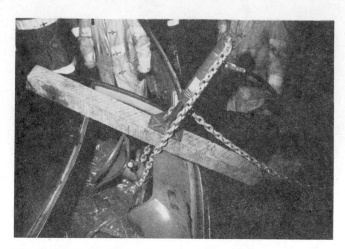

FIG. 7-63 Working four footer in place with chain, porto-power ram, flat base, and vee head attachment.

steering wheel, and taking all safety precautions. Because the task is simple, very little additional work is necessary. Positioning of the wood four footers, looping the steering column with chain, and placing the lifting tool properly completes the necessary setup work. Operating the lifting tool accomplishes the final open-up phase of the evolution.

The most important wood block, the *working* four footer, is placed across the windshield opening area of the vehicle, directly above and parallel to the steering column. The bottom end of the block is positioned on the area above the firewall near the base of the windshield wiper arms to pick up the structural strength of the firewall. The upper end of the working block rests on the edge of the roofline above the sun visor area. If this structural area of the roof is damaged or otherwise weak, another four footer (a roofline block) can first be placed along the edge of the roofline. The working four footer is then placed on this *roofline block*, making a formation resembling the letter "T" above the column.

A rescue chain at least 8 feet in length is then draped over the working block. The chain is looped down beneath one side of the steering column and brought up on the other side. The chain is then hooked onto itself to form a loop. There should initially be a slight

slack in the loop of chain. It is important to remember that there is no need for cradling the steering column with chain as in the methods discussed earlier. This particular evolution works best with just a simple loop of chain. However, it is vitally important that when it passes under the steering column, this loop be kept as low on the column as possible, below the knuckle joint and close to the dashboard instrument panel.

To complete the evolution, rescue personnel place a lifting tool on top of the working four footer and under the top of the loop of chain. The chain loop is then adjusted to accommodate the lifting tool's length and snugged relatively tight (Fig. 7-63). With all personnel ready and all necessary safety measures in place, the lifting tool is operated. The rescue equipment lifts the loop of chain, which quickly lifts the steering column. If for some reason the bottom end of the working four footer begins to crush into the vehicle, there are two options. The first is to allow the block to crush the metal, anticipating that after several inches of crush the block will settle onto the strong structure of the firewall. The second is to place another four footer under the bottom end of the working block parallel to the firewall so that the three wood blocks now form a sideways letter "H." This extra *base block* spreads out the load and minimizes further crushing of the top firewall area.

Rescue equipment that can be used with the four footer over the windshield includes hand tools such as the mechanical jack (Fig. 7-64), the standard hydraulic jack with a temporary vee-head attachment, or the porto-power ram with vee head. Power rescue tool rams, spreader units, and air bags or cushions can also perform this column lift. Power

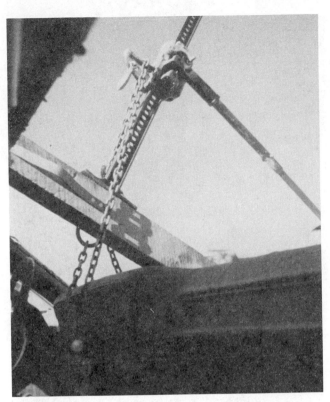

FIG. 7-64 Quick column movement uses a mechanical Handyman jack, an 8-foot length of chain, and at least one 4-foot-long block.

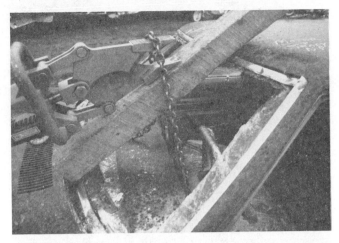

FIG. 7-65 Power rescue spreader with tips inserted under loop of the chain can move a steering column away from the driver's area very effectively in the across-the-windshield mode.

rescue system spreaders can be used with the standard automotive tips on both arms placed under the chain loop (Fig. 7-65) or be set up in the crane-lifting mode described earlier. For ease of operation and to prevent any pinching damage to the base end of the spreader units, rescuers should place the spreader units in position facing down from the top or roof side of the working four footer, with the tip end pointing down toward the front of the vehicle. This puts the rescue tool operator, all hydraulic hoses, and the bulk of the spreader unit up and out of the way during the actual column-lifting procedure.

When air bags or air cushions are used for this task, several specific safety precautions must be taken. Enough 4-foot blocks must be brought into the working position to support the underside of the bottom air bag or cushion totally. There should also be two parallel loops of chain around the column and air bag to minimize shifting of the bag and a 70% to 80% limit set on the inflation height of the bag or cushion so that the rescue chains or straps will trench into the rubber bag surface. Any rescue tool that will lift can in some way be used for this particular evolution.

If the driver's side front roof post should buckle or

fail while moving the column, there is a solution. As if constructing a stud in the wall of a building, personnel can prop another 4-foot block vertically in the driver's door area to support the underside of the roofline. When the *stud four footer* is placed at the three-way junction of the windshield, roofline, and front "A" post, it braces the roof area and takes the reaction of the column-lifting job. In training, this setup has been used for a successful column lift with the stud block, roofline block, and working block even after the entire front "A" post has been completely removed.

All things being equal, no other method can move a column as quickly, safely, and simply as the lift across the windshield with a four footer. Given an unlimited choice of tools, this author's personal choice for moving a column is a four-footer, a 7000-lb capacity mechanical jack, and an 8-foot length of rescue chain. With one rescuer and about 30 seconds, the column will be history.

INSIDE COLUMN MOVEMENT EVOLUTIONS

In certain situations, none of the three methods of column movement discussed so far can be used. If, for example, an accident vehicle has been involved in a head-on collision, the front structural area ahead of the firewall may be so distorted that there is no way to use horizontal pulling tools across it. This may also be the case if the accident vehicle is a convertible (or has been made into a convertible by rescue personnel). Lifting across the windshield can also be ruled out if the vehicle has rolled and is now on its roof.

A fourth basic column movement evolution designed for just these situations involves working rescue equipment from either alongside or inside the passenger compartment of the damaged vehicle. The seesaw effect produced with horizontal pulling tools on the split steering column on late-model automobiles can be virtually eliminated with this technique. Working directly on the column from the inside is a good method for vehicles that have been severely damaged and can be used whenever vehicle and patient conditions permit. Total dashboard, firewall, and column movement is detailed later in the chapter.

In these cases, size up of the inside column evolution reveals that the injured person is trapped by the steering column despite cutting, bending, or completely removing the steering wheel. Evolution setup requires taking all necessary safety precautions. Both the choice of equipment and its placement will be strongly influenced by the position of the trapped occupants and the current configuration of the vehicle. Rescue equipment does not have to be placed in direct contact with the column to move it, nor does every column have to go straight forward. The goal in column movement is to increase the distance between the steering wheel and column assembly and the trapped person. As long as the column can be moved away from the patient, the needed clearance can be gained. The person who is trapped really does not care how or at what angle the column moves, as long as no further injury occurs and freedom can be attained.

Accordingly, the fourth basic column-moving method is accomplished by rescue personnel using rescue equipment positioned inside the passenger compartment or along one side of the vehicle to move the column directly. A rescue tool capable of lifting or pushing is necessary. Mechanical jacks, hydraulic jacks, the porto-power ram, and power rescue system spreaders or rams can be used.

Deciding where to best place the equipment if the push is directly on the column depends on the position of the injured persons (particularly their legs and feet), the size and length of the pushing or spreading tool being used, and the position of the tool against the steering column itself (Fig. 7-66). It is recommended that the tool be placed against a low point on the column. Generally a push right on or at the brace or bracket that secures the column to the dashboard is preferred. This places the force of the equipment below any tilt column knuckle joints that may be present and centers the push low on a front wheel drive split steering column, reducing or eliminating the potential

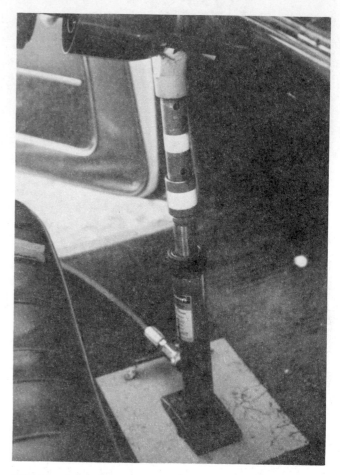

FIG. 7-66 The 10-inch square base plate is used to spread the load of the tool across a larger surface area of the floorboard during a column lifting or pushing evolution.

seesaw effect. A secondary benefit of a low column push is that it enables rescue personnel to move a major portion of the dashboard near the column simultaneously, including the bottom of the front "A" post and the brake, clutch, and accelerator pedals if both "A" posts have been disconnected from the roof structure.

If the injured patient is not in the way, rescue personnel can get directly under the column for a forward lift or push. Any tool used in this position will have its lower end on the driver's floorboard area. Because this area of the automobile is very weak and will generally not support the action of the push on the column, cribbing must be placed between the base end of the pushing tool and the floorboards to minimize collapse or tearing of the floor. If there is no room inside the vehicle at the floorboards for the blocking, the wood can be placed underneath the vehicle directly under the end of the pushing tool. While the column is pushed, the reaction crushes the

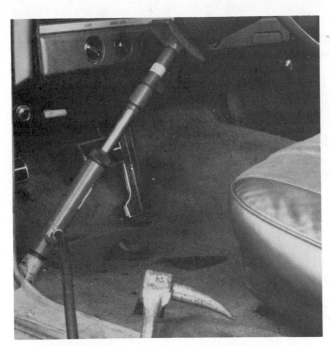

FIG. 7-67 Porto-power ram with extension tubing is positioned with the lower end on the driver's floorboard and the upper end low on the column.

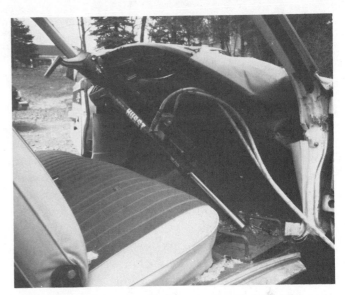

FIG. 7-68 Power ram is positioned to work from the passenger side rocker panel area to move the column. Columns *do not* always have to move forward, but they *must* move away from the trapped occupant.

floorboards onto the wood blocking below, which absorbs the reaction force.

A 7000-lb capacity mechanical jack can be used quite effectively for direct column lifting. The jack is brought into the passenger compartment, and the lifting toe of the jack is placed directly under the column and as low as possible. The handle of the jack faces the passenger side of the vehicle, leaving room for rescue personnel to operate it from this side. Rescuers should be aware that as the column moves, the toe of the jack may slip up the column into the driver's lap area. Due caution should be exercised.

A modification of this jack technique adds a short length of rescue chain to the evolution. In cases where the jack toe cannot be placed under the column for a direct push or lift, a loop of chain is formed low around the column. The toe of the jack is placed above the top of the column. The loop of chain that is around the column is then placed over the toe of the jack. While the jack operates, the toe lifts the small chain loop and the chain loop pulls the column up. Blocking is definitely required at the floorboards or under the vehicle for this technique.

Another technique uses a power rescue system spreader or ram or a porto-power tool (Fig. 7-67). With the spreader, the bottom tip of one arm is positioned to work from the driver side rocker panel at the junction of the "A" post or at a strong point on the passenger side floorboard area. The tip of the upper arm is placed at the proper low point on the column. While the arms open, the column is lifted up and toward the opposite side. As with the spreader, the power ram can be positioned to work from the rocker panel area to the column. The operation of either tool in this manner moves the column up and off to one side, away from the trapped patient (Fig. 7-68).

Some common problems are associated with this technique. As the column moves, the rescue tool has a tendency to slip, usually falling suddenly toward the driver's lap. The positioning of the driver can also increase the risks associated with this technique. The legs and feet of a driver trapped by the column may be extremely close to the column, leaving no safe working room for operation of the power rescue tools. If the trapped patient is in close proximity to the column and rescue personnel still desire to use a pushing or lifting tool, a sideways push coming from the passenger side rocker panel near the junction with the passenger side front "A" post may be the solution. Shorter length pushing or lifting tools that cannot reach the column from the passenger side rocker panel may be positioned to work off the transmission tunnel or hump at the floorboards. In front wheel drive automobiles in which a floorboard tunnel does not always exist, it may be possible to find an adequate push point at the front edge of a seat adjustment track. If the need arises and the front seats are bucket seat units, it may be possible to remove the entire passenger seat. With the seat gone, rescue personnel have a better chance of locating the pushing tool while they work from the passenger side to move the column up and to the driver's left.

When placing a pushing tool such as a ram, power spreader, or jack along either rocker panel area, rescuers must locate a suitable anchor point for the tool (Fig. 7-69). Good anchor points on most automobiles include the seat belt retractor mechanism and anchor bolt or the bottom edge of the "B" post. If the seat belt retractor unit is located on the front door as with some late model cars or the "B" post on the driver's side cannot be the anchor, rescue personnel must make their own base of support. A tool such as a power cutter, air chisel, air gun, or reciprocating saw tool can be used to remove a pie-shaped piece of the

rocker panel. Blocking must be placed directly under this cut area of the rocker panel between the vehicle and the ground. The base of the pushing tool can then be placed into the pie cut. The force of the tool as it operates compresses the cut area of the rocker panel, giving it the strength needed to accomplish the column movement. Caution is advisable whenever the driver side rocker panel area must be cut through because this area may contain fuel lines running from the tank to the engine.

Another way to produce a suitable anchor point is to use a power rescue spreader or cutter itself as the anchor point. With a power spreader, the unit is converted to a squeezer by closing the arms onto the driver side rocker panel at the desired push location. When a power cutter is being used as an anchor point, the tool would partially cut through the rocker panel area at the point where the anchor is needed. The cut-

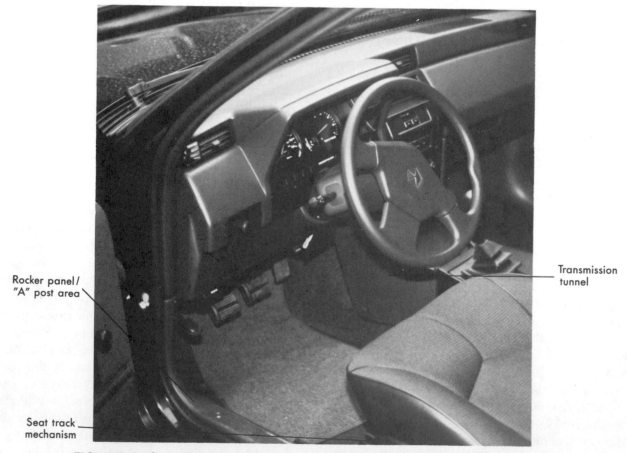

Rocker panel/
"A" post area

Transmission
tunnel

Seat track
mechanism

FIG. 7-69 Anchor points for tools that push directly against the steering column include the lower "A" post area, front of the front seat track mechanism, seatbelt anchor bolt or recoiler unit, and transmission tunnel area of floorboards.

ting action is then stopped, and the cutter unit acts as a stationary push point. The column-pushing tool (whatever it might be) is then placed against either the cutter or the spreader serving as the anchor point, and work is undertaken to move the column up and forward. Because this use can damage the anchor tool, it is not endorsed by all tool manufacturers. Each organization should therefore check with their particular manufacturer's representative before training in this technique. However, it is advisable for rescue personnel to know about the procedure in case it should be needed in a life-or-death situation, in which the urgency of the need would far outweigh the risk to the equipment.

When the steering column is pushed from inside, it is possible for the reaction force of the column moving to cause unwanted movement of portions of the vehicle. A common problem with this inside technique is that when the column moves away from the driver, the floorboard is actually pulled upward toward the driver. When the floor buckles, the roof may also be drawn inward and down into the passenger area. When lifting or pushing directly against a column, rescue personnel working the equipment and medical personnel attending to the trapped driver must constantly remain alert for structural vehicle movement. Rescue personnel should anticipate both the action and the reaction forces that can occur during the column evolution and move to disconnect the vehicle. Selected relief cuts must be made in its structural areas with saws, chisels, or power cutter units to allow the column to move without drawing portions of the vehicle into the passenger area. Ideal locations for weakening the structure of the car include cuts at the "A" post near the bottom front door hinge, the "A" post near the junction of the top of the dashboard, the floor sheet metal of the vehicle, and the vehicle's rocker panel.

Any tool used directly under the column for pushing or lifting can also be an obstruction when it is time to extricate the occupants. Therefore once the column is moved to the required position, additional steps must be taken to secure the column in the raised position. One way to allow for tool removal is to move the column past its intended position to allow for some slight return travel. Another quick way to secure the column in the raised position is to take a safety chain and secure the column to a solid point along the vehicle's front or outside structure (Fig. 7-70). A four footer can also be placed over the windshield above the column if the roof is still intact. The safety chain

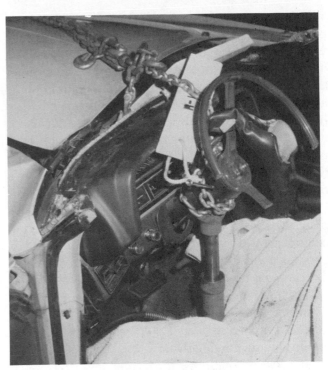

FIG. 7-70 Tool that moved a column now obstructs patient extrication pathway. A length of chain and chain binder tool across the front hood will maintain the column in position once the primary tool is removed.

can loop the column and the wood block. When the rescue equipment is released, the chain loads onto the four footer, holding the column in its raised position. The rescue equipment can then be removed, clearing the patient extrication pathway of any obstructions.

Although pushing or lifting the steering column from inside the vehicle may bring rescue personnel and operating tools close to injured patients, with proper safety precautions and a controlled, deliberate effort to operate safely, the inside push or lift technique of column movement is very effective.

STEERING COLUMN REMOVAL

The final method of releasing a person trapped by the steering column is to remove a portion of the column. Although it is the last to be discussed, this technique should by no means be the last to be tried at a rescue incident. The circumstances of each individual accident should determine the specific techniques that should or could be used. Column removal can be a very successful disentanglement technique when done *correctly*. If accomplished with improper tools or in an unsafe manner, this technique can also do more harm than good.

Column removal size up work begins with appropriate safety precautions taken. Initial setup follows with bending or removing the steering wheel. The initial setup work also includes having personnel attempt to expose the column housing and shaft assembly at a low point near the dashboard brace or bracket area. To accomplish this, rescuers may have to remove portions of the dashboard and instrument panel by manually pulling or breaking away the plastic components and cutting or sawing some of the other dashboard materials.

Once the column shaft has been exposed at a low point, it may be possible to remove portions of the column shroud that surrounds the shaft. Removing or bending away any of this thin-gauge metal decreases the amount of material that must be cut through during the removal process.

The steering column shaft on an automobile is generally made of ¾-inch cold-rolled steel. Rescue equipment for sawing through this shaft includes the hand hacksaw or the reciprocating saw (Fig. 7-71). The blades of the saw should be lubricated because the lubricant serves to cool the blade and aids in removing the cut particles. Sawing work can be done without lubrication, but the blade may wear out prematurely and the saw operator may experience greater difficulty.

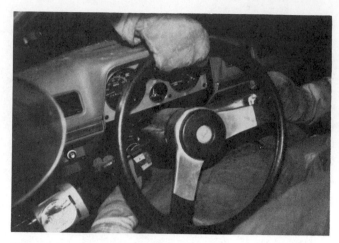

FIG. 7-72 The most efficient method of sawing through a column is to saw from the underside while applying a slightly forward pull from the top. Column will bend and break off before the saw cuts completely through the shaft, reducing the total time needed to complete the evolution.

Although not always possible, the most efficient method of cutting the column with a sawing tool is to start the cut on the underside of the column (Fig. 7-72). A second rescuer holds onto the top of the steering wheel ring, steadies the vibration of the column, and is responsible for applying a slight upward force. When applied properly, this upward force eases any binding of the saw in the cut. While the cutting proceeds along the underside of the column, the column begins to bend; when approximately 50% of the thickness of the shaft is cut through, the column can be bent upward. This moves the steering wheel and column away from the trapped occupants and may eliminate the need to completely cut the column shaft.

Use of a shearing action cutting tool is another removal option (Fig. 7-73). Generally accomplished with the cutter units of power rescue systems, this method has some serious safety concerns that must be fully understood. Some manufacturers of power rescue tools recommend against performing this task with their brand of power cutters. Cutting an object by shearing actually compresses a part of the object to the point at which a failure occurs: the object's shear point (Fig. 7-74). Rescue personnel using cutting tools must be aware of the distinct differences between shearing and sawing. Sawing is the removal of a selected portion of the object by the cutting action of serrated teeth on a saw blade. Sawing an object imparts only enough energy into the object being cut to warm the saw blade and the object on both sides of the cut itself.

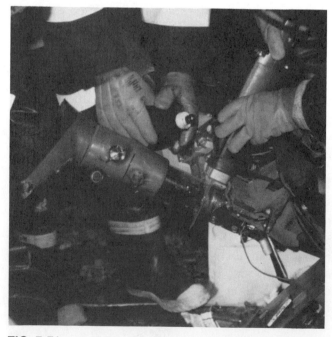

FIG. 7-71 A reciprocating saw severs the steering column housing and cold-rolled steel shaft. The blade needs lubrication with soapy water or lightweight oil during operation.

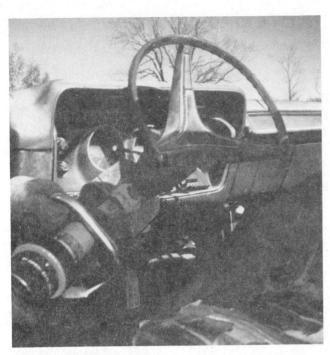

FIG. 7-73 Use of power cutter is to be employed as an option only if all conditions indicate this evolution and the patient is not close to the column.

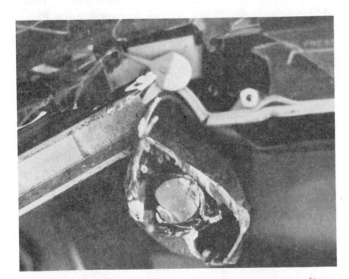

FIG. 7-74 Shearing action of power cutter units must be powerful enough to cut through sheet metal housing, inner wiring, and the solid center shaft.

However, cutting with a power rescue tool that works on the shearing principle can result in great amounts of energy being imparted to both the object being cut and the power tool doing the shearing. If the energy that builds up within the cutting tool is too

---

CHECKLIST FOR COLUMN REMOVAL

1. The manufacturer of a particular cutter tool approves of the use of the tool for cutting columns.
2. Rescue personnel are trained in operating the approved cutter tool in this removal evolution.
3. There is sufficient space to properly position and operate the cutter unit.
4. Trapped occupants are not in direct contact with any portion of the steering column, steering wheel ring, or any of the supporting spokes.
5. Trapped occupants can be well protected with covers and wooden boards.
6. The free end of the steering column can be restrained or captured as it is severed.
7. Any risk associated with this evolution can be justified as being worth the end result.

great, the tool or portions of it may fail. Shearing of an unsupported end, such as the steering column, may result in a sudden release of energy, causing the free end to launch itself at the instant of shearing. It is generally recommended not to use power cutters to completely cut through an object with an unsupported end.

Cutting the column off by use of a power rescue cutter tool may be next to impossible under actual field situations due to the positioning of an injured patient. The size of the cutting tool itself may prevent maneuvering it into the proper position for the cut. Even if the tool can be properly placed on the column shaft, the operation of the cutter may move it into a position that would compromise the patient's safety.

To improve safety and lessen the chance of an unsupported end becoming an unguided missile, rescue personnel should attempt to cut into the steering column shaft but not completely through it. By fatiguing it and creating a weak point, they may be able to bend it and break it off manually.

Shearing rescue tools should be used to remove the steering column of a vehicle only if *all* of the conditions in the above box are met.

With training in this evolution, rescue personnel will be prepared to work as safely as possible. Cutting a steering column with a power rescue tool cutter unit can be a risky evolution. The danger of injury to personnel may well be unjustified; a better, safer method to free a trapped occupant can often be found. Think twice about cutting columns in two with power cutters, then think again.

Summary of Column Movements

Each of the basic methods of disentangling persons trapped by steering columns affords the opportunity to use a great many different rescue techniques and a large variety of tools. Rescue personnel should be aware of each of the basic techniques, know a primary and a backup procedure for each, and practice it in training. Each technique should be practiced with the right tools for the assignment, both primary and backup. Only through this type of over-kill of redundancy rescue tools and techniques can safe and efficient rescue evolutions be achieved under real-world rescue conditions.

INTERIOR COMPONENT EVOLUTIONS
Pedal Evolutions

If the driver's feet are trapped by the clutch or brake pedals, moving or totally removing the pedal can free them of the entrapment. When confronted with this situation at an accident and using available vehicle rescue equipment, the rescuer, as a member of a two-person team, should be able to do the following:

- Recognize that a pedal entrapment situation presents an unsafe environment at the accident scene for the trapped and injured patient.
- Determine to what degree the pedal is contacting or trapping the vehicle occupant.
- Determine the presence of any safety problems or hazards that exist or may arise during the fulfillment of the pedal disentanglement evolution.
- Determine the most appropriate disentanglement tools, equipment, and techniques necessary for accomplishing the evolution.
- Safely and efficiently move the pedals as necessary in 2 minutes or less to allow for proper extrication of the patient, or safely and efficiently remove the pedals as necessary in 2 minutes or less to allow for proper extrication of the patient.

PEDAL ACCESS OPENING FROM EXTERIOR

Access to the patient's lower legs and feet area may be obstructed (Fig. 7-75). To determine the location of the extremities and the degree of entrapment, rescuers may need to gain access to the floorboard and pedal area directly through exterior portions of the vehicle. This can be accomplished by strategically cutting and spreading an opening in the exterior to provide physical or visual contact with the pedals themselves.

The most direct access pathway from outside the

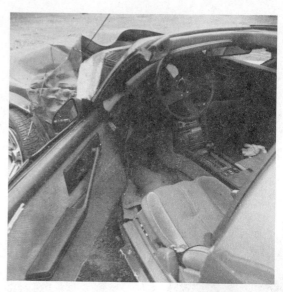

FIG. 7-75 T-bone collision with power pole has crushed the passenger leg and foot area. Under these accident conditions, access to the trapped driver's lower extremities will be severely obstructed.

vehicle to the pedal area can be gained by opening up the vehicle's front quarter panel area on the driver's side. Located behind the front wheelwell and in front of the front door hinge area, this area is actually an end of the vehicle's firewall structure. A five-door evolution can be accomplished, completely removing the "A" post or firewall structure, or an opening can simply be made through all layers of material in this vicinity. Beginning from the outside, rescue personnel must first make an opening in the outer fender and quarter panel skin (Fig. 7-76) or remove that portion of the fender completely. The front door does not necessarily have to be opened for this evolution to be done. If the door is opened, however, it is beneficial to consider removing the door completely because this opening will then provide unrestricted access to the exterior quarter panel area.

Penetration of the outer skin exposes the interior structure of the vehicle. Rescuers will find metal bracing and reinforcement material, as well as a relatively heavy-gauge metal firewall area. The inner skin may have a louvered vent opening for fresh air intake into the lower passenger compartment area, particularly if the vehicle is not equipped with air conditioning. If this vent opening is present, personnel can forcibly remove the louvered cover to gain quick access to the pedal area. If no vent is present, efforts must be undertaken to penetrate and remove the inner firewall and decorative plastic trim of the

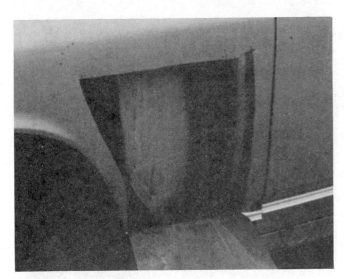

FIG. 7-76 Removal of outer fender skin front quarter-panel area is an initial step in gaining access to the pedal area from outside the vehicle.

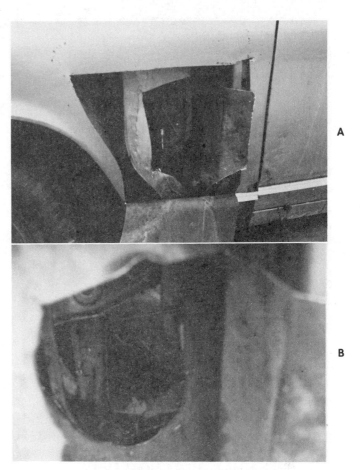

FIG. 7-77 A, Opening of inner firewall and fender area followed by removal of the air vent duct. **B,** This action yields direct access to the area where the patient's feet and legs may be trapped.

vehicle to provide access to the pedal area (Fig. 7-77). Extreme caution must be exercised in the final stages of this evolution to prevent any direct contact with the trapped patient.

In most entrapment situations, access to the pedal area from either the outside or the interior of the vehicle is readily available to rescue personnel that then have a multitude of tools and techniques available to move the offending pedal. A clutch or brake pedal assembly consists of a solid metal shaft with the foot pad welded perpendicular to it. The pedal's design gives it a relative degree of strength when moving front to rear but makes it considerably weaker when stressed sideways. This weakness is an advantage when rescuers must move the pedal.

Force can be applied either against the pedal directly or by a remote means. Direct force requires positioning sufficiently small rescue equipment inside the vehicle to push or lift the offending pedal free from the patient. Remote movement of a pedal (the more realistic evolution) requires securing rope, strap, or chain to the pedal and operating pulling or lifting equipment. The pull can be by manual means or from a rescue vehicle winch, a tow truck cable, a power spreader, a come-along tool, air bags or cushions, or mechanical or hydraulic jacks. The rope, strap, or chain at the pedal must be adequately secured to the shaft of the pedal. An additional wrap around the foot pad will improve the efficiency of this evolution, although this is not always possible due to the location of the patient's legs and feet.

After being securely fastened to the pedal, the pulling line should pass from underneath the bottom side of the pedal foot pad. This positioning maximizes the mechanical advantage when a sufficient force is applied. Remaining setup procedures and equipment positions for pedal pulling resemble those of the steering column movement evolution. In fact, Holmatro, Inc. has developed a device trademarked as their Rescue Boot that is specifically designed to move the steering column, steering wheel, and offending pedal in one operation with only one pulling or lifting tool placed in service.

Among the many available possibilities for using rescue equipment to move the pedal, the simplest and most effective evolution involves a strong rope or strap and a tug-of-war pull by rescue personnel themselves. A 12- to 15-foot length of ½-inch diameter or larger rope or 1-inch wide strapping is first secured to

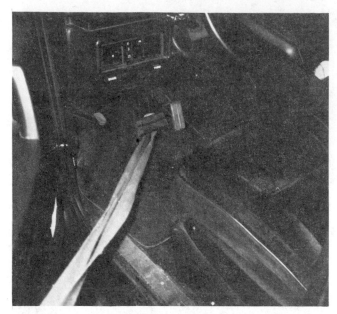

FIG. 7-78 Pedal can be moved away from the column by positioning a rope or strap securely around the pedal shaft and footpad and then exerting pull from an angle.

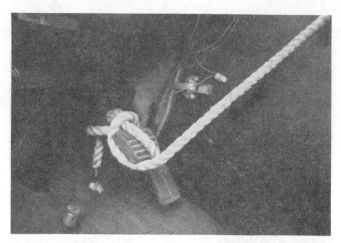

FIG. 7-79 Tug-of-war evolution will lift pedal if a rope or strap is secured to the pedal shaft and positioned to pull from underside of the pedal footpad.

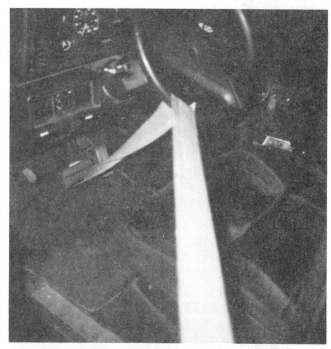

FIG. 7-80 Running a strap or rope through the lower portion of the steering wheel ring allows rescuers to pull the strap from the side of the vehicle while actual lifting the pedal. One rescuer must steady the steering wheel ring as the pulling effort is initiated.

the pedal shaft and the foot pad, passing under the pedal if possible. Several rescue crew members properly position themselves and exert a steady pull on the rope, thus developing a side stress on the pedal shaft (Fig. 7-78). This force will cause the pedal and its shaft to bend, moving it away from the trapped occupant. It is very important that this pull be directed at moving the pedal away from the steering column shaft. It is not possible to bend the pedal shaft around the steering column by brute force.

If a rope is to be used for pedal pulling, the placement of large knots at 16- to 18-inch intervals along most of the length of the rope will enable rescue personnel to obtain firm grips when pulling. It is also possible to increase the mechanical advantage of the evolution by securing the equipment to the latch end of an operable door; opening the door exerts a pull on the pedal. In lieu of a door, a long pry bar, mechanical jack, or other lifting tool can be positioned horizontally, working off the rocker panel to provide the pulling force.

Using the same tug-of-war technique, rescuers can lift the pedal away from the patient. If a rope is to be used, the rope is secured to the pedal (Fig. 7-79) and then laced through a portion of the steering wheel ring before going to the outside of the vehicle (Fig. 7-80). When the rescuers exert a pulling force, they are in the same position as before, but the forces against the

pedal change. While the rope pivots about the steering wheel ring, the lifting force is sufficient to pop the pedal upward. An additional crew member is necessary in this evolution to steady the steering wheel while the pull is being accomplished.

If pedal movement is not possible, removal can

generally be accomplished with the application of sawing tools. Power cutting or shearing equipment can only be used for this task if it can be guaranteed that the unsupported pedal *will not* fly about as it is cut and if there is sufficient room to operate these larger tools without injury to the patient.

Dashboard Evolutions

During a head-on collision between two vehicles or a vehicle and a stationary object, the front of the vehicle is deformed. The greater the vehicle collision speeds, the greater the momentum released during the collision. Greater momentum moves more portions of the vehicle in front of the occupants rearward while the rear portions of the vehicle crush forward. If front seat passengers are unrestrained at the moment of collision, they are propelled forward, their legs bend, and their bodies momentarily move off the front seat. Depending upon the energy involved in the collision and the relative size and weight of the individuals, their knees tuck toward their chest as they crush into the floorboard area under the dashboard and glove compartment. This is known as *submarining* of the front seat passengers. Their entrapment may be simply from contact with the glove compartment and the outer areas of the dashboard, or they may be totally crushed within the structure of the dashboard and firewall. Their mid to lower torso area and lower extremities are most commonly pinned. Under collision circumstances such as these, those inside the vehicle are truly caught in the middle.

When confronted with an entrapment situation and using vehicle rescue equipment as necessary, the rescuer, working as a member of a two-person team, should be able to do the following:

- Recognize that the patient or patients are trapped by the dashboard and firewall structures and the environment at the accident scene is unsafe for these trapped individuals.
- Determine the extent of dashboard and firewall entrapment.
- Determine the presence of any safety problems or hazards that exist or may arise during the fulfillment of the dashboard evolution.
- Determine the most appropriate tools, equipment, and techniques necessary for accomplishing the dashboard and firewall movement evolution.
- Safely and efficiently move the dashboard and firewall structure of a vehicle away from individuals trapped by them in 5 minutes or less.

Two vehicle rescue evolutions that release trapped front seat occupants involve moving or removing the dashboard. Although the goal of both evolutions is to disentangle the trapped patients from the collapsed structure pinning them, each is based on two completely different rescue strategies.

When a conservative rescue strategy is indicated (as with a relatively simple entrapment incident), the rescue officer decides that it is necessary to move or remove only a portion of the dashboard. This simple objective is met by either disassembling components of the dash, lifting the lower portions of the dash structure, or pulling the dash forward in a fashion similar to steering-column movement.

The components of the dash are generally plastic, cardboard, or styrofoam and contain small wires and lightweight metal framing. This makes disassembly possible with hand or power tools that can cut, pry, or disconnect. Necessary patient protection includes use of wood shortboard or longboard devices for insulation and covering with blankets or tarps.

Lifting of the lower portions of the dash on either side of the vehicle can best be accomplished by positioning the working end of mechanical or hydraulic lifting or spreading equipment on the bottom of the dashboard at the very inside edge of the front "A" posts. The only substantial metal frame component of the dashboard is located in this area (Fig. 7-81). A lift properly applied directly at this point will generally move the dashboard more than 50% of its length. The base of the lifting tool rests on either the floorboard or rocker panel area. To ensure that this area is solid enough to support the stress of the lift, rescuers should position cribbing directly under the tool or underneath the floorboards of the vehicle. The vehicle will settle onto the blocking under the vehicle while the load is applied from the tool.

The dashboard on the passenger's side can also be pulled up and away from trapped patients by treating it much like a steering column. With the patient properly protected, a long pry bar tool can be used to open a hole down through the dashboard, initially pushing through the defroster vent feature of the dash. The bar then moves through the dash components and breaks out of the dash at the bottom of the glove compartment. Caution must be exercised during these setup procedures because of the close proximity of the patient. Rescue chain of suitable size and rating to work safely with a 2- to 3-ton pulling force is laced down through this dash opening, passed completely under the dash and glove compartment structure, and

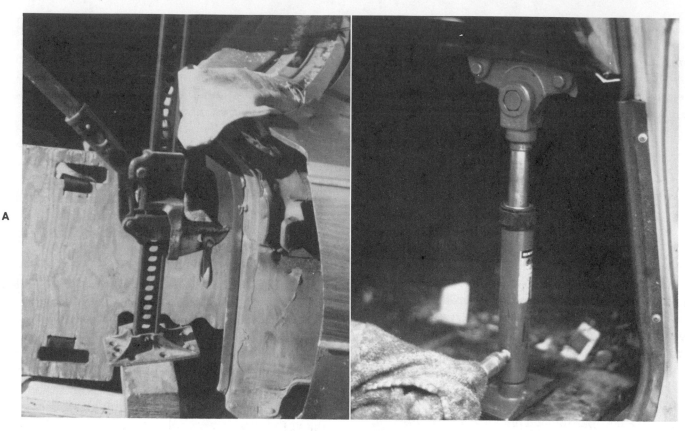

A   B

FIG. 7-81 The dashboard can be lifted by applying force from **A,** a mechanical jack or **B,** a porto-power and wide-angle head attachment.

joined back onto itself. This forms a loop of chain that can be pulled forward or lifted by using procedures similar to those of steering column evolutions (Fig. 7-82).

A recently developed dashboard disentanglement evolution uses modern rescue equipment to its fullest advantage. Its aggressive strategy is designed to solve several entrapment problems simultaneously. In this evolution, *total dashboard and firewall movement* can be accomplished as a major effort is undertaken to literally break the vehicle into distinct front and rear sections. The patient remains stationary while the sections of the vehicle are disconnected. This total dash movement is simultaneous with movement of the steering wheel, column, pedals, and the bottom sections of the "A" post. To set up for this evolution, rescuers must first accomplish complete stabilization of the vehicle, with particular attention paid to the rocker panel area between the "A" and "B" posts. Both front doors must be opened and widened or removed. In addition, the patient must be properly immobilized and all those inside insulated from the work that is to be accomplished.

Rescue equipment capable of cutting into the relatively heavy-gauge metal of the rocker panel, firewall, and roof posts must be available. This can include power cutter units, air chisels, air guns, reciprocating saws, or manual sheet metal cutters. Specific relief cuts provide for separating or disconnecting the structural areas of the vehicle (Fig. 7-83). The roof is disconnected from the lower portions of the vehicle by cutting through the "A" posts at the dashboard level and is then either flipped rearward or removed entirely. The floorboard area of the vehicle is separated from the firewall and "A" post by either slicing horizontally into the "A" post just above or below the lower door hinge area or cutting vertically into the rocker panel immediately next to the base of the "A" post. Cutting horizontally into the lower "A" post area typically allows the dash and firewall structure to be lifted or rolled forward. Cutting vertically into the rocker panel along the front door area typically separates or stretches the vehicle while the dash and firewall structure are pushed. If small-size rescue equipment that has a relatively short opening or spreading distance is used, the preliminary cuts should

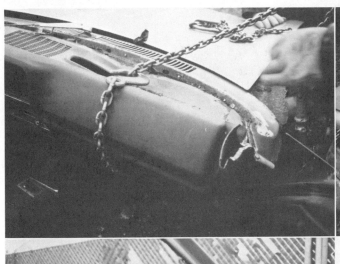
A

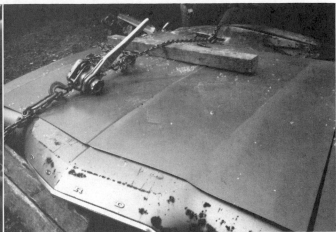
B

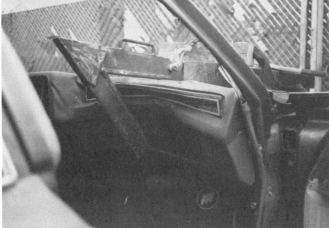
C

FIG. 7-82 A, Pulling of a dashboard can be achieved in much the same manner as pulling a steering column. When wrapping chain, rescuers must push the chain through the defroster area first and then bring it around the dashboard from the underside. **B,** If the chain has been wrapped through the dash properly, the come-along will crush and lift the dashboard up and away from the patient area. **C,** Homemade dash pulling hook is most effective when there is insufficient working room to secure the chain completely around and through the dash.

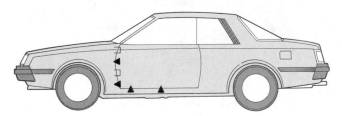

FIG. 7-83 Relief cuts must be made at strategic points before the dashboard and firewall structure can be moved forward (*rolling*) or lifted upward (*jacking*).

be made horizontally into the "A" post below the hinge. This is the five-door area described earlier. The equipment is then placed in the pie-shaped cut to act as a firewall jack. While the unit opens or spreads vertically, the "A" posts, five-door area, and dashboard are lifted. While the end of the firewall moves on the driver's side of the vehicle, the steering wheel, column, and pedals also move up and away from the passenger area (Fig. 7-84). Power ratings of 5 tons or more are required for each side of the evolution. The spread or push distance necessary depends on the location of the relief cuts, the position of the vehicle

and its occupants, and the extent of collision damage.

If available rescue equipment can open over a long spread or push distance (up to or exceeding 60 inches), the equipment can be angled to not only lift the dashboard but actually roll the dash and firewall forward. A suitable base area must be located along the rocker panel near the base of the "B" post. Rescue personnel may have to reinforce this base area to support the forces applied while the rescue equipment operates. A suitable anchor point can be created along the rocker panel if there is no natural push point by using the cutter as a clamp or the spreader as a squeezer or by opening a pie-shaped cut in the rocker panel structure. Mechanical or hydraulic equipment is then positioned to contact either the top front door hinge-mount area or the "A" post near the top of the dash (Fig. 7-85), or equipment is placed directly on the dashboard or steering column. Equipment to perform this task must again have a power rating of 5 tons or more and a long spread distance. Hydraulic ram units of power rescue systems are most effective in accomplishing this pushing and spreading evolution. With

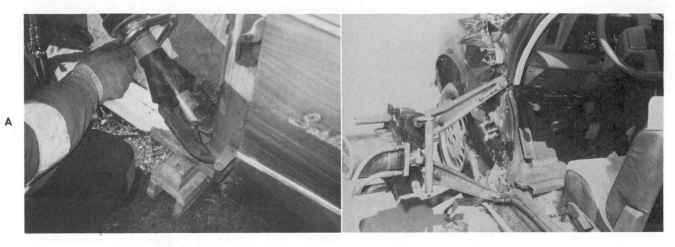

FIG. 7-84 A, Power cutter is disconnecting structural areas of the vehicle low along the "A" post in preparation for a dash lift evolution. **B,** Power spreader used to lift the dashboard and firewall structure in a jacking evolution.

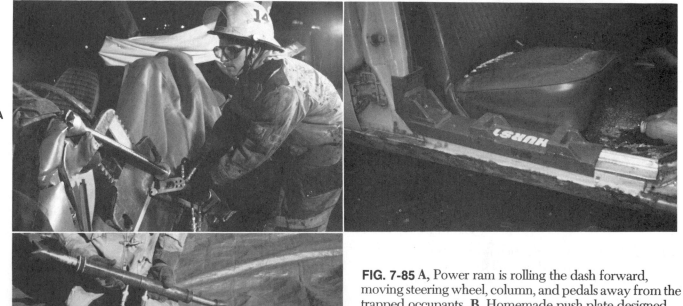

FIG. 7-85 A, Power ram is rolling the dash forward, moving steering wheel, column, and pedals away from the trapped occupants. **B,** Homemade push plate designed to support pushing tool as dash moves forward is in place. The plate straddles the rocker panel and braces off the lower portion of the "B" post. Note the presence of several notches to position the pushing tool to its best advantage. **C,** Dash can also be moved forward with mechanical jacks or a porto-power tool. Twin porto-power rams and pumps supply additional travel distance during the pushing evolution.

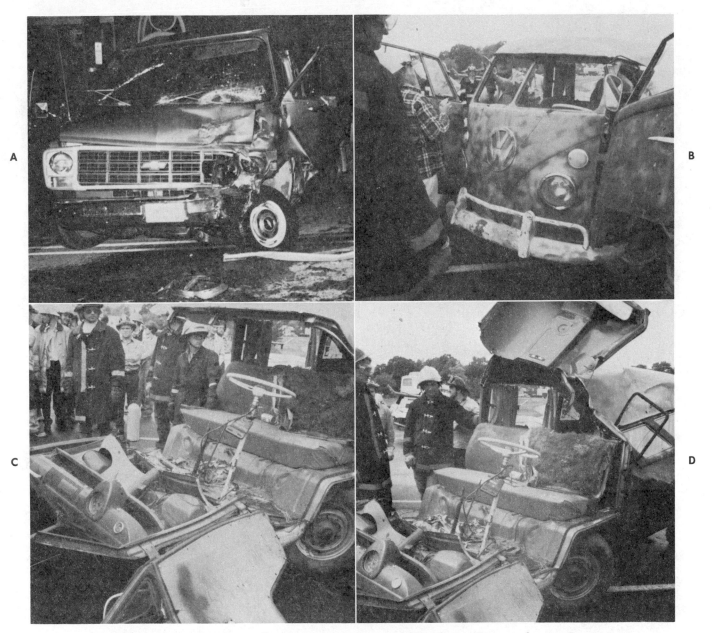

FIG. 7-86 A, A head-on collision presents rescue problems for occupants of a van. It may require moving the steering column, pedals, floorboards, dash, doors, and "A" post structure. Dash and firewall movement evolution is well suited for these situations. **B,** Disconnecting begins by stabilizing the vehicle, opening doors, and cutting through "A" posts at the top and bottom. **C,** Rolling the dashboard and firewall forward provides increased access to front seat occupants. **D,** Additional working room is provided by roof removal above the patient area.

their powerful pushing capacities and their ability to extend up to 5 feet or more, the rams can quickly and efficiently disconnect the vehicle.

Simultaneous dash movement from both sides of the vehicle is a new and important disentanglement evolution. Equipment is again positioned and operated simultaneously at each end of the firewall and dashboard. The front grille and headlight area of the vehicle is nosed downward to the point where it is touching the ground in front of the vehicle. Simultaneous pushing action moves the complete front end of the vehicle and all its components away from the trapped occupants in one smooth, efficient motion (Fig. 7-86). Blocking is then placed in the newly opened area at the "A" post or rocker panel to secure portions of the vehicle in their new position.

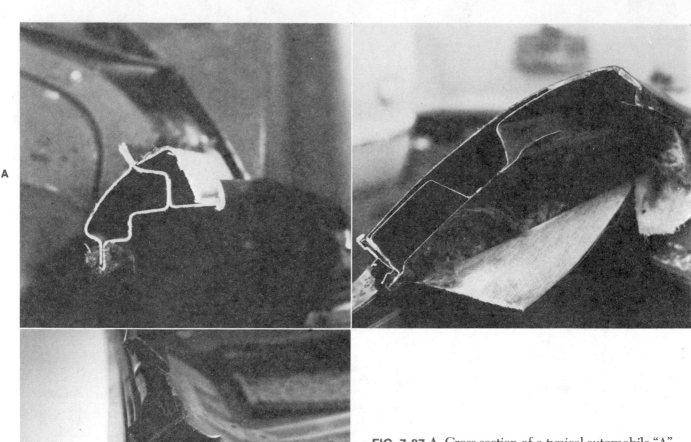

FIG. 7-87 **A,** Cross section of a typical automobile "A" post. The lowest area may be thicker due to overlapping of metal where the post joins to the firewall structure. **B,** Cross section of automobile "C" post reveals multiple layers of metal that are corrogated for strength. **C,** Detailed view of the rain gutter area of the roof.

ROOF EVOLUTIONS

Rescue evolutions that involve the roof of a vehicle range from moving or removing a portion of the roof to total removal of the roof structure itself. Each evolution has its proper time and place in the realm of vehicle rescue, and each is designed to accomplish a specific goal. Total roof removal is the least appreciated yet possibly the most important rescue evolution available to operating personnel today. A close and honest look at today's vehicles will confirm that the length, diameter, and total mass of material making up a roof post is diminishing (Fig. 7-87). The huge roof pillars of the "iron" cars of yesterday are disappearing at the same time that contemporary rescue equipment

and techniques are increasing our abilities to cut through roof post structures rapidly.

Unfortunately, many people in the rescue and medical service have resisted realizing their true rescue potential when it comes to roof evolutions. Too often in the past, rescuers struggled to extricate a patient from a wreck because they were hesitant to damage the vehicle any more than it already was by removing a portion of the roof. Medical personnel laboring under a crushed vehicle roof to immobilize injured patients inside increase their overall operating time and sacrifice the quality of their patient care (Fig. 7-88). In essence the vehicle has been allowed to work against ongoing efforts to produce a successful rescue. The vehicle rescue philosophy today must be rededi-

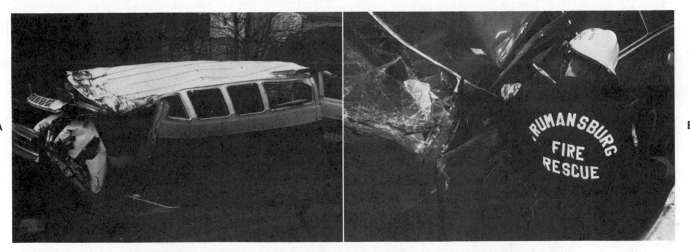

FIG. 7-88 A, Six teenagers died on high school graduation day when their van rolled over. Two fatalities occurred when the front seat occupants were pinned between the top of the seats and the underside of the roof. **B,** A crushed roof complicates patient access. A medic works to determine the status of a trapped patient.

cated to removing the vehicle from the victim before the victim is removed from the vehicle. More than any other single task rescue personnel can perform, roof removal is *the* rescue evolution that provides maximum access to the interior areas of a damaged vehicle and the patients located there.

When confronted with an entrapment situation at a vehicle accident and using vehicle rescue equipment as necessary, the rescuer, working as a member of a three-person team, should be able to do the following:

- Recognize that the damaged roof of the vehicle presents an unsafe and inefficient working environment for medical and rescue personnel at the accident scene.
- Determine whether the damaged roof should be moved, partially removed, or totally removed.
- Determine the presence of any safety problems that exist or may arise during the fulfillment of the roof evolution.
- Determine the most appropriate rescue tools, equipment, and techniques for accomplishing the desired roof evolution assignment.
- Safely and efficiently perform the desired roof evolution in 4 minutes or less.

Collapsed Roof Evolution

It may be necessary for rescue personnel to raise a portion of a collapsed roof. Mechanical, air-powered, or hydraulic-lifting or spreading equipment with a rated capacity in excess of 4000 lb is necessary to complete the evolution. Rescue personnel should take advantage of existing damage to the roof when placing their equipment. Just as repetitive bending weakens a wire, the part of the crushed roof that has bent the most becomes the weakest. A force applied at this point will yield the most efficient results. An alternative to lifting a crushed roof is removal of the collapsed portion. This can be accomplished with cutting or sawing rescue equipment.

Three-Sided Sunroof Evolution

The three-sided sunroof opening has its roots in the early days of vehicle rescue. Designed primarily for use when a vehicle is on its edge, this evolution uses sheet metal cutting equipment to open the individual layers of metal skin of the roof. The sides, edges, and posts of the roof are generally not cut during this assignment. In its day, this rescue evolution was a fairly revolutionary method of patient access. Its development came about at a time when the air chisel tool had just become available to vehicle rescue personnel; it was the most sophisticated piece of rescue equipment then in use. Early air chisels could cut through the sheet metal skin with amazing speed as compared to the speed of the crude hand tools of the 1960s rescue era. The major problems that accompanied air chisel use, which are still a concern today, were the high noise and vibration levels transmitted throughout the vehicle as the air chisel operated.

The change in production technology produced the dual-layer sheet metal roof. Still used today on certain

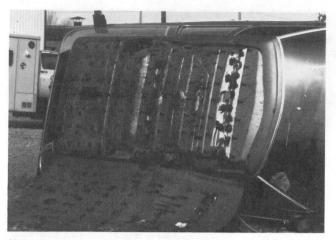

FIG. 7-89 The manufacture of vehicles with double solid layers of sheet metal in their roof structures makes the sunroof opening evolution more difficult and time consuming.

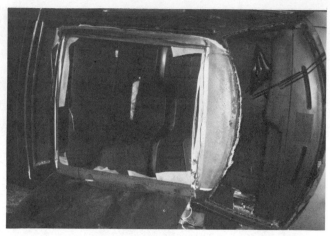

FIG. 7-90 Final result of a three-sided sunroof evolution yields an opening with all exposed, sharp metal edges made safe by taping or tarping.

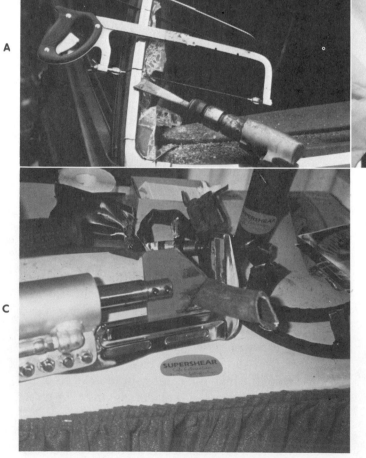

FIG. 7-91 A, Examples of tools that will cut through roof posts or a rain gutter include a standard hacksaw, carbide rod saw, or air chisel. **B,** Examples of patient insulation during roof post cut include a soft cover wool blanket and a rigid cover wooden shortboard. **C,** A new addition to the power rescue tool family is the Super Shear, a unit designed to sever metal with a moving blade functioning like a ram on a miniature log splitter machine.

vehicles, this manufacturing technique joins two distinct layers of sheet metal to compose the roof structure. The layers are bonded together with a strong adhesive compound, which doubles the time needed to do the sunroof evolution with sheet metal cutting equipment (Fig. 7-89). For effective sunroof evolutions, rescue personnel must also remove roof-framing members that may inhibit patient extrication (Fig. 7-90). In a recent accident involving a mini van that had rolled onto its driver side, all occupants were extricated safely through the large opening created by rescue personnel. With the latest generation plastic-bodied mini vans, opening a plastic roof may be an easy and relatively rapid evolution.

Progressive rescue personnel rarely consider the sunroof evolution. It has little merit on today's downsized automobile rescue environment and has largely been replaced by partial or total roof removal procedures. These evolutions take less time to complete, are less disturbing to the injured patient, and permit a safer and more efficient extrication.

Flip-Top-Box Roof Opening

When rescue personnel cut through the two front "A" posts of a vehicle and make cuts through the edges of the roofline, they are able to completely remove the front portion of the roof above the patient area. This evolution is referred to as the *flip-top-box* or *roof-flapping* evolution. The complete front roof structure and the layers of metal composing the roof are lifted and completely flipped rearward. Preparation work that must precede flipping a roof includes patient insulation, tempered glass removal, and complete severing of the seat belt shoulder harness strapping. The windshield may be removed first or flipped with the roof.

Cutting equipment for flipping a roof includes hand hacksaws, reciprocating saws, air chisels, air guns, and power rescue system cutter units (Fig. 7-91). The front roof posts should be cut completely through at a point relatively close to the top surface of the dashboard. When the roof section is flipped, the major portion of the post moves with the roof, away from the patient work area. The cuts along the roofline must be at approximately the same point on each side of the vehicle. Rescue personnel must size up the situation to determine the most appropriate location for these cuts, which *must* be made completely through the shaped metal channel composing the structural frame edge of the roof. These cuts should also be planned to avoid cutting into roof-mounted seat belt recoiler units

or belt attachment bolts. The location will vary depending on whether the vehicle is a two-door or four-door model, the amount of vehicle damage, the vehicle resting position, and the location and extent of entrapment of the patients inside. The edge cuts, which become the hinge when the roof is flipped, should be made as far to the rear of the roofline as possible without becoming bogged down in the structure of the "C" post. The largest possible portion of roof can then be flipped clear of the patient work area.

If the vehicle is a four-door model, the "B" posts are attached and will limit the size of the roof that can be flipped. The solution is to incorporate a "B" post evolution along with the flip-top-box assignment. While the cutting work is being accomplished, the top of each "B" post should be cut through relatively close to the roofline. After the "A" post and roof edge cuts are finished, the roof can be flipped rearward, and a wide body "B" post evolution can follow. These posts and any attached side doors are either moved down and outward or completely removed from the vehicle, providing maximum access (Fig. 7-92).

Once roof and post cuts have been made, the front portion of the roof must be flipped. Rescuers must fold the sheet metal top of the roof like a hinge. This roof area often buckles upward because of the compression forces generated by the impact, hindering or even preventing the flipping of the roof. Rescue personnel have several options available to them for making the metal hinge function as needed. If the roof is only slightly bowed, personnel may be able to place a pike pole or long-length cribbing block across the roof at the point where the hinge is needed. A steady downward pressure may buckle the sheet metal enough to allow the roof to flip. In severe buckling situations, the sheet metal may have to be cut completely open in a line from one roof edge cut to the other. This complete separation of the sheet metal makes the flipping work progress smoothly. Personnel should *not* take an axe or Halligan forcible entry tool and slam it across the roof. This is a dangerous act that causes unwarranted distress to the patient and medics inside the vehicle.

Mandatory safety work that must follow the flip-top-box roof evolution includes taping or tarping the exposed sheet metal edges left by the cuts and immediately securing the roof in its flipped position. Tying off with a rope or strap can reduce the likelihood of the roof section moving back toward its original position. To prevent any problems, rescuers must secure the roof.

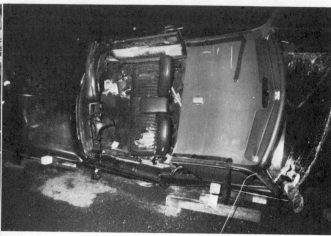

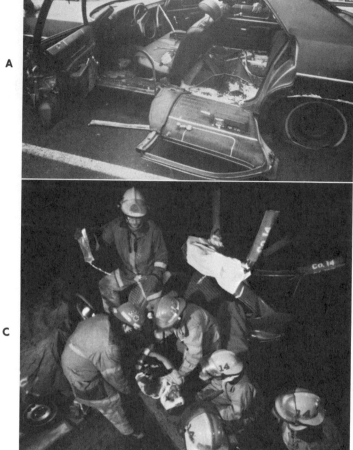

FIG. 7-92 A, Flip-top-box assignment combined with a wide body evolution results in a more efficient extrication pathway for an occupant trapped in the driver's seat area. **B,** It is possible to perform this evolution with a vehicle on its side as long as the roofline is not in contact with the ground. **C,** Roof evolution is not considered complete until exposed metal cuts have been taped or tarped and the roof secured in the flipped position.

A-B-C Evolution

The A-B-C evolution involves cutting completely through all roof posts on just one side of the vehicle. If the accident vehicle has been stabilized on its side, this evolution provides improved patient access, facilitating patient extrication.

The presence of a pressurized or compressed lifting cylinder typically near the "C" post of an automobile and the "D" post of a mini van must be investigated (Fig. 7-93). The cylinders of hatchback vehicles and the lifter assemblies on large-size tailgates present serious safety concerns when cutting evolutions take place near them. In some cases the cylinder can be quickly and safely removed from its mounting bolt or knob. A hatchback or tailgate can also be opened before the cutting of rear posts, reducing the compressive forces of the lifting cylinder.

Rescue equipment capable of cutting through the roof posts is necessary for the A-B-C cutting operation. Power rescue system cutters with a relatively small cutter blade opening may have difficulty completely cutting through a large-size rear post. There are several methods by which these large posts can be attacked with the power cutters. The first few cuts can remove a pie-shaped piece of the roof post, allowing the cutting tool to move deeper into the throat of the vee cut, penetrating further into the post itself. A series of cuts made into the post from the front may be joined by cuts made from the rear side, completely severing it. Another method involves making a continuous cut with the power cutter by sinking one blade of the tool down through the cut and closing the top blade down through the post. Continuous cutting allows the post to be completely severed.

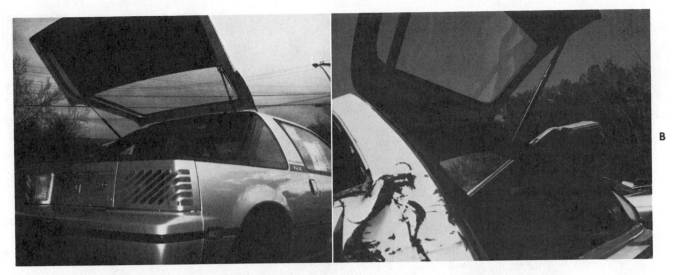

FIG. 7-93 **A** and **B**, Vehicles such as mini vans, hatchbacks, and station wagons must have rear hatches opened before total roof removal. Cutting into or through a pressurized lift cylinder can be like the explosive release of a jack-in-the-box.

One of the most effective cutting tools for severing any and all vehicle roof posts is the reciprocating saw. When equipped with a bimetal, break-resistant saw blade at least 6-inches long and used by a competent operator, this tool will slice smoothly through the large roof post in one steady cutting motion. If manual or air-powered sheet metal cutting equipment is to be used to cut roof posts, the mass of the post should first be reduced. Trim material, even inner layers of light-weight metal, should be pried off where possible before the cutting is started. The thick posts should have portions individually cut away, starting with the outside layer and working through the reinforced intermediate structure to the innermost layer of the post.

Air-powered cutting tools used to cut through a roof post must be used with the appropriate flat chisel bit in place. The tool operator should continually work the chisel bit around the exterior of the post as much as possible, pressing the tool into the post during the operation. This action slices the post equally from all sides and will accomplish the cutting task quickly. Burying the chisel bit into the post from just one attack point may not be successful because the mass of metal being cut may bunch up, resisting the cutting effort of the chisel. The chisel bit is also very susceptible to jamming deep into the cut in the post when forced in this manner.

Rescue personnel operating with Amkus power rescue spreaders are advised by the manufacturer that they can use the arms of their spreader tool as squeezers. In this case the arms of the tool are opened and placed so that they straddle the entire rear post. While the arms close, the structure of the "C" post is compressed from front to back, making cutting through the post easier because of the narrower shape. Crews operating with power rescue spreaders should check with their factory representatives for the appropriate endorsement before operating their equipment in this way.

Unlike any other roof post cut evolution, when performing an A-B-C cut on the top side of a vehicle stabilized on edge, rescuers should cut the posts at the roofline. This allows the major portion of the roof post to remain out of the way as the entire roof structure is laid down to the ground (Fig. 7-94).

Total Roof Removal Evolution

The final roof evolution is that of total roof structure removal. This task is simply an extension of the A-B-C evolution, although all roof posts are cut through at approximately dashboard level. The entire roof structure and all roof posts are removed simultaneously, making the accident vehicle resemble a convertible. When cutting all roof posts, rescuers should cut through the largest rear "C" posts first. Keeping the other posts intact helps to steady the roof structure during the evolution. Once all seat belts and any electric wires running through the roof posts or structure have been cut through, the roof can be lifted and moved off the vehicle (Fig. 7-95). This evolution also requires concern for the presence of compressed lifting cylinders and necessitates the taping or tarping of

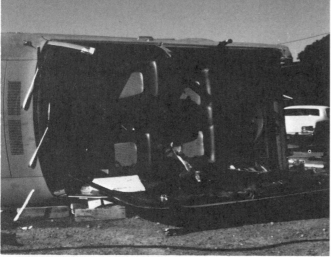

FIG. 7-94 **A,** A-B-C roof cut evolution with a vehicle on edge is the one time that posts should be cut near rain gutter/roof channel area. **B,** As roof structure is moved away from patients, the long top side roof posts remain high and out of the way of rescuers and the patient below. **C,** Safety work for A-B-C roof evolution involves taping or tarping all exposed sharp metal edges and insulating the patient.

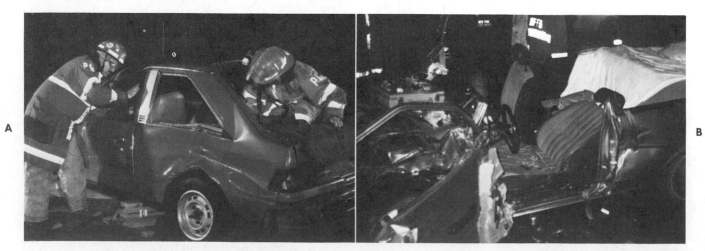

FIG. 7-95 **A,** Roof structures present the largest obstacle to having sufficient space to access and stabilize patients. **B,** Serious trauma injuries and entrapment can make rapid patient extrication a lifesaving evolution. Total roof removal permitted rescue crews to longboard this trauma patient out over the back of the front seat.

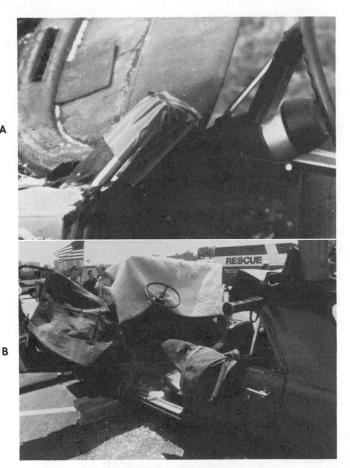

FIG. 7-96 A, Front "A" posts do not have to be cut flush with the dashboard if they are taped before patient extrication. **B,** All sharp metal cuts must be taped or tarped to prevent injuries to operating personnel or patients during the rescue process. This demonstration reveals the value of heavy canvas salvage covers or furniture blankets used by moving companies.

all the exposed metal cuts (Fig. 7-96). The roof shell that is removed should be placed in an appropriate location and with the cut roof posts facing the ground. Total roof removal is an extremely valuable rescue evolution because it allows for total access to the passenger compartment. Consideration should be given to fulfilling this important evolution early in a rescue incident.

VEHICLE SEAT EVOLUTIONS

Many interior components of a vehicle can and do come in contact with vehicle occupants during a collision. Of all the interior components, it is the seat that remains in the most direct contact with the patient

after the collision has occurred. For this reason, evolutions involving the seat of a damaged vehicle require a coordinated rescue and medical effort and high regard for some important safety considerations.

Although rescue personnel must be fully capable of moving or removing any vehicle seat the state of the art in vehicle rescue today is to do whatever is possible to leave the patient as the central focus area and *not* move the seat. The object is to move the necessary portions of the vehicle away from the patient while keeping the patient in a fixed location. Moving a seat holding an injured patient can both cause additional patient injuries and aggravate existing injuries, especially of the spinal column. Even when the patients are immobilized and attended to by EMS personnel, erratic movement of seats can quickly and needlessly compromise their medical condition.

When confronted with an entrapment situation at a vehicle accident scene and using vehicle rescue equipment as necessary, the rescuer, as a member of a two-person team, should be able to do the following:

- Recognize whether the location of an automobile seat presents an unsafe situation for the patient or an inefficient working environment for medical and rescue personnel at the accident scene.
- Determine to what degree the seat in its present location is restricting the extrication of the trapped patient.
- Determine to what degree the seat should be moved or removed or whether other evolutions are more appropriate for accomplishing the desired overall rescue strategy.
- Determine the presence of any safety problems or hazards that exist or may arise during a seat-movement evolution.
- Determine the most appropriate vehicle rescue tools, equipment, and techniques necessary for accomplishing the specific seat evolution.
- Safely and efficiently perform the desired seat evolution in 3 minutes or less.

Vehicle rescue evolutions that involve working with the automobile seat include forward or rearward movement within the passenger compartment and total seat removal. Two styles of seats can be encountered, the bench seat or bucket seat. Both consist of a metal frame attached to two adjustment tracks mounted to the floor of the vehicle. At least two bolts secure each individual mounting track to the floor, making a total of at least four bolts per seat.

During the seat evolution size up the rescuer must determine the position of the seat on its adjustment track, whether the seat will move manually, and whether there is damage to the seat structure, the track mechanisms, or the floor beneath the seat itself. During the dynamics of a head-on collision, it is possible for the seat and the patient to slide forward on the adjustment track. This forward position can temporarily hold the front seat occupants in contact with the dashboard, steering wheel, steering column, or other objects. Once the patient has been properly packaged, rescue personnel may be able to simply move the seat rearward by use of its normal operating mechanism. If there is damage to the seat adjustment tracks, seat frame, or floorboard area below the seat, it may not be possible to move the seat manually in this manner. Under these circumstances, alternative techniques involving the use of rescue equipment to push or pull the seat or procedures to completely remove the seat have to be considered. Regardless of appearances, try the normal mechanism first; it just may work.

Seat Movement Evolutions

The most commonly performed seat evolution generally involves rearward movement of the driver side front seat and is performed primarily to disentangle the driver from the many objects in the wreckage. This seat evolution can be accomplished by either pushing or pulling the seat. Initial evolution work involves providing for the safety of the injured patient through immobilization and stabilization and insulating the individual from the work to take place. Next, evolution setup work requires rescue personnel to select the exact locations for the pushing tool. One push point will form a base at a solid point along the bottom of the front "A" post of the vehicle near the door hinge area. The second tool push point, the seat contact point (Fig. 7-97), is crucial to the success of the evolution. The seat push point should be on the movable frame of the seat, *not* on the floor-mounted tracks and *not* on the seat springs or the seat cushion itself. Only the front outboard corner of the seat frame

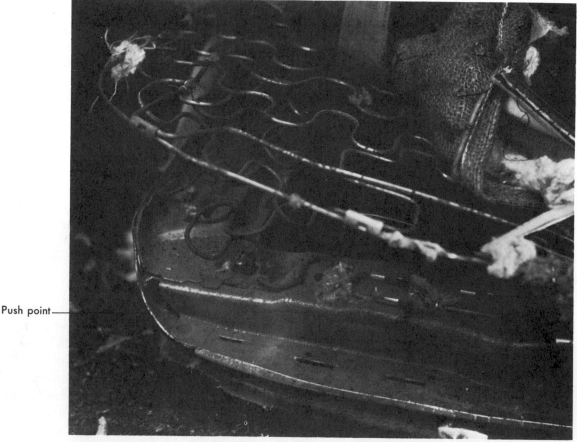

Push point

FIG. 7-97 Front seat push point should be on the movable frame of the seat and *not* on the seat springs or cushion material.

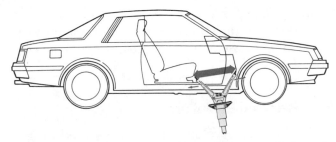

FIG. 7-98 Pushing effort must be angled to match that of the front seat structure regardless of the tool being used. Proper angle ensures that the seat will move down and back. If the pushing angle is too horizontal, the seat will be lifted or tilted.

offers the strength to resist crushing long enough for the seat to be pushed rearward.

With proper push points located, a pushing tool can then be selected. Hydraulic or mechanical tools capable of developing in excess of 4000 lb of force are required to move one side of a standard vehicle seat rearward. If the seat has an electric adjustment mechanism, equipment exerting in excess of 8000 lb of force may be required. The exact angle of placement of the pushing tool is vitally important to the efficiency of this evolution. The pushing tool *must* be angled exactly as the seat bench is (Fig. 7-98). This requires that the forward end of the tool be located at a point slightly higher than the tip at the point where the tool contacts the seat frame. This inclined angle will cause the seat to move down and to the rear. Positioning the pushing tool lower than this can cause the front of the seat to tip upward and roll rearward.

During all seat movement evolutions, an additional rescuer should hold the seat release adjustment mechanism in the neutral position. This may allow for a slightly smoother seat movement evolution. All seat movement evolutions also require that personnel watch the action and the reaction as the work is being performed. Although one side of a seat moves rearward, the opposite side may be forced forward. This reaction must be anticipated and monitored. While the evolution continues, rescuers may hear a popping sound and see a slight jerking action of the seat as it moves. This is caused by the adjustment teeth being stripped when the manual release lever is forced past them. The evolution should stop before the seat frame is moved completely off the end of the floor-mounted seat track. When the evolution ends, personnel must check the status of the large return spring that has been stretched by this rearward seat action. The spring may

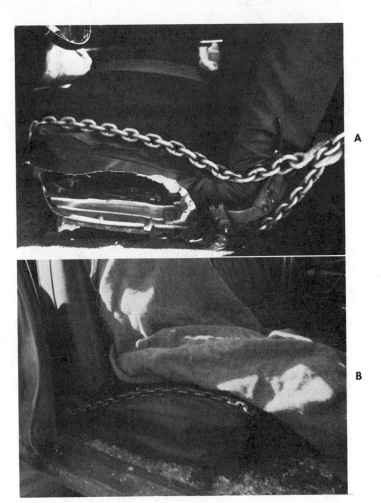

FIG. 7-99 A, When rescuers are pulling the front seat rearward, the chain should come from behind and move under the seat, wrap around the front edge, and lay over the top of the cushion. The top section of the chain can be placed under the patient's leg or thigh and still function properly. **B,** With a proper chain wrap, the seat cushion initially crushes down, and then the seat structure moves rearward.

require disconnecting from its mount to prevent an unexpected release that could cause injury.

If rescue personnel decide to move a seat rearward by employing a pulling action, a minimum 2-ton effort is again required for conventional seats, and 4 tons is needed for electric models. After the evolution size up has been conducted, chain is wrapped around the end of the seat that is to be moved. The chain wrap is begun by passing the chain in from behind the seat, moving it under the seat initially and then around the front edge. The chain continues over the top of the seat cushion along the outboard side of the seat to join back onto itself, forming a loop (Fig. 7-99). Pulling equipment is then located across the rear trunk area of the vehicle and positioned in as straight a line as possible. The same precautions for patient and evolution safety apply as before. The benefit of this chain wrap on the seat becomes evident as soon as the slack begins to be taken up by the pulling tool. With the chain coming around the bottom of the seat first, the seat cushion crushes down in the early stages of the evolution. This action will begin to lower the patient, possibly providing release at this point. Once the seat cushion has been compressed, the entire seat frame then begins its rearward travel. The success of pulling a seat rearward is strongly dependent on proper use of this chain-wrapping technique.

If rescue personnel determine that it would be advantageous to move the entire seat rearward simultaneously, either a multiple push can be performed on each side or multiple chain loops with dual-pulling tools can be employed. A single pulling tool can move an entire bench seat rearward if the chain loops from each side of the seat are joined into a single line attached to the one pulling tool. The lone tool must have sufficient pulling power and adequate travel distance to accomplish total seat bench movement evolution.

Rescue personnel at the scene of an accident may decide that one side or both sides of a seat have to be moved forward. This unusual evolution can be necessary when back seat passengers are trapped with a portion of their body under the front seat. They may have moved forward at the moment of collision and had their legs become twisted in the floorboard area under the seat in front of them. This evolution may also be required as a means of affording additional clearances for patients being extricated from the rear seat area. The seat will not be moved forward with a patient located at any point on the front seat.

Again, pushing or pulling equipment can be used usually with the pushing method being far superior to any pulling attempts. When forward movement is desired, the push point on the seat is the rear outboard corner of the frame of the seat near the point where the vertical seat back joins the horizontal seat cushion component. Pulling can be accomplished by locating pulling equipment at the front hood or fender area of the vehicle. This time, the chain first passes under the seat from front to back. The chain then forms a large vertical loop up over the entire seat back when it joins to the pulling chain near the dash. This allows the seat back to fold forward and away from any rear seat patients and causes the seat cushion to bend upward

as the pulling force is applied. The most efficient operation is produced when the forward-pulling loop of chain is as close to the outboard seat track mechanism as possible.

Seat Removal Evolution

The final seat evolution that can be used to free trapped persons involves total bucket seat or bench-seat removal. This specific evolution may be required as a means of creating additional access to trapped occupants, clearing an extrication pathway, or removing a bucket seat with the patient immobilized to it.

Rescuers can simply and effectively remove a vehicle seat if they are able to unbolt the seat floor tracks (Fig. 7-100). If the bolts are not accessible, the metal floorboard material around the bolts can be cut or chiseled through, allowing the seat, floor tracks, and bolts to lift off the floor as a complete unit. Depending on the collision damage to the seat and the track mechanism, rescuers may be able to cut through the seat mount bolts with a hammer and cold chisel, air chisel, or air gun tool. The flat chisel bit should be used for this procedure. If no patient is located on or in close proximity to the seat, it may be possible to use spreading or lifting equipment to pry the seat upward (Fig. 7-101), either moving it off its track mechanism or causing the bolts to pull free of the floorboards. It is advisable to pry the rear mounts of the seat free initially and then attack the front bolts. This action causes the seat to move forward and away from the passenger area while it is being removed.

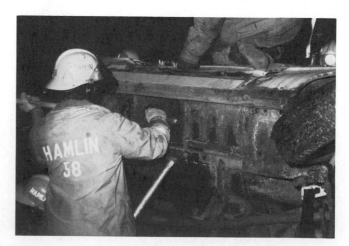

FIG. 7-100 Total seat removal is possible by cutting or unbolting the bolts securing the seat to the floorboard.

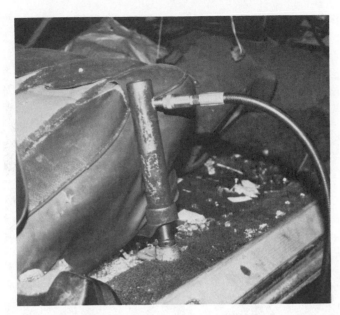

FIG. 7-101 Porto-power ram with cylinder and plunger toes in position to either pry seat away from floor-mounted track or force entire seat and track mechanism out of the floorboard. This evolution is practical only when no patients are on the seat.

SPECIALIZED VEHICLE ACCESS SITUATIONS

Real-world accident situations can present rescue personnel with the need to open or remove portions of the floor of the vehicle. This undercarriage opening may be necessary to assist in removing portions of the vehicle that are trapping the patients, provide access to the patients inside the vehicle, or provide an extrication pathway for patient removal from the passenger compartment of the vehicle.

In a Long Island, New York, incident the driver of a station wagon was trapped deep within the wreckage. The vehicle, found on its driverside, had slammed roof first into a power pole, severing the pole in several places and crushing the roof down into the passenger compartment. During the rescue process the undercarriage area was opened piece by piece and portions of the floor, driveshaft, front seat, and the seat-mounting tracks were removed. Eventually there was sufficient space to permit extrication of the patient from the vehicle. The work of opening the undercarriage was largely responsible for this safe and efficient patient extrication. Several weeks later the driver, on crutches, visited the local fire station to say thanks for a job well done.

When confronted with an entrapment situation at a vehicle accident scene using vehicle rescue equipment

as necessary, the rescuer, working as a member of a two-person team, should be able to do the following:

- Recognize that the vehicle's floor and undercarriage structure hinders safe and efficient patient care and extrication.
- Determine to what degree selected portions of the undercarriage should be moved, opened, or removed.
- Determine the presence of any safety problems that exist or may arise during the fulfillment of the undercarriage evolution.
- Determine the most appropriate vehicle rescue tools, equipment, and techniques necessary for accomplishing the desired undercarriage evolution.
- Safely and efficiently perform the desired evolution in 5 minutes or less.

Undercarriage Opening

The metal undercarriage of a vehicle is generally composed of a slightly heavier gauge metal than the side or roof body panels. Tools and techniques that effectively cut body sheet metal also function well to cut through the flooring. Additional equipment may be necessary to remove any vehicle components located underneath the floor that obstruct the floor-opening evolution. The hollow metal driveshaft can be removed by cutting through it or disconnecting it at its attachment to the transmission. Electrical wiring and the steel cable of the emergency brake system can be cut or disconnected. Fuel lines may need to be disconnected and crimped or plugged to prevent leakage.

The actual area of the floor to be opened depends on the intent of the evolution, the damage to the vehicle, and the location and condition of the patients inside the vehicle (Fig. 7-102). Initial floor opening work should concentrate on single-thickness metal areas where no interior obstructions are anticipated. Working directly under the front or rear seats or the dashboard should be avoided initially because these areas hinder the evolution. When the floor opening is made, the flooring can be either completely removed or cut on three sides and folded outward (Fig. 7-103). Once the opening of the metal is completed, the vehicle's carpeting and underlayment must be opened. This cloth or rug material can be cut with a sharp knife or saw. Once the opening is finished, exposed sharp metal edges should be taped or tarped to provide additional safety.

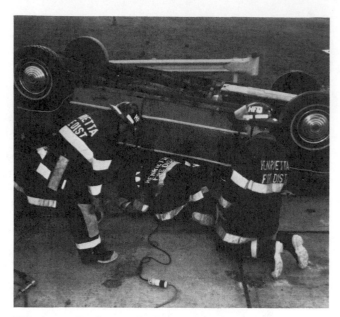

FIG. 7-102 Realistic vehicle rescue training must be conducted with vehicles in different positions. A vehicle's physical position can significantly change the complexity of a rescue scenario.

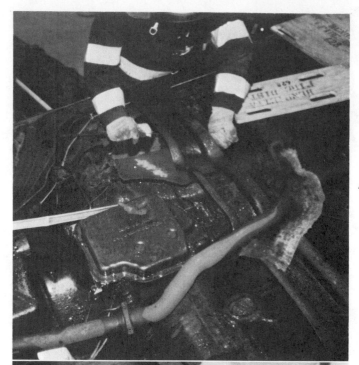

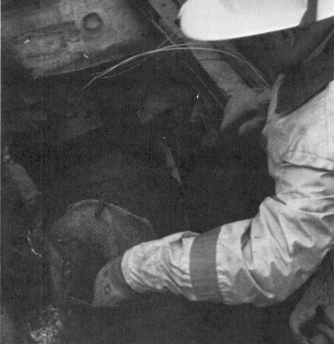

FIG. 7-103 A, Rescue crews must be familiar with procedures for working with the undercarriage. **B,** In real-world incidents, access into or through the floorboards may be required to reach the patients.

The opening in the vehicle floor may be sufficient to remove the portions of the vehicle, such as the seats, that are trapping the occupants. The opening may also provide access to injured patients in interior areas of the passenger compartment. In most difficult entrapment situations, the opening in the floor may be used as an extrication pathway for patient removal. Emergency service personnel must have the skills and the ability to open any portion of the undercarriage of any vehicle involved in an accident situation.

Trunk Evolutions

In certain special rescue situations, access to the interior passenger compartment is severely restricted. Rescue personnel must be prepared for these unique circumstances because conventional interior access is not always possible at every incident. Unique vehicle position or collision damage can easily eliminate all normal access means.

When confronted with an entrapment situation at a vehicle accident scene and using vehicle rescue equipment as necessary, the rescuer, working as a member of a two-person team, should be able to do the following:

- Recognize that conventional access to the passenger compartment through a vehicle's doors, windows, windshield, or roof is not possible.

- Determine that access to the passenger compartment is possible by forced entry into the trunk area and subsequent access to the interior of the vehicle is possible from the trunk compartment.

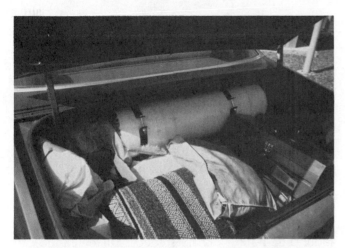

FIG. 7-104 Standard operating procedures requiring the trunk of every vehicle involved in an incident to be opened are valuable in situations such as when a vehicle is dual fueled and the shutoff valve is located under a plastic shroud on the cylinder.

- Determine the presence of any safety problems or hazards that exist or may arise during the trunk opening and passenger compartment access evolution.
- Determine the most appropriate vehicle rescue tools, equipment, and techniques for accomplishing the trunk-opening and passenger compartment access evolution.
- Safely and efficiently force entry into the trunk compartment of a vehicle in 60 seconds or less.
- Safely and efficiently gain access to the interior passenger compartment area of a sedan type of vehicle from the trunk area in 8 minutes or less.

Access to the trunk compartment of a vehicle may be necessary for several reasons. Routinely, trunk access is necessary at an early point in the incident as a means of detecting potential vehicle safety hazards (Fig. 7-104). Fire and rescue-oriented organizations should adopt a standard operating procedure, such as is shown in the box, for their response to each and every motor vehicle incident.

Numerous hazards may be found in the trunk area of any vehicle at any time. A gasoline can for the lawn mower, a propane cylinder for the backyard grill unit, or chemicals for the garden are just some of the potential hazards that can threaten the health and safety of operating personnel at the emergency scene. Fire and rescue personnel may also discover human beings inside the trunk areas. People may be inside the trunks of vehicles for a variety of reasons. A recent incident in upstate New York carries with it a very important safety message for fire, medical, and rescue

STANDARD OPERATING PROCEDURE

- Effective immediately, all fire and rescue command personnel shall fulfill the requirements of this standard operating procedure by ensuring that a determination is made about the presence of occupants or of health or safety hazards within the trunk compartment area of every vehicle involved in an emergency incident to which fire or rescue personnel are summoned. This shall include, but not be limited to, all vehicle fire or vehicle accident emergency incidents.
- Command personnel shall direct their operating members to take such reasonable and prudent action that may be necessary to open the trunk of the motor vehicle, assess any relative safety hazards presented by the contents of the trunk, and initiate proper action to render any potential hazards safe for operating personnel.
- The trunk shall be opened and the interior areas of the trunk surveyed as soon as it is practical during the incident. If present at the emergency scene, law enforcement personnel shall be requested to observe the trunk-opening evolution, verify the exact contents of the trunk, and provide security for the contents.

personnel. The story began when a woman who had just purchased a new automobile returned it to the dealership complaining of a rattling sound while the automobile was being driven. To survey the problem and isolate the exact location of the noise, two mechanics from the garage were assigned to check it out. After a short time, the mechanics realized that the noise was coming from somewhere in the rear area of the vehicle. One of the mechanics climbed in the trunk with a flashlight, and his partner drove the vehicle around the city streets. During the process the vehicle was involved in a collision that rendered both the driver and the mechanic inside the trunk unconscious. Only because the fire department had a standard operating procedure for trunk hazard survey work was the trunk opened and the second accident victim located.

Teenagers sometimes place friends inside the trunk of a vehicle to smuggle them into a drive-in movie theater without paying the admission fees. Other situations can be a matter of life or death. A young woman from Rochester, New York, was abducted by two men, raped, and then stuffed in the trunk of her own vehicle. The two criminals then torched the vehicle, hoping to dispose of their victim in the inferno. Firefighters who arrived to extinguish the vehicle fire discovered the woman in the trunk in time to save her life. The trunk of every vehicle being worked on must be opened to determine exactly what or who is inside.

If undamaged by fire or collision, the trunk can generally be opened by using the proper key or the inside electric-powered trunk release button. If the trunk is physically damaged, opening with the key or electric release should be attempted first, although forcible entry procedures will generally be necessary if the trunk latch mechanism or electrical system is inoperative. Such forcible entry work can be accomplished without causing undue additional damage.

Forcible entry to the trunk area can be accomplished by spreading the latch apart, performing a through-the-lock entry evolution, or cutting the trunk lid sheet metal. If rescue personnel decide to force the trunk lid open with spreading equipment, the goal is to spread or pry the upper and lower trunk latch mechanisms apart. This evolution begins by applying the spreading equipment a short distance away from the latch. The trunk lid is forced upward at that point, and wedge blocking or pry bars are placed to hold the lid in its "up" position. The prying action continues while the force is applied closer to the latch mechanism. The spreading effort continues to concentrate on the latch mechanism until a complete release is accomplished (Fig. 7-105).

Personnel must be prepared for sudden upward movement of the lid during the release. A physical restraint may be necessary to minimize the sudden opening of the trunk lid. If personnel are forcing open the trunk of a vehicle stabilized on its side, gravity no longer keeps the power of trunk-lifting cylinders or springs in check. When opened in this position, the trunk lid will instantly fly open. Personnel must clear the immediate area around the trunk lid and provide a positive restraint to minimize the hazard associated with the lid being opened.

The through-the-lock forcible entry method involves moving or removing the trunk key lock cylinder (Fig. 7-106). The most successful technique is to

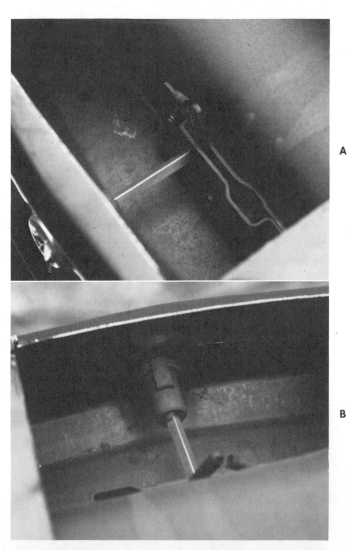

FIG. 7-106 A, Cut-away view shows trunk latch mechanism connected to the exterior key cylinder by a square metal rod assembly. **B,** Key cylinder is secured into trunk lid with a horseshoe-shaped metal clip.

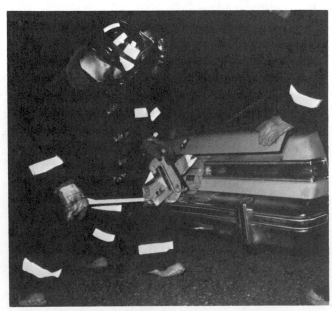

FIG. 7-105 Trunk is forced open by using a hand-operated hydraulic spreader.

drive the cylinder inward. This can best be accomplished by placing the pointed end of a Halligan type of forcible entry bar against the cylinder, driving it inward by striking with a flat-headed axe or hammer (Fig. 7-107). The key cylinder moves inside the trunk lid, leaving a hole in the trunk lid. A second through-the-lock entry method involves the use of a heavy-duty, automobile body dent puller tool. The screw end of the tool is threaded deep into the key cylinder. The sliding weight is then rammed rearward, actually pulling the key cylinder out of its mounting in the trunk lid. To open the trunk, rescuers insert a flat-bladed tool such as a screwdriver into the hole of the lid and mate it into the small vertical slot of the trunk latch mechanism (Fig. 7-108). When the bladed tool is turned from the five o'clock to the seven o'clock position, the trunk latch operates, releasing the lid.

A final trunk forcible entry method involves use of a sheet metal cutting tool to open the area of the trunk lid near the latch and key cylinder. With the lid opened, the interior latch is exposed. A bladed tool is then inserted into the operating slot and turned to operate the latch release.

Opening the trunk can provide an emergency means of accessing the interior areas of the passenger compartment. The unique style of vehicle collision that occurs when an automobile rams into the side or rear of a tractor-trailer truck is known as an *underride*.

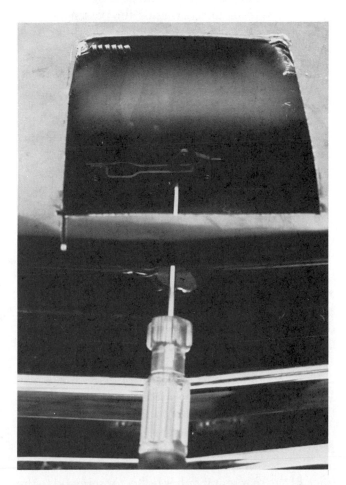

A

B

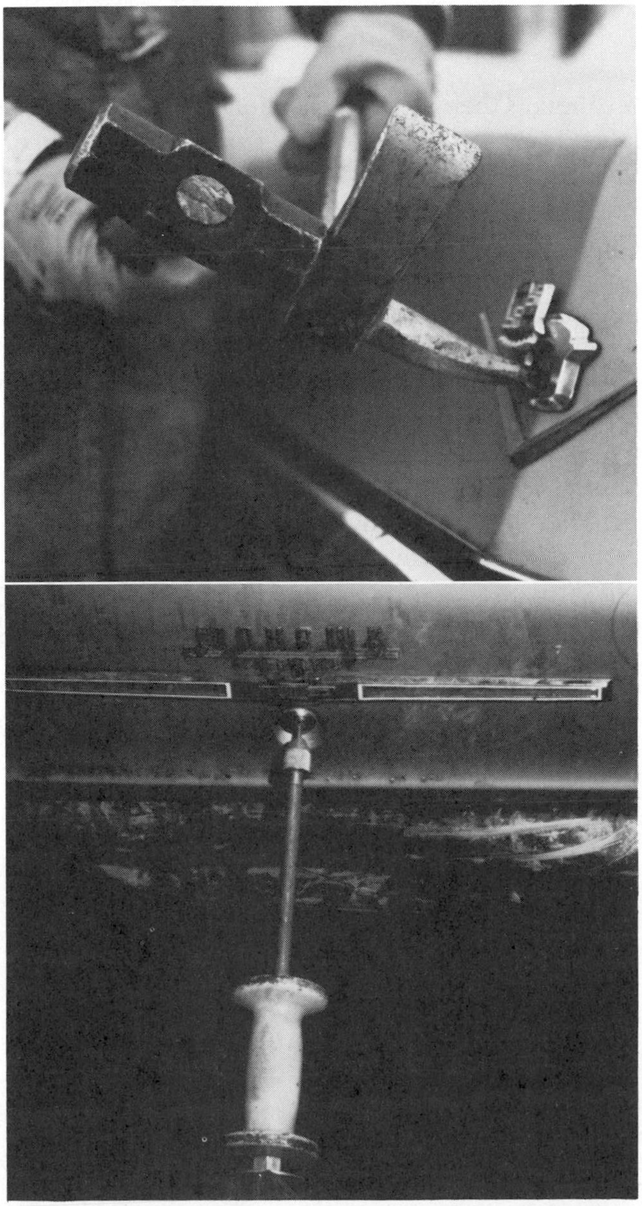

FIG. 7-107 Through-the-lock forcible entry into a trunk area can be accomplished by **A,** driving the key cylinder into the trunk lid or **B,** pulling the cylinder out with a heavy-duty, body dent puller.

FIG. 7-108 With key cylinder removed, thin, flat-bladed screwdriver can be inserted into the slot originally occupied by the square rod linkage. Turning the screwdriver slightly will release the interior latch mechanism.

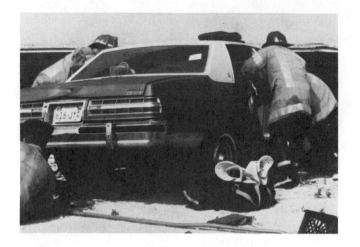

FIG. 7-109 Vehicle underride results when the front of a vehicle is crushed into and under a much larger vehicle such as a tractor-trailer truck. (Courtesy Steve Kidd, Orlando, Fla.)

The momentum of the automobile propels it into and actually under the large truck. The vehicle can be jammed so completely under the trunk that only the rear trunk portion remains accessible (Fig. 7-109). When passenger compartment access is necessary, opening the trunk and accessing the passenger compartment from that area may be the only option available. Rescue personnel must ensure that vehicle hazards, particularly those related to the fuel system, have been accounted for and neutralized. The vehicle must also be properly stabilized to prevent movement.

The passenger access evolution size up continues after the trunk is opened. Any contents of the trunk that obstruct working room in that area must be unloaded. The forward partition wall of the trunk compartment must be studied with emphasis on its construction and the location of any fuel system components. The vehicle fuel tank may be located horizontally or on its edge across the front or sides of the trunk, or the stainless steel vapor recovery lines from the fuel system may be installed inside a metal tube in this area. When confronted with any of these fuel system components, the rescue officer may decide to remove them, work the evolution around them, or halt the evolution and attempt a different access method.

If the evolution is to be accomplished, rescue personnel must either move or remove the front wall of the trunk area. Any metal bracing, sheet metal partitions, or cardboard material must be moved or removed. With the initial wall opening made, the attachments of the rear seat are then attacked. The back of the rear seat is either bolted or screwed to the metal rear window deck or the metal partition separating the trunk from the passenger compartment. The seat can be cut free from these mounts, or

the mounts themselves can be attacked to release the rear seat back. Concentrating efforts along the top of the seat back works well, allowing the lower seat bracket attachments to remain attached. With the top connections released, the back of the seat can be pivoted forward. A pass-through truck feature available on selected new autos may make this evolution relatively rapid (Fig. 7-110).

Once the rear partition wall has been opened sufficiently and the back of the rear seat moved forward, rescue personnel can attempt physical entry into the passenger compartment. If the location of occupants prevents the back of the rear seat from being moved forward, rescuers must then leave the seat in place and physically disassemble it piece by piece. The springs and wire structure must be cut, the cloth opened, and the cushion material removed. This operation prolongs the total time necessary to accomplish passenger compartment access. The thin metal composing the rear window speaker decking may also be removed to facilitate a larger access opening to the passenger compartment.

HAZARD CONTROL AND SAFETY EVOLUTIONS

Emergency service personnel may have to perform several activities at the scene of an incident that are related more to safety than to patient rescue or extrication. These important hazard and safety-related evolutions include the following:

- Opening a vehicle hood
- Opening a vehicle trunk
- Opening a vehicle tailgate
- Plugging a leaking fuel system
- Removing a vehicle fuel tank

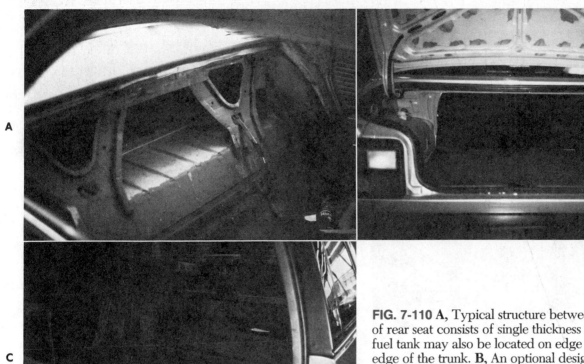

FIG. 7-110 A, Typical structure between trunk and back of rear seat consists of single thickness metal bracing. The fuel tank may also be located on edge at forwardmost edge of the trunk. **B,** An optional design on newer vehicles provides a trunk pass through, allowing for easy access from the trunk to the rear seat area of an automobile. **C,** The back of the rear seat is laid forward.

Hood Evolutions

Standard operating procedures for an emergency fire or rescue organization should require that on-scene personnel disable the battery of every vehicle they work on if the vehicle has been involved in an accident or fire and has been damaged. Safety teams must therefore be able to open the hood of the vehicle. Once it is open, emergency personnel can check for fluid leaks or other potential safety hazards under the hood, take action to control any problems, and perform overhaul work in the engine compartment portion of a vehicle that has burned.

Attempts should be made to first use the normal inside or outside hood release mechanism. If that mechanism fails to release the hood latch, opening the hood can become a very difficult and sometimes complex evolution.

The first major design change in vehicle hood-release mechanisms occurred when they were moved from their original exterior release position to the inside release location by automobile manufacturers attempting to make their vehicles more theft deterrent. The inside hood release mechanism uses the same basic front hood latch assembly, but its release action is accomplished by pulling on a thin wire cable running from the front hood area to the inside of the passenger compartment (Fig. 7-111).

The problems presented by this inside release assembly occur primarily when a fire occurs in the engine compartment of the vehicle. The aluminum release cable is susceptible to damage from heat despite being encased in a protective shroud. Because of the thin diameter of the aluminum cable and the routing of the release cable along the very top of the driver side front fender area (Fig. 7-112), any heat evolving from an engine fire will quickly heat the wire cable to the point that it burns or melts completely. When this occurs, any attempt to pull the inside hood release cable results in the plastic pull handle and a length of wire coming completely out of its assembly. The hood remains latched because the cable has been severed by the fire.

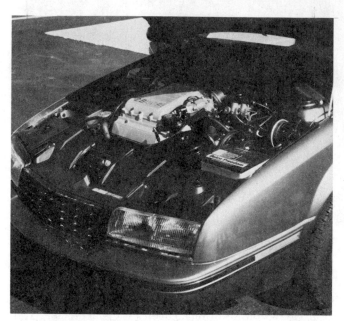

FIG. 7-111 The engine compartment of a modern vehicle shows the inside hood release mechanism surrounded by lightweight metal and plastic body components.

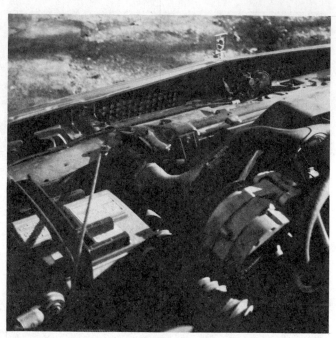

FIG. 7-112 Thin-gauge wire hood release cable is secured high along the top of the driver side fender area within the engine compartment. This location makes the cable vulnerable to effects of heat from an engine compartment fire.

A second problem resulting when the inside hood release is exposed to a vehicle engine compartment fire is that attempts to physically force the front hood latch and release mechanism apart are generally derailed by the nature of the material that now surrounds the front hood area. What was once metal on older vintage vehicles, that offered a strong prying point to force the hood open is now a mass of plastic derivatives, and fiberglass. The material located near the hood release mechanism softens and melts when exposed to the heat of a fire or disintegrates on collision impact (Fig. 7-113). The popular all-plastic front end offers no assistance when fire service personnel attempt to pry or force the hood release open. Lack of a strong leverage point frustrates virtually all attempts to force the hood open. Methods to get the hood open require a good size up, proper application of equipment and techniques, and some common sense in solving individual problems when they are found.

In an engine compartment fire situation the initial fire knockdown must be accomplished before attempting to open the hood. Water can be applied into the engine compartment by sweeping the nozzle under the vehicle or bouncing the water off the roadway to suppress the fire burning under the hood. An effective knockdown attack may also be accomplished by directing the water into the wheelwell area of the burning vehicle. The inner fender in most modern vehicles is plastic and melts through quickly. This allows the water spray shot into the wheel area to reach the seat of the fire. The hood should not be opened during the initial vehicle fire attack because this action would allow additional oxygen to fan the flames. The cooling water spray must also be directed at reducing explosion potentials from components such as the energy-absorbing bumper system and the front shocks or components in the engine compartment or undercarriage of the vehicle.

Personnel must not approach the burning vehicle fire from the front. Fire suppression personnel may, however, be able to stand close to the vehicle at the side once the fire has been knocked down. From this location, they may be successful in prying the edges of the hood away from the fender. With the hood edge bent upward, additional water or other fire extinguishing agents can be directed onto the smoldering fire.

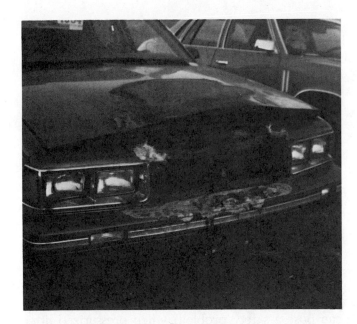

FIG. 7-113 Melted plastic and fiberglass front area can make prying or pushing hood open at the latch a difficult and time-consuming task. Personnel may be able to open the hood using pliers to pull on the stub of wire cable still remaining at the latch.

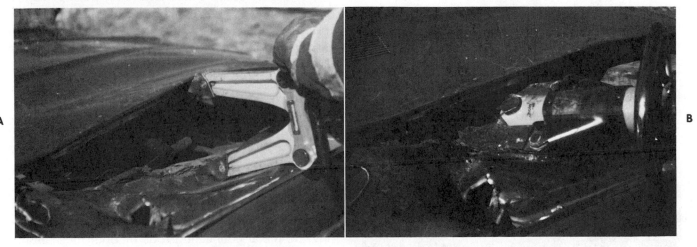

A
B

FIG. 7-114 A, Prying hood open may be possible if work is initiated from the side. B, This presents a safer position for personnel and allows access to hinges for cutting. This is *not* a technique for forcing hoods open while a vehicle is burning.

However, the hood must still be opened for final fire extinguishment. At this point the fire has been knocked down, and the urgency of the emergency has subsided. Personnel can continue to work from each front fender area to open the hood. Most hoods open from the front and hinge at the upper rear corners near the firewall. Working from the sides, personnel can force the hood up, exposing the hinge assembly (Fig. 7-114). The hinges can be severed with sawing or cutting equipment. With both hinges cut completely free of the hood, personnel can lift the entire hood up and forward, opening it from rear to front. This allows complete access to the engine compartment for fire

extinguishment and hazard control. Another method of opening the hood involves the use of sheet metal cutting equipment to cut the hood and upper hood latch assembly away from the remaining portion of the hood. Using an air chisel tool or manual sheet metal cutting equipment can be very frustrating and time consuming for this task because the upper hood latch area consists of several layers of sheet metal, each of which must be cut through individually. Cutting the upper hood latch away from the lower latch mechanism can be most effectively accomplished by three well-placed cuts of a rotary power saw. Working from above the hood and latch mechanism, rescuers make a deep cut across the back of the latch assembly and parallel to the front of the vehicle. Two parallel cuts are then made (one on each side of the latch assembly) to form a horseshoe-shaped flap of hood metal that surrounds the upper latch assembly. All cuts must be deep enough to penetrate all the layers of the sheet metal of the hood. When the final cut has been made, the hood can be opened fully. The upper and lower latch assemblies remain connected, but the hood has essentially been cut away from them. A different application of the same rotary saw involves using it to make a horizontal cut just under the lip of the hood itself. If deep enough, this cut will sever the rod latch mechanism, releasing the upper hood from the latch. Portions of the front grille or trim components of the vehicle may have to be removed to allow the saw blade to penetrate deep enough into the hood latch assembly to sever it.

If fire damage is minimal but the inside hood-release cable has been burned completely through, it may still be possible to get the hood latch mechanism to release somewhat normally. Even though the release cable may have burned through, a short stub of cable generally remains attached directly to the front hood latch assembly (Fig. 7-115). With access to the latch mechanism gained by removal of the front grille and trim materials, personnel may locate this cable stub and manually release the hood latch by pulling on the cable with a pair of pliers. This action simulates normal cable operation and, if successful, releases the hood quickly and efficiently.

Tailgate Evolutions

When fire or rescue personnel must open the tailgate or hatchback of a vehicle, many of the techniques used for trunk opening can be employed. Personnel can use the key or inside release mechanisms, or forcible entry can be accomplished by either spreading at the latch, using the through-the-lock entry technique, or cutting away the tailgate or hatchback sheet metal to expose the inner latch mechanism. As mentioned previously, work with vehicle hatchbacks or tailgates can pose a safety problem when pressurized lifter devices are present. These lifters may be large coiled springs tightly compressed inside the lifter tubes or pressurized piston units. Rescuers should never apply heat or cut into or through any style of lifter for any reason. It may be possible to safely remove the lifter unit, preventing any potential injury while work progresses with the hatchback or tailgate.

If personnel open a station wagon tailgate by cutting the sheet metal to expose the inner latch assembly, they can expect to find dual-control rods and latch mechanisms (Fig. 7-116). If the tailgate opens as a door and also opens outward to a flat position, both release mechanisms located at the extreme right and left sides inside the tailgate must be accessed. Operating the metal connecting rods of both mechanisms simultaneously will allow the tailgate to open.

Fuel System Evolutions

Plugging a leaking vehicle fuel system can become a necessary emergency incident evolution. Using technology learned from advancements in fire service handling of hazardous materials incidents, personnel may either successfully stop a fuel leak, minimize the flow, contain and neutralize the spill, or remove the vehicle fuel source completely. In all cases, adequate fire safety measures must be in place before, during, and after any work is attempted with the vehicle's fuel or any components of the fuel system.

Stopping a liquid or vapor fuel leak may involve the use of a plugging or sealing material fitted into the source of the leak (Fig. 7-117). If a fuel line has broken, for example, a small wooden cone or a golf tee may be

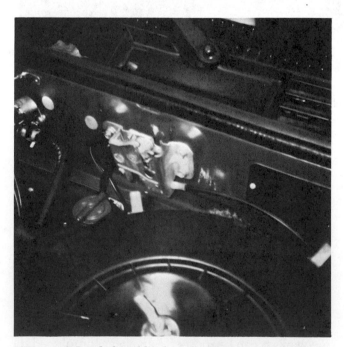

FIG. 7-115 Inside hood latch and release mechanism mounted at top center portion of the firewall. Note cable exposed inside latch assembly.

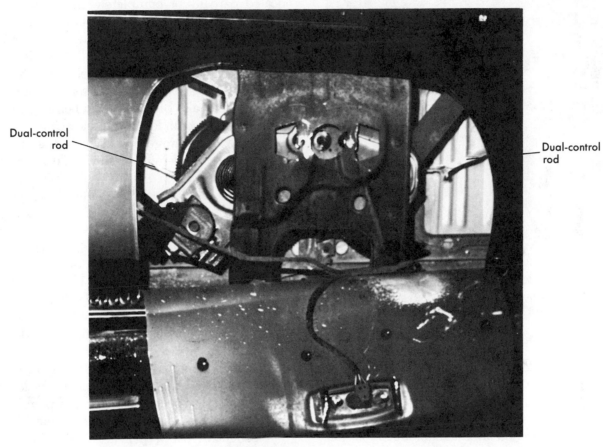

Dual-control rod

Dual-control rod

FIG. 7-116 Cut-away view shows cloth-covered dual-control rods deep inside the panel on both sides of a station wagon's rear gate.

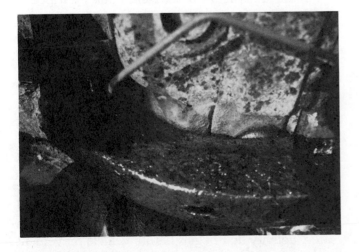

FIG. 7-117 Fuel leaks can originate from broken fuel lines, damaged filler necks, punctured fuel tanks, loose gas caps, or another component of the fuel system. Emergency procedures and equipment must be available for promptly dealing with fuel leak incidents safely and efficiently.

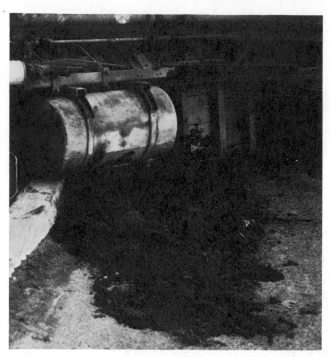

FIG. 7-118 Once diesel fuel leak has been stopped, the spilled product must be dealt with at an accident scene.

successfully fitted into the open end of the line to stop the leak. A leak from a line can also be stopped or reduced by clamping the line shut.

Liquid fuel spillage can be contained by use of absorbent materials and adequate diking of the spill. Commercially available absorbent materials or simple clay absorbent compound can be used for this purpose (Fig. 7-118). The spilled fuel may also be neutralized by deploying special hydrocarbon-neutralizing agents.

Depending on the final resting position of the vehicle that is leaking fuel, it may also be possible to accomplish a total fuel tank removal evolution. When a vehicle is stabilized on its edge or roof, the gasoline or diesel fuel tank is often readily accessible to rescue personnel. Most fuel tanks are secured to the vehicle by two parallel thin metal banding straps. These straps can simply be cut through, releasing the tank from its mounting. Some vehicle models use an enlarged lip located around the fuel tank to secure it to the vehicle with sheet metal screws. These fuel tanks would be difficult to remove at an accident scene. It is now common to find vehicle fuel tanks on smaller size automobiles mounted inside the trunk or the passenger-compartment area of the vehicle. It may not be practical to consider fuel tank removal under these circumstances.

Jacking and Shoring Evolutions

Emergency service personnel may be confronted with an entrapment situation in which an individual is located partially or completely under the accident vehicle. In a not uncommon collision scenario, an unbelted occupant is ejected during the dynamics of the collision and is trapped beneath the vehicle. This rescue problem is particularly likely if a vehicle rollover accident has occurred. The services of a rescue company may also be requested when a homeowner becomes trapped under the vehicle being repaired in the driveway or garage. Typically, the cinder blocks or lone bumper jack fail suddenly while the mechanic is under the vehicle. At a bank drive-in window a rescue company recently responded to a report of a person trapped under a vehicle. The medical and rescue personnel found an elderly woman crushed under the rear axle of an automobile that had been waiting at the drive-in window. The vehicle had suddenly moved into reverse, backing over the elderly pedestrian walking behind it. These are only a few examples of the many possible real-world entrapment problems that require jacking and shoring of a vehicle to extricate the patient.

When confronted with a person fully or partially trapped under a vehicle and using vehicle rescue equipment, the rescuer, working as a member of a three-person team, should be able to do the following:

- Recognize that a person is partially or fully trapped under a portion of a vehicle and an unsafe working environment exists for all emergency service personnel at the scene.
- Determine to what degree the person is trapped under the structure of the vehicle and what area of the vehicle is in contact with the patient.
- Determine the presence of any safety problems that exist or may arise during the fulfillment of the jacking and shoring evolution.
- Determine the most appropriate vehicle rescue tools, equipment, and techniques necessary for accomplishing the desired jacking and shoring evolution.
- Safely and efficiently perform the desired jacking and shoring evolution within 5 minutes or less.

Jacking is the action of moving the object away from the trapped person. This is generally an upward movement. Shoring or blocking is the companion safety activity that begins before vehicle movement and continues during the jacking evolution. It is completed after the desired jacking evolution has ended. Whenever an object is lifted, it must be blocked

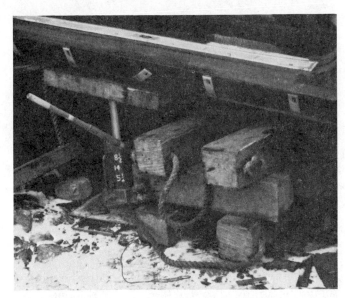

FIG. 7-119 Blocking must be used before, during, and after any jacking or lifting evolution.

before, during, and after the lift to provide safety to the trapped person and to operating personnel (Fig. 7-119). We do not want anything to get worse after the arrival of the emergency services personnel. Therefore as a general rule, every inch of lift receives an equal amount of shoring. When rescuers run out of blocking, the jacking action must stop. Experienced rescue personnel that have been involved in the service for quite some time commonly refer to this process as *jacking and packing*. The intent is the same, to prevent any unwanted movement while the rescue evolution takes place by blocking the load securely over every inch of travel.

The jacking and shoring evolution size up includes consideration of the position of the patient under the vehicle and the present condition of the patient. The victim may have received fatal traumatic injuries during the crushing accident or be alive and in relatively stable condition, especially if only an arm or leg is trapped by the vehicle. Rescue and medical personnel must anticipate that the physical and mental condition of their conscious and alert patient may rapidly deteriorate when pressure from the heavy load is removed. Because of this compensated shock condition, the rescue effort must be coordinated closely with the activities of medical crew members, who would typically have patient IV lines flowing and anti-shock trousers readied and in place if possible.

Rescuers working to lift the object, scene command safety personnel, and the medical crew must all be fully prepared before any lifting action is undertaken. Once the lifting begins and the pressure is released, the physical condition of the patient can and often does turn into a critical life or death situation. Time cannot be lost once the lift has begun. The trapped patient must be rapidly extricated and transported to a medical facility within as short a timeframe as possible.

Rescue size up for a jacking and shoring evolution also involves determining the exact location of the patient under the structure of the vehicle. The individual's proximity to heat sources such as the catalytic converter or the exhaust system must be ascertained. An acceptable patient extrication pathway must be determined, and a wide enough area for the patient to be moved onto a longboard and away from the accident scene must be maintained. The patient is generally moved out from under the vehicle head first. This allows medical personnel the opportunity to maintain contact with the patient's head to monitor vital signs and maintain an adequate airway. No rescue tools or wood blocking should be placed to obstruct this extrication pathway.

One of the three possible solutions to extricating a person trapped under a vehicle is to raise the object. Second, if for some reason the object cannot be lifted, it may be possible to lower the ground under the trapped person. This is a particularly valuable technique in agricultural entrapment settings where a farmer can be pinned in freshly tilled soil by a tractor that has rolled over. Stabilizing the tractor and digging out the ground under it can lead to a successful rescue. A third method of extricating a trapped patient that is particularly valuable when only a small portion of the vehicle is trapping the patient is to remove that part of the vehicle. If a rod or post, for example, is contacting the patient's arm, the vehicle can be stabilized and the post or rod removed, thereby releasing the patient (Fig. 7-120).

If an object is to be lifted to free a person, lifting points for rescue equipment and safe and effective locations for blocking must be chosen during the evolution size up. The load must be blocked as it is found to prevent the development of problems that might further crush the load onto the patient. The action and reaction movement of the object being lifted must also be anticipated. While one side or one portion of a vehicle moves upward, the opposing unstabilized side of the vehicle will react by moving downward. This unwanted movement must be anticipated and prevented by adequate blocking efforts. If

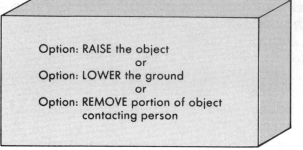

FIG. 7-120 Tactical options for freeing a person trapped by an object depend on resources available to rescue personnel and conditions found at entrapment.

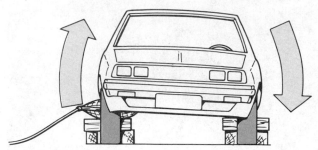

FIG. 7-121 Single-point tilting lift of vehicle produces desired action as one side is raised. Unwanted reaction, lowering of the opposite side, must be controlled with sufficient blocking.

one side of a vehicle is to be lifted to free a person under the vehicle, for example, the opposite side must be securely blocked in its present position. This reaction side must be blocked to take the load of the vehicle while it is being lifted (Fig. 7-121).

Blocking that is used to stabilize the vehicle in its present position and the blocking that will be continued as the object is lifted must be arranged as a box crib. This blocking arrangement requires two wood blocks of equally thickness to be placed parallel to each other to form each layer of the box crib. Additional equal-thickness wood pieces are arranged on top of the layer below by being placed in a crisscross pattern. This box crib design uses a lot of wood but ensures the most stable pattern of wood blocking for supporting a lifted load.

While constructing a box crib under an object, rescue personnel must remember never to place themselves in the position of being between the top layer of the crib and the underside of the object being lifted. Rescuers must resist the tendency to grab a wood block with their hand, reach under the vehicle, and attempt to place the block on the box crib. Hands must remain below the working surface of the top wood blocks at all times. Wedge blocks are used to take up distances less than the full thickness of a wood block.

Lifting equipment that can accomplish the lifting evolution includes one or more 7000-lb capacity mechanical jack tools, standard hydraulic jacks, or the porto-power ram used as a basic ram or with its toe attachments in place. Power rescue system spreaders, rams, air bags, or air cushions may also be used for this lifting operation. All these types of tools should be placed on large-area baseplates to minimize crushing into the ground when a load is applied to the tool. If conventional 4-inch wide by 18-inch long blocks are

all that is available to serve as a baseplate, the blocks should be arranged so that they do not roll out from under the tool.

Although the tool is functioning as a jack and should be lifting vertically, rescuers must remember that the tips of a spreader tool do not open in a straight line. Measured at the tips, the arms open in a curve or arc pattern. This action can actually move or push the object in an off-angle direction. Personnel must constantly be on the lookout for this unwanted potential movement. The spreader tool can suddenly and violently fail if the tool kicks out from under the load (Fig. 7-122).

Personnel must also be aware of any operating peculiarities inherent to their particular brand of power spreader. Several models of the Hurst rescue system spreaders, for example, act in an unexpected manner when the tool is being used to lift a load because of the design of their hydraulic valve operating system. If pressure is exerted on the arms of the tool, they initially move closer together rather than spread or open when the trigger is moved in the opening or spreading direction. This inward movement is due to unbalanced hydraulic pressure inside the tool and the hydraulic valving assembly, which allows the pressures to equalize. This action of the tool can cause a real problem at a rescue scene. The tool operator who believes the hydraulic trigger of the spreader is positioned in the correct direction sees the arms of the tool actually begin to close rather than open. For a brief moment, the rescue tool operator thinks that an error has been made in the operation of the trigger and may actually move the trigger in the opposite direction. This causes the arms of the tool to close even farther, allowing the load to drop closer to or onto the patient.

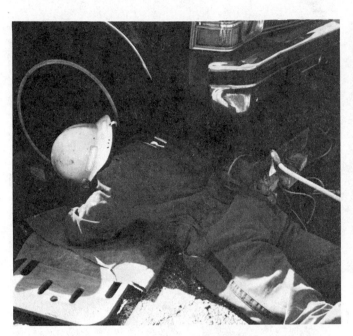

FIG. 7-122 Personnel working at any jacking and shoring evolutions should *never* place themselves in a position or location that prevents them from immediately escaping a dangerous situation.

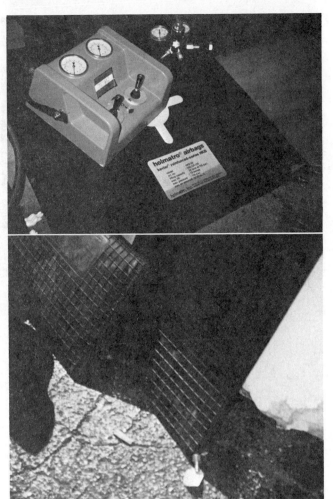

A

B

FIG. 7-123 A, Crew member assigned to operate air bag system controller should be in a position to observe the team leader's instructions and most of the action occurring. **B,** Brass air coupling of an air bag should always be protected from contamination and physical damage.

To prevent this possibly dangerous scenario, the tool operator and the rescue team working with this equipment must anticipate the downward operation of the selected Hurst spreaders under these conditions. The downward action can be minimized by ensuring that the trigger is initially being moved in the correct direction. The tool operator can also quickly move the trigger from its neutral position to the open position without hesitation. This equalizes the hydraulic pressure quickly and minimizes any closing action of the tool. Blocking must also be completely in contact with the vehicle so that there is no downward movement of the vehicle.

Air-operated rescue equipment that can lift portions of a vehicle includes air bags or air cushions (Fig. 7-123). When operating in the lifting mode, air bags can be stacked for added height. Safe, sturdy locations for the bags or cushions that maintain the equipment away from damaging heat sources or sharp objects must be chosen. Rescue personnel should also be capable of using air bags to lift a vehicle in one uncommon and unique way. By forcing air bags into the front and rear sides of an inflated tire and inflating

both bags simultaneously, personnel can lift a vehicle at its tires (Fig. 7-124). Once the tire is lifted by these *wheel chock* air bags, a third bag can be inserted directly under the center of the tire that is off the ground. Inflating the third air bag allows for additional lifting of the vehicle. This tactic works only on wheels and tires that do not rotate freely, for example, the tires on the drive axle of a truck.

Rescuers must remember that air bag or air cushion rescue tools allow the object being lifted to actually float on a pillow of air. The bags or cushions provide the lift. However, they do not provide the safety of a stable object. This can only be accomplished with proper box crib arrangements of blocking at strategic

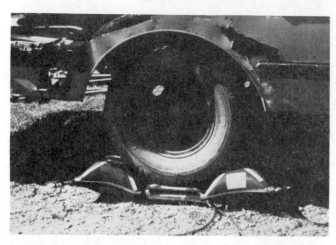

FIG. 7-124 Wheel chock lift with high-pressure air bags is accomplished by inflating bags in front of and behind the tire and then placing the third bag under the center of the lifted tire. This evolution should not be used on free-rotating wheels or tires (for example, the front tire of large bus or truck vehicles).

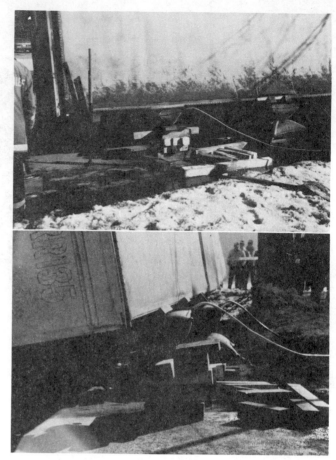

FIG. 7-125 A, Rear portion of tractor-trailer truck involved in a rollover is being lifted by fire department rescue personnel. **B,** During jacking evolution, load shifting and lack of proper vehicle stabilization caused air bags and box cribbing to explosively release from their location. A rescue officer standing within the dangerous strike zone was injured. His fire department helmet was gouged deeply by a flying block of wood.

locations on the object. Air bags or air cushions *do not* stabilize a lifted load. They simply aid in the overall stabilizing effort.

During air bag or air cushion operation, rescue personnel must continually be aware of the possibility of load shift. This action may cause the bags or cushions to instantly and violently pop out from their location (Fig. 7-125). Personnel should be positioned at strategic observation points to monitor any movement of the cribbing, the air tools, or the load during lifting. Unless they are on their feet at all times, they may not be in a position to escape a dangerous situation. The higher the load is lifted, the greater the chance of a sudden load shift occurring. During jacking and shoring evolutions, rescue personnel should maintain a location and physical body position that allows for rapid escape should an unforeseen load shift occur. Crew members should not kneel, sit, or lay flat during the action.

Personnel must remember to have a solid layer of wood cribbing directly under the cushions or bags if it is necessary to support that area (Fig. 7-126). A hollow box crib arrangement of wood is acceptable for all the intermediate layers of the crib, but the layer of wood in contact with the actual tool must be solid. In addition, cribbing should not be placed between the top bag or cushion and the object being lifted. The bag or cushion should be allowed to contact the object directly and form or mold itself around the shape of that object. This maximizes the adhesion capability between the rubber bag or cushion and the object being lifted.

Once the vehicle is lifted sufficiently to allow the patient to be removed, the final blocking efforts are performed, the longboard positioned, and the patient extricated from the entrapment. This action requires a coordinated effort by all the rescue and medical personnel operating on the scene.

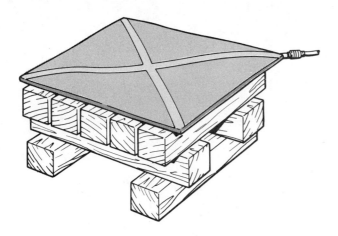

FIG. 7-126 Box crib design with a solid top layer used with a high-pressure air bag for a jacking evolution.

SUMMARY

As this chapter points out, actually operating the specific rescue tools and equipment is only one aspect of the total realm of vehicle rescue. Ideally, every emergency service provider fulfilling any role at the scene of a vehicle accident should have a working knowledge of today's new technology features, be familiar with accepted accident scene command and control procedures, fully understand accident scene safety hazards and precautions, and possess an understanding of basic patient medical practices and procedures. Emergency service personnel who refer to themselves as vehicle rescue technicians find the field of vehicle rescue complex and challenging. These technicians train in all related fields of knowledge in addition to learning to operate the vehicle rescue equipment effectively to accomplish the specific evolutions.

Only by developing this well-rounded foundation of knowledge of vehicle rescue practices and procedures can the vehicle rescue technician safely and efficiently become a working member of a team. Proper training in all aspects of the vehicle rescue field, coupled with the experience of working under "combat" conditions on the streets in the response district, will produce the top quality rescue personnel demanded by our ever-changing world.

The tools must be continually worked with and studied. The rescue evolutions must be practiced and practiced again until they become second nature. In the field of vehicle rescue the individual's skill level can deteriorate quickly if training is not a routine element in the career of the emergency provider. Continually striving to master the tools and techniques and the practices and the procedures of today's vehicle rescue enables rescue technicians to perform at the peak of their ability. The challenge at an accident scene should not come from trying to figure out the proper way to hook up or use a specific rescue tool. The time for training with the tool has passed once the accident has occurred. The accident scene is no place for on-the-job training. Your life, the lives of your fellow crew members, and the well being of the patients we strive to serve truly rests with you and your ability to rise to the challenges presented by the accident itself.

Training is our most important asset. It is the means by which we can assure ourselves that we will be able to meet and master these challenges each and every time we respond to an emergency scene. Be serious about your work. Strive to do your best. Take pride in your ability to serve your fellow men, women, and children at these critical moments in their lives.

The difference between training and no training can be the difference between life and death.

Bibliography

CHAPTER 1

Air bag tests, Insurance Institute for Highway Safety Status Report 23:1, 1988, newsletter.

Air bag: trooper's shield for life, Insurance Institute for Highway Safety Status Report 21:2, 1986, newsletter.

Automakers gear up to produce millions of air-bag-equipped cars, Insurance Institute for Highway Safety Status Report 23:1, 1988, newsletter.

Burnley proposes new side impact standard for better protection, Insurance Institute for Highway Safety Status Report 23:1, 1988, newsletter.

Butterbaugh WH, National LP-Gas Association: Personal communication, Jun 10, 1986.

Davis L: Rural firefighting operations — Book 1, Ashland, Mass, 1985, International Society of Fire Service Instructors.

Federal Register 43:3598, 1978.

Fire Service Information: Stay clear of potential tire explosion, Fire Service Extension of Iowa State University of Science and Technology 12:2, 1982.

Gage-Babcock and Associates, Inc: Automobile burn-out text in an open-air parking structure, Rep No 7328, Scranton, Pa, Jan 1973, Scranton (PA) Fire Bureau and Underwriter's Laboratories, Inc.

Garner R: A common car fire poses uncommon hazards, Fire Command 53:35, 1986.

Jackson HCL Jr: Personal communication, Dec 23, 1986.

Jackson HJ and Philbin PA: Muffler ignites plastic fuel tank, Fire Engineering 129:34, 1976.

Manufacturing Technical Bulletin: Safety, packaging, storage, and security of driver air bags, Series SMI, No 100, Detroit, 1987, General Motors Corp.

NHTSA expands study of fuel tank defects, Insurance Institute for Highway Safety Status Report 13:1, 1978, newsletter.

NY analysis indicates 9% drop in crash deaths, Insurance Institute for Highway Safety Status Report 21:1, 1986, newsletter.

Propane — engine fuel of tomorrow...here today! Pamphlet No. Pefot-15, Jan 1980, Suburban Propane.

Small passenger vehicles a problem, Insurance Institute for Highway Safety Status Report 22:1, 1987, newsletter.

Supplemental air bag restraint system, Booklet No FPS-12035-87A, 1986, Ford Motor Co.

US Department of Health, Education, and Welfare, Office of Human Development Services: Auto safety and your child, DHEW Pub No (OHDS) 78-30123, Washington, DC, 1978, US Government Printing Office.

CHAPTER 3

Conrad MB: Principles of extrication, EMT 2:48, 1978.

Elling R: Dispelling myths on ambulance accidents, JEMS 11:60, 1989.

IAFF International Fire Fighter: DOT emergency response guidebook: use with caution, IAFF 71:11, 1988.

Mann E: Course held in saving lives of persons trapped in autos, Decatur Daily Democrat, p 7, Aug 16, 1971.

National Fire Protection Association: Fire protection guide on hazardous materials, ed 9, Quincy, Mass, 1986, National Fire Protection Association.

New York State Police: Annual report, 1981, Albany, NY, 1981, Division of State Police.

NHSTA expands study of fuel tank defects, Insurance Institute for Highway Safety Status Report 13:1, 1978.

State University of New York Agricultural and Technical College: Industrial control theory information sheet, Canton, NY, 1982, State University of New York.

Summary of motor vehicle accidents, No. MV-144, Albany, NY, Jan-Dec 1988, State of New York Department of Motor Vehicles.

Washburn AE and others: U.S. fire fighter deaths, 1984, Fire Command 52:21, 1984.

CHAPTER 4

Burnley proposes new side impact standard for better protection, Insurance Institute for Highway Safety Status Report 23:1, 1988, newsletter.

Butman AM and McSwain, NE Jr: Emergency patient removal, Journal of Pre-Hospital Care 1:23, 1984.

Helmet removal from injured patients, Akron, Oh, 1980, American College of Surgeons Committee on Trauma.

National Association of Emergency Medical Technicians: Pre-hospital trauma life support course, Akron, Oh, Dec 1984.

National Fire Academy: Incident command I course, Emmitsburg, Md, 1982.

National Transportation Safety Board: Safety study: performance of lap belts in 26 frontal crashes, Pub No 917006, Washington, DC, 1986, US Government Printing Office.

Pre-Hospital Trauma Life Support Committee: Pre-hospital trauma life support, Akron, Oh, 1986, National Association of Emergency Medical Technicians and Committee on Trauma.

Rapid patient extrication, EMS Program No 87-40, Albany, NY, Dec 1987, NY State Department of Health.

Root HD: A guide to the evaluation and treatment of serious head injuries, recommended guidelines, Akron, Oh, 1983, American College of Surgeons Committee on Trauma.

The rapid takedown: an alternative to backboarding the standing patient, No. 87-11, Albany, NY, 1987, NY State Department of Health.

US Department of Transportation National Highway Traffic Safety Administration: The automobile safety belt fact book, DOT No HS 802 157, Washington, DC, 1982, US Government Printing Office.

CHAPTER 6

Hurst RT-23/Aerosafe 2300 data sheet, Conshohocton, Pa, 1987, Hale Fire Pump Co.

Material safety data sheet: Shell Tellus T Oil 23, Houston, Shell Oil Corp.

National Fire Protection Association: Investigation report: flammable liquid tank explosion with fire fighter fatality, Fire Command 52:24, 1985.

Office of the Fire Marshall: Auto extrication, Ontario, Canada, 1984, notes.

Technical information: Allied Tool Corp, Sharpes, Fla.

Technical information: Amkus, Inc, Downers Grove, Ill.

Technical information: Bahco Kraftverktyg, Enkoping, Sweden.

Technical information: Enerpac, Milwaukee.

Technical information: FM Brick, Inc, Horsham, Pa.

Technical information: Hale Fire Pump Co, Conshohocken, Pa.

Technical information: HK Porter, Inc, Somerville, Mass.

Technical information: Holmatro, Inc, Millersville, Md.

Technical information: Kinman of Indianapolis, Indianapolis.

Technical information: Lampe-Lifter, Zumro Co, New Bern, NC.

Technical information: Lancier, Inc, Pittsburgh.

Technical information: Lincoln Safety Products, St Louis.

Technical information: Lukas of America, Inc, Stamford, Conn.

Technical information: MatJack Indianapolis Industrial Products, Indianapolis.

Technical information: Orion World, Inc, Melbourne, Fla.

Technical information: Paratech, Inc, Frankfort, Ill.

Technical information: Special Services and Supply, Inc, Chenoa, Ill.

Technical information: Superior Pneumatic & Manufacturing, Inc, Cleveland.

Technical information: Sweed Machinery, Inc, Gold Hill, Ore.

Technical information: Vetter Systems, Pittsburgh.

Technical information: Viking Rescue System, Villa Park, Ill.

Index